LAHEY CLINIC NUMBER

THE MEDICAL CLINICS OF NORTH AMERICA

VOLUME 56 / NUMBER 3
MAY 1972

SYMPOSIUM ON
THERAPEUTIC PROBLEMS

Henry E. Zellmann, M.D., *Guest Editor*

W. B. SAUNDERS COMPANY — Philadelphia · London · Toronto

W. B. Saunders Company: West Washington Square
                         Philadelphia, Pa.   19105

                         12 Dyott Street
                         London, WC1A   1DB

                         833 Oxford Street
                         Toronto 18, Ontario

The Medical Clinics are also published in other languages,
by the following:

Spanish   Nueva Editorial Interamericana, S. A. de C. V., Cedro 512,
               Apartado 26370, Mexico 4, D.F., Mexico

Italian   Piccin Editore, Via Porciglia, 10,
               35100 Padua, Italy

Portuguese   Editora Guanabara Koogan, S.A., Rua do Ouvidor,
               132 ZC 21, Rio de Janeiro, Brazil

Greek   John Mihalopoulos and Son,
               Thessaloniki, Greece

THE MEDICAL CLINICS OF NORTH AMERICA
May 1972   **Volume 56 — Number 3**

The Medical Clinics of North America is published every other month by W. B. Saunders Company,
West Washington Square, Philadelphia, Pennsylvania 19105, at Hampton Road, Cherry Hill, New Jersey
08034. Subscription price is $21.00 per year. Second class postage paid at Cherry Hill, New Jersey 08034.
This issue is Volume 56, Number 3.
The editor of this publication is Albert E. Meier, W. B. Saunders Company, West Washington Square,
Philadelphia, Pennsylvania 19105.

Library of Congress catalog card number 17-28505

Contributors

Internal Medicine

SIDNEY ALEXANDER, M.D.
GEORGE O. BELL, M.D.
DONALD J. BRESLIN, M.D.
ROBERT A. ENGLAND, M.D.
RICHARD M. FINKEL, M.D.
RICHARD A. OBERFIELD, M.D.
ARTEMIS G. PAZIANOS, M.D.
DAVID I. RUTLEDGE, M.D.
NEIL W. SWINTON, JR., M.D.
HENRY E. ZELLMANN, M.D.

DHIROOBHAI C. DESAI, M.D.[1]
PHILIP I. HERSHBERG, M.D.[2]

Department of Allergy and Dermatology

SAMUEL L. MOSCHELLA, M.D.
JOHN M. O'LOUGHLIN, M.D.
E. LAURIE TOLMAN, M.D.

Department of Anesthesiology

ANDREW E. ST. AMAND, M.D.

Department of Gastroenterology

ROBERT E. CROZIER, M.D.
MAMIGON GARABEDIAN, M.D.
JAMES A. GREGG, M.D.
VICTOR M. ROSENOER, M.D.

GEORGE M. GILL, M.D.[3]
GUALBERTO GOKIM, JR., M.D.[4]

Department of Gynecology

ROBERT W. CALI, M.D.

---

[1]Fellow in Internal Medicine (Cardiology).
[2]Assistant Professor of Medicine, Harvard School of Public Health; Research Associate, Lahey Clinic Foundation.
[3]Clinical Assistant Professor of Pediatrics, New Jersey College of Medicine and Dentistry; Attending Physician, Children's Hospital, Newark, New Jersey.
[4]Fellow in Gastroenterology.

Department of Neurology

H. Stephen Kott, M.D.
Stephen L. Wanger, M.D.

Department of Psychiatry

Walter I. Tucker, M.D.   Richard C. Lippincott, M.D.[5]

Department of Radiotherapy

Ferdinand A. Salzman, M.D.

Department of Surgery

Blake Cady, M.D.

---

[5]Assistant Professor of Psychiatry, University of Vermont Medical College, Burlington, Vermont; Psychiatric Consultant, Stoma Rehabilitation Clinic, New England Deaconess Hospital, Boston.

Contents

Foreword.. 583

    Henry E. Zellmann

Drug Interactions in Clinical Medicine.. 585

    Victor M. Rosenoer and George M. Gill

Interaction of drugs in man may give rise to therapeutically important modifications of action in duration, intensity, or even type. In order to use drugs safely and effectively, the physician must be aware not only of reported interactions, but also of the possibility of those not yet described. Absorption, distribution, excretion, and metabolism of various agents of particular clinical interest are examined.

Treatment of Severe Angina Pectoris 599

    Dhiroobhai C. Desai and Sidney Alexander

The presence of angina pectoris usually implies significant diffuse coronary atherosclerosis. The majority of these patients, nevertheless, can be treated adequately by properly applied medical therapy. Coronary surgery should be considered in the small proportion who do not respond to medical measures. Indications for aortocoronary saphenous vein bypass are outlined.

The Management of Paroxysmal Atrial Fibrillation............................. 611

    David I. Rutledge

Attention should first be directed to the probable cause of paroxysmal atrial fibrillation, and this eliminated or controlled when possible. Sedation will control many episodes; digitalis should be considered in cases of atrial fibrillation of recent onset. Propranolol and quinidine are useful agents; cardioversion is discussed, as well.

Treatment of Ventricular Arrhythmias in
Ambulatory Patients... 615

> Robert A. England
>
> Ventricular arrhythmias are frequently seen in pa-
> tients who have no serious disease. In such patients
> with ventricular ectopic beats, the goal is sympto-
> matic relief, and various treatment modalities are out-
> lined. Paroxysmal ventricular tachycardia presents
> problems in both diagnosis and treatment. Suggestions
> to aid in diagnosis are presented, as well as a dis-
> cussion of the various choices for therapy.

Prevention and Treatment of Sudden Cardiac Death........................... 625

> Philip I. Hershberg and Sidney Alexander
>
> Data indicate that lethal arrhythmias rarely occur
> without warning and that most deaths early in the
> course of myocardial infarction can be prevented by
> proper drug therapy. While prevention is the best
> treatment, patients who are at high risk for acute myo-
> cardial infarction must be instructed properly so that
> the time between onset of symptoms and arrival at
> the hospital can be reduced. The authors suggest and
> discuss the possibility of instituting drug therapy
> before the patient reaches the hospital.

Therapy of Complicated Arterial Hypertension.................................... 633

> Donald J. Breslin and Neil W. Swinton, Jr.
>
> Effective treatment of the hypertensive patient de-
> pends on a comprehensive initial evaluation. Hyper-
> tension may be labile, complicated by the patient's
> emotional status, secondary to disorders of the kid-
> neys, adrenals, or ischemic disease of the brain or
> heart, or present in the preoperative patient. Some
> systemic disorders may be affected adversely by anti-
> hypertensive therapy. The use of specific agents in
> these various situations is discussed.

Hyponatremia 645

> Richard M. Finkel
>
> Difficulties in treating patients with hyponatremia
> usually arise because consideration has not been
> given to the underlying pathophysiology. It is usually
> possible on the basis of simple laboratory and clinical
> observations to determine whether the hyponatremia
> is the result of depressed serum water content, solute
> accumulation in extracellular fluid, water overload,
> sodium depletion, or "resetting of the osmostat."

A Multidisciplined Approach for the Management of
Metastatic Breast Cancer 651

Richard A. Oberfield, Blake Cady,
Artemis G. Pazianos, and Ferdinand A. Salzman

Intelligent therapeutic management in patients with
advanced breast cancer offers useful control and prolongation of a comfortable life. An aggressive, multidisciplined approach involving surgeons, radiotherapists, endocrinologists, and medical oncologists can
be of significant value in designing an appropriate
sequential long-range plan of therapy for each patient.

Practical Aspects of Investigation and
Treatment of Colorectal Cancer... 665

Richard A. Oberfield

A review of three aspects of colorectal cancer: basic
problems relating to primary treatment of the disease, the present chemotherapy program for systemic metastatic disease, and management of liver
metastasis, the latter involving a regional form of
chemotherapy which has produced increased remission rates and possibly prolonged survival for this
most difficult form of metastasis.

The Physician's Responsibility to the Dying Patient............................ 677

Richard C. Lippincott

Both the patient's and the physician's attitudes about
dying greatly influence the quality and compassion of
care. Three areas of psychologic conflicts associated
with dying are identified: the patient's intrapsychic
process, the relationship between patient, physician,
and entire health team, and the patient's family relationships.

The Effectiveness of Lithium Carbonate in the
Prevention of Manic and Depressive Episodes 681

Walter I. Tucker and George O. Bell

The purpose of this article is to indicate the effectiveness, safety, and practicability of prophylactic lithium
carbonate treatment in office and general hospital
practice. Results reported are based on experience in
the treatment of private patients, but nevertheless
do corroborate the findings reported in more controlled hospital studies and indicate that effective
treatment can be carried out in such a patient population with minimal risk.

The Role of Hypnotherapy in Clinical Medicine 687

Andrew E. St. Amand

While hypnotherapy is not a panacea for all patients, and enthusiasm for its use must not replace good clinical judgment, in the properly selected patient it can be an effective adjunct to conventional modes of therapy.

The Management of Parkinson's Syndrome 693

Stephen L. Wanger

Current methods for the treatment of Parkinson's syndrome are developing directly from basic scientific discoveries concerning catecholamines. Depending upon the severity of involvement, patients may be treated with amantadine hydrochloride with or without anticholinergic drugs or benztropine, and later with levodopa if necessary. Thalamic surgery continues to have a limited role and is reserved for patients with nonprogressive unilateral tremor and rigidity.

The Treatment of Multiple Sclerosis 711

H. Stephen Kott

At present, no drug therapy of great value in the treatment of multiple sclerosis exists. A low saturated and high unsaturated fat diet may retard the progress somewhat, and ACTH in high dose, short-term usage may be effective for acute exacerbations.

Hyperthyroidism 717

Henry E. Zellmann

Options in dealing with the various types of hyperthyroidism remain limited by ignorance of their etiology. Medical treatment, surgery, and radioiodine therapy are considered as they may be applied in Graves' disease, toxic nodular goiter, T-3 thyrotoxicosis, and iatrogenic and factitious hyperthyroidism.

The Present Status of Chemotherapy in Dermatology 725

Samuel L. Moschella

Evaluation of topical application, intralesional administration, arterial infusion, regional perfusion, and systemic chemotherapeutic agents in various types of dermatologic disorders. Systemic agents dis-

cussed include methotrexate, azathioprine, hydroxyurea, and alkylating agents.

Chemosurgery (Mohs' Technique) in the
Treatment of Epitheliomas 739
E. Laurie Tolman

Since chemosurgery has been shown to produce cure
rates higher than those usually obtained by radiation
or other excisional or destructive modalities in the
treatment of recurrent skin lesions, it should be considered first for therapy of recurrent cutaneous epitheliomas, especially basal cell epitheliomas, regardless of the previous treatment. Description of technique and discussion of its advantages and disadvantages.

Immunologic Deficiency States 747
John M. O'Loughlin

A brief review of the congenital and acquired forms
of immunologic deficiency disorders shows that if a
high index of suspicion is present, means are now
available for the diagnosis and treatment of these
disorders.

Management of Patients with Chronic Obstructive
Jaundice 759
Victor M. Rosenoer and Gualberto Gokim, Jr.

Several problems require consideration in the clinical
syndrome of obstructive jaundice: nutritional problems, which follow the deficiency of bile salts in the
intestine, and pruritus, which has been related to
increased concentrations of bile salts in the blood and
skin. Administration of drugs must be tempered by an
awareness that the duration and intensity of action of
many drugs are increased in some patients with liver
disease.

Obscure Chest Pain as a Symptom of Reflux Esophagitis 771
Robert E. Crozier, James A. Gregg, and
Mamigon M. Garabedian

Chest pains associated with esophagitis may be
chronic and at times severe, and often are difficult to
distinguish from those of coronary artery disease.
Whenever possible, endoscopy should be performed
when esophagitis is suspected, to determine its ex-

tent and severity and also to discover if associated inflammatory disease is present in the stomach and duodenum. Acid perfusion tests have been the single most helpful technique in diagnosing chest pain arising from esophagitis.

Retrograde Cannulation of the Ampulla of Vater:
A Preliminary Report 781

James A. Gregg

Indications for cannulation of the ampulla of Vater are many, and the procedure should prove valuable in diagnosing diseases of the pancreas and biliary system without the use of surgery.

Management of the Climacteric and Postmenopausal
Woman 789

Robert W. Cali

At the center of the controversy surrounding these patients is the alleged need for, safety of, and value of prolonged hormone therapy. Hormones should be used only when indicated to control distressing vasomotor symptoms, dysfunctional uterine bleeding, and senile vaginitis. It should be remembered that the climacteric and menopause are normal physiologic events in the life of a woman, and the proper aim of therapy is to facilitate the transition, not eliminate it.

ADDITIONAL ARTICLE

The Future of Tumor Immunology 801

B. Cinader

The role of immunology in various aspects of detection, treatment, and control of cancer: early diagnosis, identification and assessment of the patient's disease, evaluation and selection of chemotherapeutic agents, evaluation of short and long term consequences of excision therapy, appropriate regulation of body defense mechanisms, and preventive treatment.

Index 837

RECENT SYMPOSIA

July 1971
  DIABETES MELLITUS

September 1971
  INTENSIVE CARE UNITS

November 1971
  MODERN CONCEPTS IN RENAL DISEASE

January 1972
  HEMORRHAGIC DISORDERS

March 1972
  CLINICAL IMMUNOLOGY

FORTHCOMING SYMPOSIA

July 1972
  ENDOCRINE DISEASE
  RAYMOND V. RANDALL, M.D., *Guest Editor*

September 1972
  VENEREAL DISEASES
  BRUCE WEBSTER, M.D., *Guest Editor*

November 1972
  CLINICAL NEUROLOGY
  MELVIN D. YAHR, M.D., *Guest Editor*

January 1973
  CORONARY HEART DISEASE
  LEON RESNEKOV, M.D., *Guest Editor*

March 1973
  CLINICAL SIGNS OF BLOOD DISEASE
  ARNOLD D. RUBIN, M.D., *Guest Editor*

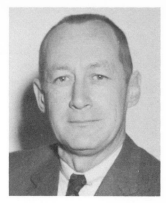

Foreword

HENRY E. ZELLMANN, M.D.

Were H. G. Wells' time machine available to us to bring back a physician of the past to view our present medical scene, which of the greats would we choose? Among many distinguished candidates, Richard Bright comes to mind. Nephrology revisited would perhaps show the most spectacular progress compared with 1840. Only the simplest anatomic pathology would be familiar to Bright. Replacing his diagnostic equipment of a spoon and a candle would be a bewildering number of ways to assess renal morphologic and pathophysiologic change. He would be astounded by the contributions of renal biopsy, electron and fluorescent microscopy, body fluid and electrolyte measurements, and achievements in radiology, angiology, and immunology.

Bright's greatest surprises, of course, would await him in therapy, the theme of our present volume. Diuretics to fit each portion of the nephron! Antibiotics tailored precisely to the organism! Blood and plasma substitutes, fluid and electrolyte replacement, and dialysis. And at the therapeutic pinnacle, that most durable of complex organ replacements – the kidney transplant. As one of my colleagues says, "the heart is just a pump and the thyroid gland can be replaced by a pill, but the kidney – there is an organ." By comparison, poor Richard could only look back upon purging, phlebotomy, sweating, and calomel.

Would he, on the other hand, think us in any way worse off than he? Omission in his era of nonspecific therapy was hardly reprehensible – it was often, in fact, a favor to the patient. Today, failure to bring to bear every available therapeutic measure can have serious moral as well as legal implications. He would see, also, the two sharp edges of our medical tools. The risk of iatrogenic disease was never greater from the widespread use of adrenocorticosteroids, potent diuretics, immunosuppressive agents, and antibiotics with subsequent opportunistic infection.

So much for the present. What if we could, with our time machine, move into the future? For nephrology, our projections are naturally limited by its narrow field, but refinements in dialysis and perfection of transplantation are almost assured. For the whole of medicine, however, the horizons seem limitless. Our social scientists tell us that we already

583

suffer from overkill in the area of research. More equitable delivery of medical service is what we anticipate for the future. From our present identity as a drug-oriented culture, therapeutically, as well as socially, we may well witness a turnabout. We should not be surprised to see emphasis on desensitization and conditioning therapy. Preventive medicine, always desirable, might extend to premarital courses in personality development to reduce the incidence of neurosis and psychosis in the offspring. And in the millenium, thought and behavioral control as well as genetic manipulations may make much of our current therapy unnecessary.

HENRY E. ZELLMANN, M.D.
Guest Editor

The Lahey Clinic Foundation
605 Commonwealth Avenue
Boston, Massachusetts 02215

Drug Interactions in Clinical Medicine

Victor M. Rosenoer, M.D., and George M. Gill, M.D.

The continual expansion of the number of therapeutic agents available in clinical practice and the frequent use of multiple medications have, over the past decade, led to increased awareness of the possible interaction of drugs. Emphasis recently has been on the effect of drugs on the activity of drug-metabolizing enzymes, located primarily in the smooth endoplasmic reticulum of the liver cell. It should be stressed, however, that this is not the only site at which drugs interact.

The pharmacologic and toxic effects of most therapeutic agents are thought to be related to the concentration of free drug at the receptors of the target cells. In the steady state, rarely achieved in practice, receptor-free drug is in equilibrium with drug free in solution in the plasma or bound to tissue or plasma constituents. The concentration of drug available to the specific effector sites is influenced by the processes of absorption from the site of administration, distribution in the plasma and tissues, metabolism, and excretion. Drugs may interact at all of these stages of their "life cycles" within the body, thus modifying the duration or intensity of their action.

DRUG ABSORPTION

The relationship between drugs and diet is so well known that few physicians give it the consideration it deserves. Marked effects have been observed. The concentration of drugs available for absorption from the gastrointestinal tract can be reduced by adsorption onto the surface of solids. Sorby and Liu[72] showed that the rate and extent of absorption of promazine were significantly reduced when a clay-pectin antidiarrheal mixture was administered concurrently. Complexing with metal ions, such as calcium, magnesium, aluminum, or iron salts in milk or antacids, may interfere with the absorption of tetracycline.[41]

The absorption of orally administered thyroxine, triiodothyronine, and sodium warfarin is prevented by the ion exchange resin, cholestyramine, which binds these drugs in the intestinal tract.[8, 49] Since cholestyramine may also decrease the absorption of dietary vitamin K by binding bile salts, an effect which would enhance coumarin action, the net effect of cholestyramine administration during clinical anticoagulation cannot be predicted. In animals, cholestyramine has been found to impair the absorption of digitoxin, aspirin, secobarbital, and phenylbutazone, as well as warfarin.[27]

Surfactants, for example polysorbate 80 (Tween 80), dioctyl sodium sulfosuccinate, and sorbitol, may affect the rate or extent of absorption or both by solubilizing the drug, possibly increasing the total amount of drug available for absorption. Thus Gwilt et al.[30] demonstrated that sorbitol will enhance the absorption of acetaminophen in man. Dietary fat will enhance the absorption of griseofulvin, while castor oil increases the absorption of extract of male fern, leading to a marked increase in both gastrointestinal and central nervous system toxicity.

Most drugs are weak organic electrolytes. The biologic barrier between the gastrointestinal lumen and the plasma behaves as if it were permeable only to the undissociated form of weak electrolytes.[61] Absorption is dependent upon the concentration of the non-ionized drug moiety—a concentration profoundly influenced by alterations of pH, for example, by antacids or by acidifiers. Thus, those drugs which are weak acids (salicylic acid, coumarin, nitrofurantoin, nalidixic acid, sulfonamides) will not be well absorbed in an alkaline medium. Those drugs which are weak bases (theophylline, antipyrine, quinidine, chloroquine, mecamylamine, amphetamines) will be absorbed better in an alkaline medium.

Clearly, drugs affecting gastrointestinal motility, such as atropine and other anticholinergic agents, may have important effects on absorption of drugs. If gastric emptying is slow, absorption from the small intestine will be delayed; reduced peristalsis may retard dissolution, and the drug may not be brought into contact with the absorbing epithelium. Hypermotility may decrease absorption of enteric-coated preparations. The effects of anticholinergic agents on drug absorption in man have not been studied in detail, although animal studies suggest that they are of importance. Consolo[17] found that imipramine and desimipramine reduce the absorption of phenylbutazone and oxyphenylbutazone in the rat—an effect possibly related to the atropine-like activity of the tricyclic antidepressants. Effects on intestinal motility may explain the delayed intestinal absorption of phenobarbital, phenytoin, and ethosuximide (Zarontin) in mice treated with amphetamine.[26]

Recently Riegelman et al.[57] tested the hypothesis that orally administered phenobarbital interferes with the metabolism of griseofulvin because of its ability to induce liver enzymes that increase drug metabolism. They used a simple random crossover study in 6 healthy men who volunteered to receive griseofulvin administered orally and intravenously both with and without phenobarbital. The elimination kinetics of griseofulvin for a given subject were identical with or without the administration of phenobarbital. Thus, no evidence of enzyme induction was observed. The amount of orally administered griseofulvin absorbed was decreased, however, when phenobarbital was given, implying that phenobarbital reduced the absorption of the drug. Dicumarol absorption in man is apparently inhibited by heptabarbital and allopurinol and enhanced by nortriptyline hydrochloride.[52, 77]

Specialized processes for the transport of various organic acids and bases, inorganic ions, sugars, and amino acids occur in the gut. Drugs such as neomycin[35, 36] and phenformin[73] affect intestinal absorption and reduce d-xylose excretion. Aspirin, phenylbutazone, and indomethacin have been shown to inhibit the active transport of L-tryptophan,[42] and salicylates affect the passage of glucose[64] across isolated rat intestinal preparations. Recently, Kendall et al.[37] have shown that indomethacin depresses the intestinal absorption of d-xylose in man by an undetermined mechanism. Mucosal damage did not occur. Aspirin, on the other hand, reduced the urinary excretion of d-xylose without influencing intestinal absorption.

With neomycin and para-aminosalicylic acid-induced malabsorption states, absorption of other drugs is likely to be abnormal. Thus, the serum level of the powerful new tuberculostatic drug, rifampicin, is decreased when it is given with para-aminosalicylic acid. The precise mechanism remains to be elucidated, but the therapeutic implications are clear: para-aminosalicylic acid and rifampicin should be given 8 to 12 hours apart.[9]

An active transport process certainly appears to be essential for the jejunal absorption of folic acid in man,[7] although controversy exists regarding the degree of reduction and methylation of the pteridine nucleus during absorption. Natural folate occurs as the polyglutamate, and the weight of evidence suggests that the polyglutamyl form must be broken down to the monoglutamate in the intestinal wall by folic acid conjugase before absorption.[54] This enzyme is present in the stomach, small bowel, and colon, and it has been suggested that inhibition of the conjugase may be responsible for the low serum folate levels found in patients receiving diphenylhydantoin, oral contraceptives, and nitrofurantoin.[20, 33, 65, 74, 75] Hoffbrand and Necheles[33] and Rosenberg et al.[58] reported that diphenylhydantoin inhibited intestinal conjugases; however, Baugh and Krumdieck[5] found that in vitro diphenylhydantoin did not inhibit partially purified conjugase preparations from human intestine, brain, or liver. The mechanism of diphenylhydantoin-induced folic acid deficiency thus remains uncertain.

DRUG DISTRIBUTION

Many of the drugs of clinical interest are transported in the plasma and bound to the plasma proteins, particularly but not exclusively bound to albumin. It is generally accepted that the bound fraction is devoid of pharmacologic activity,[10] and the therapeutically important concentration is that of free unbound drug, which is in dynamic equilibrium with the bound protein moiety.

In some circumstances this equilibrium may be disturbed markedly, leading to clinically important changes in the concentration of the free active agent. Thus sulfonamides, salicylates, and phenylbutazone, by competing for drug-binding sites on albumin, will displace a number of albumin-bound drugs and increase the concentration of unbound active agent in a manner similar to the displacement of unconjugated bilirubin from albumin binding by these drugs.

Several studies have been made of competitive binding involving antimicrobial agents. The highly protein-bound acidic drugs, such as phenylbutazone, oxyphenbutazone, sulfinpyrazone, coumarin anticoagulants, salicylates, probenecid, tolbutamide, and iophenoxic acid, can displace sulfonamides from plasma proteins, thereby enhancing their antibacterial action.[2-4] Sulfamethoxypyridazine, sulfaethylthiadiazole, and aspirin reduce the binding of penicillin analogs, resulting in higher levels of the unbound active drug. Kunin[39] has pointed out that certain agents which will displace penicillin derivatives will not alter the activity of novobiocin and tetracycline derivatives. Probably the latter agents bind at sites other than those at which the penicillins are bound. Probenecid, although highly protein-bound, does not displace penicillin, further indicating that drugs have specific binding sites, according to their chemical configuration.[40]

In man, concurrent therapy with warfarin and a variety of drugs that bind extensively to plasma albumin has been associated with an increased anticoagulant response. Such drugs include phenylbutazone, oxyphenylbutazone, chlorophenoxyisobutyric acid (clofibrate) and chloral hydrate.[1, 23, 25, 32, 60, 67, 71, 76] Normally 98 per cent of warfarin is bound to albumin, so that only 2 per cent of the total drug in the plasma is biologically active. If the binding is reduced from 98 to 96 per cent by another drug competing for the same albumin binding sites, the pharmacologically active concentration of warfarin is doubled! It is not surprising that hemorrhagic crises have ensued, some with fatal outcomes. This potentiation of anticoagulant effects, caused by drugs which displace warfarin, occurs within a few hours or days of starting the new drug. The effect is also readily reversed when the drug is withdrawn, and the dose of warfarin should be returned to its original level if the anticoagulant effect is to be maintained.

A paradoxical result of drug displacement is that more drug is available for metabolic degradation and renal excretion, so that the biologic half-life may be reduced. This has led to a misinterpretation of data. Chloral hydrate increases the rate of clearance of warfarin from the plasma in patients receiving both drugs. This effect was ascribed to the induction of new enzymes in the hepatic microsomes with a resulting increase in the rate of metabolism of both drugs.[19] However, when enzyme induction occurs, as when barbiturates are given, the anticoagulant effect of warfarin is reduced.[43] In contrast, chloral hydrate increases the action of warfarin, and if the anticoagulant dose is not decreased, serious bleeding may follow. Sellers and Koch-Weser[60] have shown that one of the major metabolites of chloral hydrate, trichloroacetic acid, accumulates in the plasma and displaces warfarin from binding sites on serum albumin. The drug is more readily available for combination with receptors at its site of action and also for metabolism and excretion.

Hypoglycemic episodes have been reported following drug interactions with tolbutamide. However, protein displacement of the predominantly protein-bound tolbutamide does not appear to be the primary cause of this hypoglycemic effect, although it may well contribute to it. Inhibition of the metabolic inactivation of tolbutamide by phenylbutazone, sulphenazole, and bishydroxycoumarin significantly increases the half-life of tolbutamide and precipitates the hypoglycemic reaction.[13, 69]

The gastrointestinal and bone marrow toxicity of methotrexate may be enhanced by protein displacement by sulfonamides and salicylates.[22] It should be noted that salicylates also compete with methotrexate for renal excretion, thus enhancing the possibility of increased methotrexate toxicity.

Binding of drugs to tissues may be modified by the concomitant administration of other drugs. Primaquine is an antimalarial that localizes in the liver, lung, and brain. Quinacrine also binds extensively in the liver. When patients receive both drugs simultaneously, the plasma concentration of primaquine is increased fivefold to tenfold, and its rate of disappearance from the plasma is markedly reduced.[81] Quinacrine clearly alters the metabolism and distribution of primaquine in man and enhances the toxicity of the latter. As quinacrine disappears very slowly from the body, this phenomenon may be observed even when primaquine is given as long as 3 months after the last dose of quinacrine.

The cardiovascular effects of norepinephrine can be potentiated by a number of antihistaminic agents. Isaac and Goth[34] have attributed this to an inhibition of the uptake of norepinephrine by various tissues, resulting in an increase in the concentration of unbound norepinephrine. Clearly, a potential hazard exists in the administration of antihistaminic agents to patients already receiving monoamine-oxidase inhibitors (MAO inhibitors), since a hypertensive crisis may ensue.

The antihypertensive drugs guanethidine and bethanidine are actively transported to their site of action within the adrenergic neuron by the same membranous concentrating mechanism that is responsible for the uptake of norepinephrine, thus permitting the drugs to exert a selective blocking action on adrenergic neurons. The sympatholytic effect is directly proportional to the quantity of guanethidine or bethanidine that accumulates in these specific sites. Reserpine, amphetamines, and the imipramines discharge norepinephrine, guanethidine, and bethanidine from the adrenergic neurons, resulting either in hypertension (if large amounts of catecholamines are released) or loss of the antihypertensive effect of guanethidine and bethanidine if they are no longer allowed access to the receptor.[12, 29, 47, 48, 62] The reversal of the antihypertensive effect of guanethidine by desmethylimipramine is relatively slow in onset but persists for an average of 5 days after discontinuance of the antidepressant drug. In contrast, maximum antagonism of the antihypertensive effect of bethanidine by desmethylimipramine is observed within 4 hours, but the duration of antagonism is as prolonged as that of guanethidine. Recently, Misage and McDonald[46] have drawn attention to the antagonism of the hypotensive action of bethanidine by Ornade, which contains the sympathomimetic amine, phenylpropanolamine hydrochloride.

The D-thyroxine-warfarin interaction illustrates yet another potential site of drug interaction, namely, the ability of one drug to influence the affinity of the receptor by another, either by binding to its receptor sites or by changes in the receptor structure. D-thyroxine potentiates the anticoagulant effect of warfarin. Solomon and Schrogie[59, 70] have proposed that this is the result of an increased affinity of warfarin for its receptor site in the liver. Certainly, D-thyroxine does not affect the absorption, distribution, or rate of metabolism of bishydroxycoumarin, but an increased rate of clotting factor catabolism in the presence of D-thyroxine has not been ruled out.

DRUG EXCRETION

Drug excretion may be affected greatly by changes in urinary pH. If the urine is at a pH at which the drug is present primarily in the ionized form, the possibility of passive resorption is considerably reduced, resulting in diminished circulating drug concentrations. If the urine is at a pH at which the drug is not ionized, the possibility of passive resorption is enhanced, resulting in increased plasma levels. Agents such as ammonium chloride, sodium bicarbonate, and the citrates have been used to alter the urinary pH, while dietary modifications commonly are responsible for changes in urinary pH. The influence of diuretics, especially those which inhibit carbonic anhydrase, such as acetazolamide and chlorothiazide, must also be considered.

Usually, acidic drugs such as aspirin, phenobarbital, sulfadiazine, and nitrofurantoin are excreted faster when the urinary pH is alkaline. An acid pH favors the excretion of basic drugs such as atropine, perphenazine, meperidine, amphetamine, imipramine, and amitryptyline hydrochloride. These effects are of clinical significance only if the pKa of the drug is in the range of about 7.5 to 10.5 for bases and 3.0 to 7.5 for acids, and if a significant proportion of the drug is normally excreted unchanged in the urine.[44] Such interactions have a practical application in the treatment of intoxication with salicylates and phenobarbital.

Beckett et al.[6] reported the influence of urinary pH on the elimination of D-amphetamine. After a single dose, 54.5 per cent of the drug was excreted in the urine in 16 hours when the urinary pH was 5.0; only 2.9 per cent was excreted in the same period of time when the urinary pH was 8.0. Milne et al.[45] suggested that the production of alkaline urine following the administration of the carbonic anhydrase inhibitor, acetazolamide, might be in part responsible for the reduced rate of excretion of simultaneously administered mecamylamine.

Many acidic drugs and drug metabolites are actively secreted by the proximal tubular active transport mechanism, and interactions may arise from competition for this system. Salicylic acid, sulfonic acids, sulfonamides, acetazolamide, probenecid, penicillins, phenylbutazone, oxyphenbutazone, sulfinpyrazone, indomethacin, chlorothiazide, chlorpropamide, and many drug metabolites share the tubal anion secretory system, which is the same as the tubular resorption system for uric acid. This explains why these drugs may modify uric acid clearance. Probenecid, introduced into clinical practice to inhibit the active tubular secretion of penicillin, thereby raising the effective plasma penicillin concentration, is more commonly used as a uricosuric agent, and the uricosuric action of probenecid is effectively antagonized by salicylates. Oyer et al.[53]

have drawn attention to the paradoxical urate retention when salicylates and phenylbutazone are taken together. Probenecid will inhibit the renal excretion of indomethacin[63] and also the tubular transport of certain radiodiagnostic agents such as iodopyracet and related iodinate organic acids, para-aminohippuric acid and phenolsulfonphthalein, thereby interfering with the interpretation of renal function studies utilizing these agents.

Field et al.[24] have reported the potentiation of acetohexamide hypoglycemia by phenylbutazone and have attributed it to an interference with renal excretion of the active metabolite, hydroxyhexamide. Similarly, bishydroxycoumarin and phenylbutazone inhibit the renal clearance of chlorpropamide in man and potentiate its hypoglycemic effect.[21, 38]

DRUG METABOLISM

The ability of one drug to stimulate or to inhibit the metabolism of another is clearly an important factor in therapeutics today. Drugs which interfere with enzymatic pathways can enhance or prolong the effects of other drugs, or both. This is of particular concern with drugs which are extensively modified before excretion. For example, the inhibition of acetaldehyde dehydrogenase by disulfiram has been utilized in the therapy of the alcoholic. Subsequent exposure of the patient to alcohol produces the usual acetaldehyde accumulation syndrome of nausea, vomiting, headache, flushing of the face, and hypotension. Less well known are other compounds – calcium carbimide (also used in the treatment of alcoholism), chlorpropamide, tolbutamide, and metronidazole – which inhibit this enzyme and may be associated with a similar intolerance to ethanol.[56]

The effect of the MAO inhibitors, formerly widely used as antidepressants, deserve special mention. The sympathetic transmitter substances, epinephrine and norepinephrine, are monoamines, and the MAO inhibitors might therefore be expected to enhance and prolong their actions. However, in this instance the unexpected occurs, since epinephrine and norepinephrine, after their release into the circulation, are predominantly inactivated by catecholorthomethyl transferase, and the paucity of grossly observable signs following the administration of MAO inhibitors is deceptive. Conversely, within the nerve, enzymatic catabolism of the sympathomimetic amines is accomplished by mitochondrial MAO. This mechanism is necessary to regulate the tissue metabolism of catecholamines and serotonin and thus indirectly controls the concentration of pharmacologically active amines stored in nerve endings.

Certain sympathomimetic amines act indirectly by releasing stored catecholamines, and hence their actions are potentiated by the MAO inhibitors. The hazard of hypertensive crises in patients taking MAO inhibitors extends to the consumption of "cold medications" or other substances containing sympathomimetic amines (often sold without prescriptions) and foods containing tyramine, such as certain cheeses. Such drugs as ephedrine, amphetamine, methylamphetamine, phenylpropanolamine, and phenylephrine should not be given to subjects also receiving MAO inhibitors. Indeed concurrent therapy with tranylcypromine and methylamphetamine has resulted in death from intracranial hemorrhage.[62] An interesting effect of the MAO inhibitors, the reversal of the sedation and hypothermia produced by reserpine, is probably the result of this mechanism. In producing sedation, reserpine releases stored amines. The paradoxical exciting effect is the result of the release of high concentrations of stored catecholamine that follow MAO inhibitor therapy. Combinations of MAO inhibitors with imipramine have resulted in hyperthermia, convulsions, and even death, probably by a similar mechanism. It should be recalled that guanethidine, bethanidine, and alpha-methyldopa also initially release norepinephrine from the adrenergic neuron, and should not be given to individuals treated with MAO inhibitors.

When initially administered to rats, certain MAO inhibitors decrease the metabolism of hexobarbital by the microsomal drug-metabolizing enzymes, thus prolonging the duration of sleep. Chronic administration results in stimulation of the synthesis of the microsomal enzymes, enhancing the metabolism of hexobarbital. It is of interest that the pharmacologic effect of barbiturates, meperidine, phenothiazines, and alcohol are potentiated in man by the MAO inhibitors.[62, 78] Another source of potential morbidity lies in the use of other drugs whose primary action provides no hint of MAO inhibitory effect. Thus, the anti-infective agent, furazolidone, the antituberculous drug, isoniazid, and the antineoplastic drug, procarbazine, all have significant MAO inhibitory activity. Studies in man have demonstrated that furazolidone inhibits intestinal MAO, increases the urinary excretion of tryptamine, and markedly increases the pressor response to tyramine and amphetamine.[55]

In a manner analogous to the MAO inhibitors, the anticholinesterase agents inhibit the action of cholinesterase, the enzyme which inactivates acetylcholine and thus terminates transmitter activity at the cholinergic nerve endings. Hence, the cholinesterase inhibitors, both of the "reversible" type characterized by neostigmine and edrophonium and of the "irreversible" type, the organophosphate derivatives, which differ essentially only in their duration of activity, allow acetylcholine to accumulate at cholinergic sites and are potentially capable of producing an effect equivalent to continuous stimulation of cholinergic fibers. They will antagonize the muscle-relaxant effects of the nondepolarizing neuromuscular blocking agents such as d-tubocurarine and the aminoglycoside antibiotics (kanamycin, neomycin, and streptomycin), whereas they will potentiate the depolarizing skeletal muscle relaxants (succinylcholine and decamethonium) as well as those antibiotics which reputedly also produce depolarization (colistimethate, gramicidin, and polymixin). Clearly physicians should inquire about exposure to organophosphate insecticides or the use of anticholinesterase eye drops before administering succinylcholine. Such agents should be discontinued 6 weeks before operation if muscle relaxants are to be used.

The xanthine oxidase inhibitor, allopurinol, is widely used in the treatment of gout and for prophylaxis of hyperuricemia in patients receiving cytotoxic drugs for the treatment of malignant diseases. It is often forgotten that this was initially studied as an inhibitor of the metabolism of 6-mercaptopurine, and caution must be exercised when these two drugs are used together. Further, it should not be overlooked that the widely used immunosuppressive drug, azathioprine, slowly releases 6-mercaptopurine in vivo and will also be potentiated by the concomitant use of allopurinol. Vesell et al.[77] have reported that allopurinol administered for 14 days tripled the half-life of bishydroxycoumarin, presumably by inhibiting coumarin metabolizing enzymes. The gastrointestinal absorption of bishydroxycoumarin appeared to be decreased. The net effect of allopurinol on the hypoprothrombinemic action of bishydroxycoumarin has not yet been reported, although potentiation might be expected.

Less easily predictable drug interactions have also been reported. Solomon and Schrogie[66] have found that phenyramidol (an analgesic muscle relaxant) potentiates the anticoagulant effect of bishydroxycoumarin by inhibiting its metabolism. Phenylbutazone, sulfaphenazole, phenyramidol, and bishydroxycoumarin inhibit the metabolic inactivation of tolbutamide in man, an effect that can cause profound hypoglycemia.[13, 69] Phenyramidol, bishydroxycoumarin, disulfiram, and methylphenidate decrease the metabolism of diphenylhydantoin and may produce signs of diphenylhydantoin toxicity, including ataxia and nystagmus.[28, 31, 50, 51, 68]

The intensity and duration of action of many drugs are related to the rate of metabolic inactivation by the hepatic microsomal drug-metabolizing enzymes. The amount of these enzymes may be increased by a variety of foreign organic compounds that stimulate the synthesis of these enzymes.[14, 15] Several hundred compounds are now known to induce the synthesis of drug metabolizing enzymes in laboratory animals. These compounds include barbiturates, antihistamines, oral hypoglycemic and uricosuric agents, insecticides, such as DDT, and carcinogens, such as 3:4 benzpyrene. Pretreatment with phenobarbital may reduce the paralysis time in mice given a high dose of zoxazolamine, from more than 11 hours to 102 minutes, while the lethality of the drug is also significantly decreased.[16] On the other hand, it is essential to remember that drug metabolism is not synonymous with drug inactivation. The toxicity of certain organic thiophosphates, which are relatively nontoxic until they are metabolized by liver microsomes to potent anticholinesterase agents, is markedly increased by pretreating rats with stimulators of liver microsomal enzymes.

In some instances, the stimulatory effects of drugs and foreign chemicals on drug metabolism have been observed in man. Thus, phenobarbital will enhance the rate of metabolism of bishydroxycoumarin in man, with a concomitant decrease in the plasma level of the drug and a decrease in the anticoagulant activity.[18] Similar reports in man indicate that other barbiturates and griseofulvin should be used with caution in patients receiving coumarin anticoagulant therapy. While the patient is receiving an adequate maintenance dose of anticoagulant, the addition of stimulator of drug metabolism may reduce the efficacy of the therapy; when the enzyme stimulator is withdrawn and therapy with the anticoagulant is continued without an appropriate decrease in dose, the risk of hemorrhage is considerable. This aspect of drug interaction underlines the necessity for coordinated patient care and, in particular, for accurately maintained patient records.

Phenobarbital has been shown to increase the rate of diphenylhydantoin metabolism in man.[18] The plasma levels of diphenylhydantoin were distinctly lower in patients treated daily with diphenylhydantoin, 300 mg., and phenobarbital, 120 mg., than in those treated daily with diphenylhydantoin, 300 mg., alone. This particular anti-epileptic combination presents little clinical problem, but the simultaneous use of drugs which enhance dilantin metabolism but lack anticonvulsant activity may present clinical difficulties.

The metabolism of aminopyrine in man is stimulated by phenylbutazone; various barbiturates and glutethimide increase the rate of metabolism of dipyrone, a derivative of aminopyrine, and digitoxin metabolism may be increased by phenobarbital. Tolerance to such drugs as glutethimide, meprobamate, barbiturates, and antihistamines in man may well be related to their ability to stimulate their own metabolism.[11]

Recent studies in animals have suggested that the hepatic microsomal enzymes also hydroxylate steroids such as estrogens, androgens, and glucocorticoids. Various drugs, including phenobarbital, diphenylhydantoin, and phenylbutazone will enhance steroid hydroxylase activity, stimulating in man the metabolism of cortisol to the inactive 6-beta-hydroxycortisol. Werk et al.[79] have shown that diphenylhydantoin ameliorates Cushing's syndrome and produces an increased excretion of the hydroxylating metabolite in the urine. It is noteworthy that diphenylhydantoin will interfere with the plasma cortisol-dexamethasone suppression test.[80]

SUMMARY

Drugs may interact in man, giving rise to therapeutically important modifications of action, in duration, intensity, or even type. Although the principles involved are simple, it is difficult to lay down guidelines that will help the clinician to avert major problems. Certainly, many drug interactions go unrecognized, because of either the subjective nature of the clinical response or the wide margin of safety of the drugs in question.

Unfortunately, the results of animal experiments involving plasma protein-binding and microsomal enzyme induction or inhibition cannot be applied directly to man. Species differences, biphasic effects, first inhibiting and later stimulating microsomal enzymes, and the disease-diet-drug interplay modify the results of multiple drug regimens. However, it would appear that compounds that are lipid soluble at physiological pH, not normally rapidly metabolized, and moderately to strongly bound to plasma proteins, that is, compounds not readily excreted by the kidney, may be more likely to cause induction of the hepatic drug-metabolizing enzymes. Drugs which are strongly protein bound may displace, or be themselves displaced by, other protein-bound compounds, while organic anions may be expected to compete for renal tubular excretion. Acidifiers and alkalies may well modify drug absorption and excretion by altering passive non-ionic diffusion, while oral resins may be expected to alter drug absorption.

In order to use drugs safely and effectively, the physician must be aware not only of reported interactions but also of the possibility of those not yet described. He must keep a careful note of the dietary and drug therapy prescribed for his patient, as caution is necessary in the addition or deletion of any drug from the therapeutic regimen. Multiple drug therapy, although rational, is likely to become increasingly hazardous.

REFERENCES

1. Aggeler, P. M., O'Reilly, R. A., Leong, L., et al.: Potentiation of anticoagulant effect of warfarin by phenylbutazone. New Eng. J. Med. 276:496–501 (March 2) 1967.
2. Anton, A. H.: The relation between the binding of sulfonamides to albumin and their antibacterial efficacy. J. Pharmacol. Exper. Ther. 129:282–290 (July) 1960.
3. Anton, A. H.: A drug-induced change in the distribution and renal excretion of sulfonamides. J. Pharmacol. Exper. Ther. 134:291–303 (Dec.) 1961.
4. Anton, A. H.: The effect of disease, drugs and dilution on the binding of sulfonamides in human plasma. Clin. Pharmacol. Ther. 9:561–567 (Sept.-Oct.) 1968.
5. Baugh, C. M., and Krumdieck, C. L.: Effects of phenytoin on folic-acid conjugases in man. Lancet 2:519–521 (Sept. 6) 1969.
6. Beckett, A. H., Rowland, M., and Turner, P.: Influence of urinary pH on excretion of amphetamine. Lancet 1:303 (Feb. 6) 1965.
7. Bernstein, L. H., Gutstein, S., Weiner, S., et al.: The absorption and malabsorption of folic acid and its polyglutamates. Amer. J. Med. 48:570–579 (May) 1970.
8. Benjamin, D., Robinson, D. S., and McCormack, J.: Cholestyramine binding of warfarin in man and in vitro. Abstract. Clin. Res. 18:336 (April) 1970.
9. Boman, G., Hanngren, A., Malmborg, A. S., et al.: Drug interaction: decreased serum concentrations of rifampicin when given with P.A.S. Lancet 1:800 (April 17) 1971.
10. Brodie, B. B.: Displacement of one drug by another from carrier or receptor sites. Proc. Roy. Soc. Med. 58:Suppl:946–955 (Nov.) 1965.
11. Burns, J. J.: Implications of enzyme induction for drug therapy. Amer. J. Med. 37:327–331 (Sept.) 1964.
12. Chang, C. C., Costa, E., and Brodie, B. B.: Reserpine-induced release of drugs from sympathetic nerve endings. Life Sci. 3:839–844 (Aug.) 1964.
13. Christensen, L. K., Hansen, J. M., and Kristensen, M.: Sylphaphenazole-induced hypoglycaemic attacks in tolbutamide-treated diabetic. Lancet 2:1298–1301 (Dec. 21) 1963.
14. Conney, A. H.: Pharmacological implications of microsomal enzyme induction. Pharmacol. Rev. 19:317–366 (Sept.) 1967.
15. Conney, A. H.: Drug metabolism and therapeutics. New Eng. J. Med. 280:653–660 (March 20) 1969.
16. Conney, A. H., Davison, C., Gastel, R., and Burns, J. J.: Adaptive increases in drug-metabolizing enzymes induced by phenobarbital and other drugs. J. Pharmacol. Exper. Ther. 130:1–8 (Sept.) 1960.
17. Consolo, S.: An interaction between desipramine and phenylbutazone. J. Pharm. Pharmacol. 20:574–575 (July) 1968.
18. Cucinell, S. A., Conney, A. H., Sansur, M., et al.: Drug interactions in man. I. Lowering effect of phenobarbital on plasma levels of bishydroxycoumarin (Dicumarol) and diphenylhydantoin (Dilantin). Clin. Pharmacol. Ther. 6:420–429 (July-Aug.) 1965.
19. Cucinell, S. A., Odessky, L., Weiss, M., et al.: The effect of chloral hydrate on bishydroxycoumarin metabolism. A fatal outcome. J.A.M.A. 197:366–368 (Aug. 1) 1966.
20. Dahlke, M. B., and Mertens-Roesler, E.: Malabsorption of folic acid due to diphenylhydantoin. Blood 30:341–351 (Sept.) 1967.
21. Dalgas, M., Christiansen, I., and Kjerulf, K.: Hypoglycaemic episodes induced by phenylbutazone in diabetic patients treated with chlorpromazine. Ugesk. Laeger. 127:834–836 (July-Sept.) 1965.
22. Dixon, R. L., Henderson, E. S., and Rall, D. P.: Plasma protein binding of methotrexate and its displacement by various drugs. Fed. Proc. 24:454 (April 12) 1965.
23. Eisen, M. J.: Combined effect of sodium warfarin and phenylbutazone. J.A.M.A. 189:64–65 (July 6) 1964.
24. Field, J. B., Ohta, M., Boyle, C., et al.: Potentiation of acetohexamide hypoglycemia by phenylbutazone. New Eng. J. Med. 277:889–894 (Oct. 26) 1967.
25. Fox, S. L.: Potentiation of anticoagulants caused by pyrazole compounds. J.A.M.A. 188:320–321 (April 20) 1964.
26. Frey, H. H., and Kampmann, E.: Interaction of amphetamine with anticonvulsant drugs.

II. Effect of amphetamine on the absorption of anticonvulsant drugs. Acta Pharmacol. 24:310–316, 1966.

27. Gallo, D. G., Bailey, K. R., and Sheffner, A. L.: The interaction between cholestyramine and drugs. Proc. Soc. Exper. Biol. Med. 120:60–65 (Oct.) 1965.

28. Garrettson, L. K., Perel, J. M., and Dayton, P. G.: Methylphenidate interaction with both anticonvulsants and ethyl biscoumacetate. J.A.M.A. 207:2053–2056 (March 17) 1969.

29. Gulati, O. D., Dave, B. T., and Gokhale, S. D.: Antagonism of adrenergic neuron blockade in hypertensive subjects. Clin. Pharmacol. Ther. 7:510–514 (July-Aug.) 1966.

30. Gwilt, J. R., Robertson, A., Goldman, L., and Blanchard, A. W.: The absorption characteristics of parcetamol tablets in man. J. Pharm. Pharmacol. 15:445–453 (July) 1963.

31. Hansen, J. M., Kristensen, M., and Skorsted, L.: Dicoumarol-induced diphenylhydantoin intoxication. Lancet 2:265–266 (July 30) 1966.

32. Hobbs, C. B., Miller, A. L., and Thornley, J. H.: Potentiation of anticoagulant therapy by oxyphenylbutazone (A probable case). Postgrad. Med. J. 41:563–565 (Sept.) 1965.

33. Hoffbrand, A. V., and Necheles, T. F.: Mechanism of folate deficiency in patients receiving phenytoin. Lancet 2:528–530 (Sept. 7) 1968.

34. Isaac, L., and Goth, A.: Interaction of antihistaminics with norepinephrine uptake: a cocaine-like effect. Life Sci. 4:1899–1904 (Oct.) 1965.

35. Jacobson, E. D., Chodos, R. B., and Faloon, W. W.: An experimental malabsorption syndrome induced by neomycin. Amer. J. Med. 28:524–533 (April) 1960.

36. Jacobson, E. D., Prior, J. T., and Faloon, W. W.: Malabsorptive syndrome induced by neomycin: morphologic alterations in the jejunal mucosa. J. Lab. Med. 56:245–250 (Aug.) 1960.

37. Kendall, M. J., Nutter, S., and Hawkins, C. F.: Xylose test: effect of aspirin and indomethacin. Brit. Med. J. 1:533–536 (March 6) 1971.

38. Kristensen, M., and Hansen, J. M.: Accumulation of chlorpropamide caused by dicoumarol. Acta Med. Scand. 183:83–86 (Jan.-Feb.) 1968.

39. Kunin, C. M.: Enhancement of antimicrobial activity of penicillins and other antibiotics in human serum by competitive serum binding inhibitors. Proc. Soc. Exper. Biol. Med. 117:69–73 (Oct.) 1964.

40. Kunin, C. M.: Clinical pharmacology of the new penicillins. II. Effect of drugs which interfere with binding to serum proteins. Clin. Pharmacol. Ther. 7:180–188 (March-April) 1966.

41. Kunin, C. M., and Finland, M.: Clinical pharmacology of the tetracycline antibiotics. Clin. Pharmacol. Ther. 2:51–69 (Jan.-Feb.) 1966.

42. Levy, G., Angelino, N. J., and Matsuzawa, T.: Effect of certain nonsteroid antirheumatic drugs on active amino acid transport across the small intestine. J. Pharm. Sci. 56:681–683 (June) 1967.

43. MacDonald, M. G., Robinson, D. S., Sylwester, D., et al.: The effects of phenobarbital, chloral betaine, and glutethimide administration on warfarin plasma levels and hypoprothrombinemic response in man. Clin. Pharmacol. Ther. 10:80–84 (Jan.-Feb.) 1969.

44. Milne, M. D.: Influence of acid-base balance on efficacy and toxicity of drugs. Proc. Roy. Soc. Med. 58:Suppl:961–963 (Nov.) 1965.

45. Milne, M. D., Rowe, G. G., Somers, K., Muehrcke, R. C., and Crawford, M. A.: Observations on the pharmacology of mecamylamine. Clin. Sci. 16:599–614, 1957.

46. Misage, J. R., and McDonald, R. H., Jr.: Antagonism of hypotensive action of bethanidine by "common cold" remedy. Brit. Med. J. 4:347 (Nov. 7) 1970.

47. Mitchell, J. R., Arias, L., and Oates, J. A.: Antagonism of the antihypertensive action of guanethidine sulfate by desipramine hydrochloride. J.A.M.A. 202:973–976 (Dec. 4) 1967.

48. Morrelli, H. F., and Melmon, K. L.: The clinician's approach to drug interactions. Calif. Med. 109:380–389 (Nov.) 1968.

49. Northcutt, R. C., Stiel, J. N., Hollifield, J. W., et al.: The influence of cholestyramine on thyroxine absorption. J.A.M.A. 208:1857–1861 (June 9) 1969.

50. Olesen, O. V.: Disulfiramum (antabuse) as inhibitor of phenytoin metabolism. Acta Pharmacol. 24:317–322, 1966.

51. Olesen, O. V.: The influence of disulfiram and calcium carbimide on the serum diphenylhydantoin. Excretion of HPPH in the urine. Arch. Neurol. 16:642–644 (June) 1967.

52. O'Reilly, R. A., and Aggeler, P. M.: Effect of barbiturates on oral anticoagulants in man. Clin. Res. 17:153 (Jan. 30) 1969.

53. Oyer, J. H., Wagner, S. L., and Schmid, F. R.: Suppression of salicylate-induced uricosuria by phenylbutazone. Amer. J. Med. Sci. 251:1–7 (Jan.) 1966.

54. Perry, J., and Chanarin, I.: Absorption and utilization of polyglutamyl forms of folate in man. Brit. Med. J. 4:546–549 (Nov. 30) 1968.

55. Pettinger, W. A., Soyangco, F. G., and Oates, J. A.: The inhibition of monoamine oxidase in man by furazolidone. Clin. Pharmacol. Ther. 9:442–447 (July-Aug.) 1968.

56. Podgainy, H., and Bressler, R.: Biochemical basis of the sulfonylurea-induced antabuse syndrome. Diabetes 17:679–683 (Nov.) 1968.

57. Riegelman, S., Rowland, M., and Epstein, W. L.: Griseofulvin-phenobarbital interaction in man. J.A.M.A. 213:426–431 (July 20) 1970.
58. Rosenberg, I. H., Godwin, H. A., Streiff, R. R., et al.: Impairment of intestinal deconjugation of dietary folate. A possible explanation of megaloblastic anaemia associated with phenytoin therapy. Lancet 2:530–532 (Sept. 7) 1968.
59. Schrogie, J. J., and Solomon, H. M.: The anticoagulant response to bishydroxycoumarin. II. The effect of D-thyroxine clofibrate and norethandrolone. Clin. Pharmacol. Ther. 8:70–77 (Jan.-Feb.) 1967.
60. Sellers, E. M., and Koch-Weser, J.: Potentiation of warfarin-induced hypoprothrombinemia by chloral hydrate. New Eng. J. Med. 283:827–831 (Oct. 15) 1970.
61. Shore, P. A., Brodie, B. B., and Hogben, C. A. M.: The gastric secretion of drugs: a pH partition hypothesis. J. Pharmacol. Exper. Ther. 119:361–369 (March) 1957.
62. Sjöqvist, F.: Psychotropic drugs (2). Interaction between monoamine oxidase (MAO) inhibitors and other substances. Proc. Roy. Soc. Med. 58:Suppl.:967–978 (Nov.) 1965.
63. Skeith, M. D., Simkin, P. A., and Healey, L. A.: The renal excretion of indomethacin and its inhibition by probenecid. Clin. Pharmacol. Ther. 9:89–93 (Jan.-Feb.) 1968.
64. Smith, M. J. H.: Effects of salicylate on the metabolic activity of the small intestine of the rat. Amer. J. Physiol. 193:29–33 (April-June) 1958.
65. Snyder, L. M., and Necheles, T. F.: Malabsorption of folate polyglutamates associated with oral contraceptive therapy. Clin. Res. 17:602 (Dec. 12–13) 1969.
66. Solomon, H. M., and Schrogie, J. J.: The effect of phenyramidol on the metabolism of bishydroxycoumarin. J. Pharmacol. Exper. Ther. 154:660–666 (Dec.) 1966.
67. Solomon, H. M., and Schrogie, J. J.: The effect of various drugs on the binding of warfarin-14C to human albumin. Biochem. Pharmacol. 16:1219–1226 (July 7) 1967.
68. Solomon, H. M., and Schrogie, J. J.: The effect of phenyramidol on the metabolism of diphenylhydantoin. Clin. Pharmacol. Ther. 8:554–556 (July-Aug.) 1967.
69. Solomon, H. M., and Schrogie, J. J.: Effect of phenyramidol and bishydroxycoumarin on the metabolism of tolbutamide in human subjects. Metabolism 16:1029–1033 (Nov.) 1967.
70. Solomon, H. M., and Schrogie, J. J.: Change in receptor site affinity: a proposed explanation for the potentiating effect of D-thyroxine on the anticoagulant response to warfarin. Clin. Pharmacol. Ther. 8:797–799 (Nov.-Dec.) 1967.
71. Solomon, H. M., Schrogie, J. J., and Williams, D.: The displacement of phenylbutazone-14C and warfarin-14C from human albumin by various drugs and fatty acids. Biochem. Pharmacol. 17:143–151 (Jan.) 1968.
72. Sorby, D. L., and Liu, G.: Effects of adsorbents on drug absorption. II. Effect of an antidiarrhea mixture on promazine absorption. J. Pharm. Sci. 55:504–510 (May) 1966.
73. Stowers, J. M., and Brewsher, P. D.: Studies on the mechanism of weight reduction by phenformin. Postgrad. Med. J.45:12 (May) 1969.
74. Streiff, R. R.: Malabsorption of polyglutamic folic acid secondary to oral contraceptives. Clin. Res. 17:345 (May 3–4) 1969.
75. Toole, J. F., Gergen, J. A., Hayes, D. M., and Felts, J. H.: Neural effects of nitrofurantoin. Arch. Neurol. 18:680–687 (June) 1968.
76. Udall, J. A.: Drug interference with warfarin therapy. Clin. Res. 17:104 (Jan. 31) 1969.
77. Vesell, E. S. Passananti, G. T., and Greene, F. E.: Impairment of drug metabolism in man by allopurinol and notriptyline. New Eng. J. Med. 283:1484–1488 (Dec. 31) 1970.
78. Vigran, I. M.: Dangerous potentiation of meperidine hydrochloride by pargyline hydrochloride. J.A.M.A. 187:953–954 (March 21) 1964.
79. Werk, E. E., Jr., Choi, Y., Sholiton, L., et al.: Interference in the effect of dexamethasone by diphenylhydantoin. New Eng. J. Med. 281:32–34 (July 3) 1969.
80. Werk, E. E., MacGee, J., and Sholiton, L.: Effect of diphenylhydantoin on cortisol metabolism in man. J. Clin. Invest. 43:1824–1835 (Sept.) 1964.
81. Zubrod, C. G., Kennedy, T. J., Jr., and Shannon, J. A.: Studies on chemotherapy of human malarias. Physiological disposition of pamaquine. J. Clin. Invest. 27:114–120 (May) (pt. 2) 1948.

605 Commonwealth Avenue
Boston Massachusetts 02215

Treatment of Severe Angina Pectoris

Dhiroobhai C. Desai, M.D., and Sidney Alexander, M.D.

Angina pectoris is a clinical syndrome caused by myocardial ischemia.[31, 50, 60] It is produced by temporary imbalance between myocardial oxygen requirements and supply. Severe angina pectoris represents a particularly delicate state of this balance, which becomes easily disturbed by slight physiologic stress leading to frequent, often prolonged, and easily provoked anginal pain.

Angina pectoris may be stable or unstable. When stable, symptoms in a given individual are usually predictably produced; relief by rest, relaxation, and nitroglycerin or other drugs is similarly predictable. Angina becomes unstable when a change in the symptom pattern occurs; pain is more easily provoked, lasts longer, and may occur spontaneously. Previously successful methods of relieving symptoms may no longer work. The onset of unstable angina usually implies a significant change in the myocardial oxygen supply and demand relationship; further impairment of an already compromised coronary circulation may have occurred. Less commonly, increased myocardial oxygen requirements owing to such causes as emotional stress, infection, thyrotoxicosis, pulmonary emboli, or worsening of heart failure may be responsible. At times the syndrome of unstable angina pectoris may be indistinguishable from that of impending myocardial infarction.

CORONARY CIRCULATION AND MYOCARDIAL OXYGEN CONSUMPTION

Normally the heart receives about 5 per cent of the total cardiac output, approximately 250 ml. per minute. The myocardium extracts about 70 per cent of the oxygen in the arterial blood,[21] resulting in an arteriovenous oxygen difference considerably greater than that found in any other organ. The coronary circulation is unique because increased myocardial oxygen demands must be met primarily by increasing coronary blood flow rather than increasing arterial oxygen extraction. Cardiac function is thus vulnerable to disease of the coronary arteries in which coronary blood flow is limited.

Factors which chiefly influence the myocardial oxygen demands[5, 44, 53, 55, 56] are outlined in Table 1. The normal coronary arterioles are exquisitely responsive to myocardial oxygen demands, and in normal individuals, coronary flow may be increased several times the resting value by altering the resistance to flow at the arteriolar level. Resistance is mediated through a number of metabolites, including carbon dioxide, potassium, hydrogen, lactic acid, histamine, polypeptides, and adenine nucleotides, chiefly adenosine.[2, 8, 17, 21, 29, 33, 40]

Whether the diseased coronary circulation can adequately meet myocardial oxygen demands will be determined by the degree and location of the coronary disease, the perfusion pressure across the stenosed vessels, and the presence and extent of effective collateral circulation. More than 50 per cent of the lumen of a large coronary artery must be occluded before flow through the vessel is compromised.[37] When flow is inadequate, myocardial ischemia occurs. The myocardium must then resort to its limited anaerobic metabolic pathways, and lactic acid is produced.[12] The function of the left ventricle is impaired during ischemia, often accompanied by signs and symptoms of left ventricular failure.

Effective therapeutic measures should therefore be directed either toward decreasing myocardial oxygen requirements, usually by drugs, or toward increasing coronary blood flow by various surgical techniques.

PATHOLOGY OF ANGINA PECTORIS

Postmortem studies,[1, 35, 71] and more recently direct visualization of the coronary arteries during life by selective coronary arteriography,[46] have defined the pathologic anatomy of angina pectoris. Zoll and associates[71] noted one or more occlusions or narrowing of the major coronary arteries in 90 per cent of postmortem studies in patients who had angina pectoris during life. The occlusive disease was usually diffuse, but in one fourth of the cases only a single vessel was involved. Most major lesions occurred within a few centimeters of the origin of the major coronary trunks. Occasionally this syndrome may occur, in the absence of coronary atherosclerosis, in patients with severe valvular disease, hypertension, syphilitic aortitis, abnormalities in oxyhemoglobin dissociation,[20] and nonatherosclerotic disease of the small coronary vessels.

Table 1. *Determinants of Myocardial Oxygen Consumption*

Major
    Total myocardial wall tension
        Intraventricular pressure
        Intraventricular volume
        Ventricular muscle mass
    Heart rate
    Blood pressure
    Myocardial contractility

Minor
    Basal or resting metabolism of myocardium
    Electrical activation of myocardium

Some controversy exists regarding the relationship between myocardial infarction and thrombotic coronary occlusion. For years the term coronary thrombosis was synonymous with myocardial infarction in the minds of both physicians and lay persons. More recent studies[58] suggest that in some patients total occlusion of coronary vessels by thrombus may be the result rather than the cause of myocardial infarction. The exact pathogenesis of infarction without complete occlusion remains unclear.

Nonfunctional intercoronary anastomoses are present in all normal hearts.[49] In the presence of coronary disease these may become larger and more profuse and are frequently demonstrated at coronary arteriography.[27] In some patients with severe large vessel coronary disease, myocardial oxygenation and ventricular function are maintained through such collateral circulation.

In many patients with angina pectoris, large areas of functionally impaired or noncontracting myocardium are present.[21, 30] Actual aneurysmal formation may occur.[11] Compensatory hypertrophy and dilatation of the remaining functioning myocardium take place, further increasing the disparity between oxygen demand and supply.

TREATMENT

Coronary atherosclerosis takes decades to develop before becoming clinically apparent. Little evidence exists to suggest that any of the accepted methods of therapy, which may effectively treat anginal symptoms, alter the atherosclerotic process or prolong life. Obviously the best treatment is preventive. The factors which identify the "coronary-prone" individual have been well defined.[15, 16] These include hypertension, diabetes, diet and abnormalities of lipid metabolism, heavy tobacco consumption, and perhaps obesity, level of physical activity, and heredity. The possible benefit of modification of some of these factors is being widely investigated but will not be discussed further in this report.

Treatment for angina pectoris may conveniently be divided into two major areas—drugs that reduce myocardial oxygen requirements, and surgical techniques that increase myocardial oxygen supply. Each patient with angina pectoris has his own unique pain pattern; each will respond differently to therapeutic measures. All too often it has been our experience that treatment has consisted mainly of a prescription for nitroglycerin with instruction to "take it when you have a pain." Only careful definition of the patient's total problem, including the specific physical and emotional factors that produce the pain, and periodic evaluation of both the effectiveness of therapy and the status of the heart will produce successful results. Much emphasis has been placed on patient instruction in such diseases as diabetes, peptic ulcer, and hypertension. The same principle must be applied to the treatment of angina pectoris.

The Nitrites

Nitroglycerin remains the single most effective drug in the treatment and prevention of anginal symptoms. The exact mechanism by which nitroglycerin produces its beneficial effect is not completely clear.

Although nitroglycerin causes coronary vasodilatation and increases coronary blood flow in normal persons, coronary flow is not increased appreciably in patients with symptomatic coronary artery disease[3, 9, 28] whose coronary arterioles may already be dilated maximally by the potent stimulus of myocardial ischemia. More likely, nitroglycerin works by reducing myocardial oxygen consumption. The drug has a direct effect on peripheral arteriolar and venomotor tone, causing peripheral pooling of blood. Venous return falls, with a resultant decrease in diastolic and systolic volumes. Myocardial wall tension, cardiac output, and at times blood pressure, all significant determinants of myocardial oxygen consumption, are thereby reduced.[7, 34, 38, 45, 66]

In an occasional patient, particularly in the upright position, the decrease in venous return and cardiac output may significantly reduce diastolic pressure, resulting in diminished coronary perfusion and reflex tachycardia. In such patients both nitroglycerin and the long-acting nitrites, which share these effects, may be ineffective.

Doses of nitroglycerin as low as 0.15 or 0.30 mg. are usually effective. Benefit is often denied the patient because larger doses (0.4 to 0.6 mg.) are routinely prescribed, which produce such unpleasant symptoms as headaches, flushing, or palpitations. Nitroglycerin may be most effective when used prophylactically. When it is taken shortly before activity that usually provokes angina, symptoms are often prevented or decreased in severity. Many patients are reluctant to take nitroglycerin because they fear dependence on it or loss of its effectiveness. It must be pointed out carefully that nitroglycerin may be taken without harm as frequently as necessary, and that drug dependence does not occur.

Regular prophylactic use of long-acting nitrites, particularly those that can be taken sublingually, may benefit some patients. They may be particularly effective when used in conjunction with beta-adrenergic blocking agents such as propranolol hydrochloride (Inderal).[51] However, they should never be substituted entirely for nitroglycerin. They are expensive, and side-effects are common. Their onset of action is too long to abort the acute attack of angina. Recent studies show that they may, in fact, reduce the effectiveness of nitroglycerin.[54, 69, 70]

Beta-Adrenergic Blocking Agents

The sympathetic nervous system, through its beta-adrenergic action, markedly influences myocardial oxygen requirements by accelerating heart rate and enhancing myocardial contractility. A major advance in the symptomatic treatment of angina was made when clinically effective, relatively nontoxic agents such as propranolol hydrochloride, which would block these effects, became available. Myocardial oxygen requirements are decreased, resulting in increased exercise tolerance and decreased frequency of anginal attacks.[10, 18, 22, 57, 67] Improvement is obtained in about 75 per cent of patients to whom such drugs are administered; in some, complete relief from anginal symptoms occurs. Hemodynamic responses to exercise or emotional stress are blunted.

When combined with long-acting nitrites such as isosorbide dinitrate (Isordil), the effect of propranolol may be potentiated.[51] Because of its negative effect on myocardial contractility, propranolol hydrochloride must be used with extreme caution if heart failure is suspected. Because it also blocks the positive effects of the sympathetic nervous system on cardiac conduction, it may be contraindicated in patients with a high degree of atrioventricular block. It is relatively contraindicated in patients with asthma, and it should also be used with caution in diabetics who require insulin. Those patients whose diabetes is controlled with oral hypoglycemic agents or diet alone usually tolerate propranolol hydrochloride without significant disturbance of carbohydrate metabolism.

As our experience with propranolol hydrochloride has increased, we have become firmly convinced of its effectiveness and freedom from serious side-effects. We now recommend it in patients whose normal daily activities are significantly limited and those who require frequent doses of nitroglycerin.

The appropriate dose of propranolol hydrochloride may vary considerably. Since the effects of a single dose are largely dissipated in 6 to 8 hours, the drug should be taken as close to every 6 hours as possible. The usual starting dose is 10 to 20 mg. every 6 hours, increasing by increments of 10 to 20 mg. per dose every few days until the desired effect is achieved. Many so-called treatment failures with propranolol hydrochloride are the result of inadequate dosage, and we do not hesitate to use a total daily dose of 320 to 400 mg. a day if necessary. Intolerance may occasionally occur, and this is often best treated by reducing the dose or stopping the drug for a few days. Only rarely will gastrointestinal side-effects, particularly cramps and diarrhea, prevent using the drug. If possible, propranolol hydrochloride should be stopped several days before operation or cardiac catheterization.

LEFT VENTRICULAR FAILURE IN ANGINA

The majority of patients with angina pectoris have normal left ventricular hemodynamics at rest. It has now been amply documented[13, 26, 42, 65] that anginal pain is often accompanied by transient left ventricular failure. Treatment of this transient failure with digitalis and diuretics has been ineffective, and the clinical course of angina has been little altered. However, when overt congestive failure or cardiomegaly is present, digitalis and diuretics should of course be used.

NOCTURNAL ANGINA

This type of angina may be particularly difficult to treat. In such patients, coronary atherosclerosis is invariably severe and diffuse. Since nocturnal angina may be precipitated by distressing dreams,[43] the use of sedatives before retiring is recommended. The head of the bed should be elevated 3 to 6 inches on blocks, thereby diminishing venous return and cardiac work. Large doses of propranolol hydrochloride also given just before retiring may be effective either alone or in combination with long-acting nitrates. Aminophylline by rectum or mouth may be useful. Our results with a nitroglycerin-containing ointment applied directly to the chest have been disappointing. Coronary angiography and surgery should be considered in these patients.

PREINFARCTION ANGINA (CORONARY INSUFFICIENCY, INTERMEDIARY SYNDROME, IMPENDING MYOCARDIAL INFARCTION)

This diagnosis is applied to those patients with angina pectoris whose symptoms have become increasingly severe and prolonged, occur at rest or without any obvious stress, and are not relieved by the usual measures. At the same time, electrocardiographic or enzymatic evidence for acute infarction is usually not evident. Myocardial infarction eventually develops in a high percentage of such patients.[41, 48, 52] For this reason we recommend immediate hospitalization, preferably in a coronary care unit or similar facility. The patient is treated as if he had sustained a myocardial infarction. The gradual subsidence of symptoms without evidence of myocardial necrosis in many of these patients has been gratifying. The role of anticoagulants in such patients is unclear, although several authorities have recommended their use.[61, 68] In the absence of demonstrable cardiac damage, the period of intensive care and rest is abbreviated, and the patient is gradually returned to his previous level of activity.

CAROTID SINUS STIMULATION

In 1928 Wasserman[64] noted that carotid sinus stimulation may terminate an attack of angina. Levine[36] emphasized its value in the diagnosis of angina. It is well recognized that various vagal maneuvers may relieve angina by decreasing the heart rate or the blood pressure. Reflex vagal stimulation has recently been produced by electrical stimulation of the carotid sinus.

This technique was first utilized clinically for hypertension by Bilgutay and Lillehei.[4] Since then Braunwald and her colleagues[6, 23] have applied it to the treatment of severe angina with initially good results. At present, we believe it should be considered in those patients with severe angina not well controlled by drug therapy who are not reasonable candidates for direct coronary surgery.

SURGICAL TREATMENT

There is much current interest and enthusiasm in the newer surgical methods for increasing myocardial blood flow. Vineberg[62, 63] pioneered the technique of internal mammary artery implantation. A 3 year cooperative study by the American College of Chest Physicians[14] has summarized the experience of many centers with this procedure. Symptomatic improvement was recorded in 76 per cent of 2255 patients in whom a single vessel implant was performed. The mortality rate was 5.9 per cent. Multiple implants were performed on 629 patients; 63 per cent of these were symptomatically improved. The mortality rate in this group was 7.5 per cent. However, our own experience in a relatively small number of patients was somewhat disappointing. Subjective improvement sometimes occurred despite lack of patency of the implanted vessel at postoperative catheterization. Our surgical colleagues were also dissatisfied with this indirect approach to the arterial disease.

A more direct approach has recently been introduced by Favaloro[24] who utilized the technique of aortocoronary artery saphenous vein by-pass. The precise anatomy of the diseased coronary circulation is first defined by selective coronary arteriography. In the majority of patients, patency of the vessels distal to the narrowed segments allows by-pass of the involved areas by a saphenous vein graft from the aorta to the distal segment. Unlike the implantation techniques, this procedure produces immediate increase in myocardial blood flow. As experience has accumulated, and the surgical risk has fallen, this technique has become the procedure of choice in most centers.

Recent reports[19, 25, 39] suggest that excellent results can be obtained in more than 90 per cent of patients with disease in one or two vessels, with a mortality rate less than 5 per cent. Similar results have been obtained in about 75 per cent of patients with triple vessel disease, but the mortality rate has been considerably higher. Both subjective relief of anginal pain and objective increase in exercise tolerance with decrease in clinical, electrocardiographic, and hemodynamic manifestations of myocardial ischemia have been documented.[19, 25, 32, 39, 47] However, follow-up studies have shown closure of the grafts in some patients, and the long-term patency rate is difficult to predict at this time. Nor is it likely that surgical therapy will influence the underlying atherosclerotic process. Unfortunately, none of the large surgical series have been adequately controlled in a statistically acceptable fashion to allow valid comparison between medical and surgical management of these patients with severe angina.[59]

Indications for Coronary Surgery

Considerable disagreement still exists regarding the indications for coronary surgery. In a few centers the presence of clinical coronary disease is itself an indication for coronary arteriography and possible surgery if the coronary anatomy is favorable. Yet many cardiologists remain unconvinced of any lasting benefit and are unwilling to submit even their severely disabled patients to the immediate mortality, discomfort, disability, and expense of surgery. Our own position is somewhere between.

Severe disabling anginal pain, which persists despite adequate medical therapy, remains the prime indication for coronary surgery. We are particularly aggressive in younger patients with severe angina whose long-term prognosis with medical therapy alone is poor. Age, however, is not an absolute contraindication.

Significant left ventricular dysfunction can be caused by coronary disease. Increased blood flow to the ischemic myocardium may improve left ventricular function.[47] Patients with severe angina who have ventricular failure should also be considered for coronary surgery. If necessary, the saphenous vein by-pass procedure can be combined with resection of the akinetic or dyskinetic myocardium.

More recently, this technique has been utilized in patients whose angina has become unstable or in whom preinfarction angina has developed. If these patients do not respond to rigorous medical therapy, surgery should be considered. The rationale, of course, is to prevent major myocardial destruction by improving coronary flow while the ischemia is still reversible. Our experience in this area is hopeful but limited. Emergency revascularization of the myocardium in acute myocardial infarction, when resistant cardiogenic shock develops, has been performed in a few patients. The long-term effectiveness of such therapy cannot yet be evaluated.

Electrical instability, manifest chiefly by ventricular arrhythmias, has a particularly ominous prognosis in patients with severe angina. If this instability is prolonged and remains refractory to reasonable drug therapy, such patients should also be considered for surgery.

A word should be said about the indications for coronary arteriography. This technique is invaluable in defining the cause of chest pain when the etiology is unclear. The major indication in patients with known coronary disease is to define the anatomy of the coronary circulation in those patients who are being seriously considered for coronary surgery. We do not recommend coronary arteriography merely to define the extent of atherosclerotic process in patients who adequately respond to medical treatment.

As experience with this type of surgery and knowledge of the long-term results accumulate, indications will almost certainly change. It may find much wider applicability in all forms of coronary heart disease.

SUMMARY

The presence of angina pectoris usually implies significant, diffuse coronary atherosclerosis. Many of these patients, however, do surprisingly well when medical therapy is properly applied; the majority can be treated adequately by such means. However, a small proportion defy usual medical measures. In these patients coronary surgery should be considered. The long term benefit from surgery has yet to be defined, but the immediate results from aortocoronary saphenous vein by-pass are gratifying. The indications for such surgery have been outlined.

REFERENCES

1. Allison, R. B., Rodriguez, F. L., Higgins, E. A., Jr., et al.: Clinicopathologic correlations in coronary atherosclerosis. Four hundred thirty patients studied with postmortem coronary angiography. Circulation 27:170–184 (Feb.) 1963.
2. Berne, R. M.: Regulation of coronary blood flow. Physiol. Rev. 44:1–29 (Jan.) 1964.
3. Bernstein, L., Friesinger, G. C., Lichtlen, P. R., et al.: The effect of nitroglycerin on the sys-

temic and coronary circulation in man and dogs: myocardial blood flow measured with xenon. Circulation 33:107–116 (Jan.) 1966.

4. Bilgutay, A. M., and Lillehei, C. W.: Surgical treatment of hypertension with reference to barospacing. Amer. J. Cardiol. 17:663–667 (May) 1966.

5. Bing, R. J.: Cardiac metabolism. Physiol. Rev. 45:171–213 (April) 1965.

6. Braunwald, E., Epstein, S. E., Glick, G., et al.: Relief of angina pectoris by electrical stimulation of the carotid-sinus nerves. New Eng. J. Med. 277:1278–1283 (Dec. 14) 1967.

7. Braunwald, E., Oldham, H. N., Jr., Ross, J., Jr., et al.: The circulatory response of patients with idiopathic hypertrophic subaortic stenosis to nitroglycerin and to the Valsalva maneuver. Circulation 29:422–431 (March) 1964.

8. Braunwald, E., Sarnoff, S. J., Case, R. B., et al.: Hemodynamic determinants of coronary flow: effect of changes in aortic pressure and cardiac output on the relationship between myocardial oxygen consumption and coronary flow. Amer. J. Physiol. 192:157–163 (Jan.) 1958.

9. Carson, R. P., Wilson, W. S., Nemiroff, M. J., et al.: The effects of sublingual nitroglycerin on myocardial blood flow in patients with coronary artery disease or myocardial hypertrophy. Amer. Heart J. 77:579–584 (May) 1969.

10. Chamberlain, D. A.: Effects of beta adrenergic blockade on heart size. Amer. J. Cardiol. 18:321–328 (Sept.) 1966.

11. Cheng, T. O.: Incidence of ventricular aneurysm in coronary artery disease. An angiographic appraisal. Amer. J. Med. 50:340–355 (March) 1971.

12. Cohen, L. S., Elliott, W. C., Klein, M. D., et al.: Coronary heart disease. Clinical, cinearteriographic and metabolic correlations. Amer. J. Cardiol. 17:153–168 (Feb.) 1966.

13. Cohen, L. S., Elliott, W. C., Rolett, E. L., et al.: Hemodynamic studies during angina pectoris. Circulation 31:409–416 (March) 1965.

14. Coronary surgery surveyed. J.A.M.A. 206:1010 (Oct. 28) 1968.

15. Dawber, T. R., and Kannel, W. B.: Susceptibility to coronary heart disease. Mod. Concepts Cardiovasc. Dis. 30:671–676 (July) 1961.

16. Doyle, J. T., Heslin, A. S., Hilleboe, H. E., et al.: A prospective study of degenerative cardiovascular disease in Albany: report of three years' experience. I. Ischemic heart disease. Amer. J. Public Health (Part 2) 47:25–32 (April) 1957.

17. Driscol, T. E., Moir, T. W., and Eckstein, R. W.: Autoregulation of coronary blood flow: effect of interarterial pressure gradients. Circ. Res. 15:103–111 (Aug.) 1964.

18. Dwyer, E. M., Jr., Weiner, L., and Cox, J. W.: Effects of beta-adrenergic blockade on left ventricular hemodynamics and the electrocardiogram during exercise-induced angina pectoris. Circulation 38:250–260 (Aug.) 1968.

19. Effler, D. B., Favaloro, R. G., and Groves, L. K.: Coronary artery surgery utilizing saphenous vein graft techniques. Clinical experience with 224 operations. J. Thorac. Cardiovasc. Surg. 59:147–154 (Jan.) 1970.

20. Eliot, R. S., and Bratt, G.: The paradox of myocardial ischemia and necrosis in young women with normal coronary arteriogram. Relation to abnormal hemoglobin-oxygen dissociation. Amer. J. Cardiol. 23:633–638 (May) 1969.

21. Elliott, W. C., and Gorlin, R.: The coronary circulation, myocardial ischemia, and angina pectoris (I). Mod. Concepts Cardiovasc. Dis. 35:111–116 (Oct.) 1966.

22. Elliott, W. C., and Stone, J. M.: Beta-adrenergic blocking agents for the treatment of angina pectoris. Progr. Cardiovasc. Dis. 12:83–98 (July) 1969.

23. Epstein, S. E., Beiser, G. D., Goldstein, R. E., et al.: Treatment of angina pectoris by electrical stimulation of carotid-sinus nerves. New Eng. J. Med. 280:971–978 (May 1) 1969.

24. Favaloro, R. G.: Saphenous vein graft in the surgical treatment of coronary artery disease. Operative technique. J. Thorac. Cardiovasc. Surg. 58:178–185 (Aug.) 1969.

25. Favaloro, R. G., Effler, D. B., and Groves, L. K.: Severe segmental obstruction of the left main coronary artery and its divisions: Surgical treatment by the saphenous vein graft technique. J. Thorac. Cardiovasc. Surg. 60:469–482 (Oct.) 1970.

26. Friesinger, G. C., Conti, C. R., and Pitt, B.: Observations on left ventricular pressure during angina pectoris. Abstract. Circulation 36 (Suppl. 2):115 (Jan.) 1967.

27. Gensini, G. G., and Bruto da Costa, B. C.: The coronary collateral circulation in living man. Amer. J. Cardiol. 24:393–400 (Sept.) 1969.

28. Gorlin, R., Brachfeld, N., MacLeod, C., and Bopp, P.: Effect of nitroglycerin on the coronary circulation in patients with coronary artery disease or increased left ventricular work. Circulation 19:705–718 (May) 1959.

29. Gregg, D. E.: Coronary Circulation in Health and Disease. Philadelphia, Lea and Febiger, 1950, 227 pp.

30. Herman, M. V., Heinle, R. A., Klein, M. D., et al.: Localized disorders in myocardial contraction. Asynergy and its role in congestive heart failure. New Eng. J. Med. 227:222–232 (Aug. 3) 1967.

31. Hunter, A.: Heart in anaemia. Quart. J. Med. 15:107–124 (April) 1946.

32. Johnson, W. D., Flemma, R. J., Manley, J. C., et al.: The physiologic parameters of ven-

tricular function as affected by direct coronary surgery. J. Thorac. Cardiovasc. Surg. 60:483–490 (Oct.) 1970.

33. Kattus, A. A., and Gregg, D. E.: Some determinants of coronary collateral blood flow in the open-chest dog. Circ. Res. 7:628–642 (July) 1959.

34. Lee, S. J. K., Sung, Y. K., and Zaragoza, A. J.: Effects of nitroglycerin on left ventricular volumes and wall tension in patients with ischaemic heart disease. Brit. Heart J. 32:790–794 (Nov.) 1970.

35. Lenegre, J., and Himbert, J.: Critical study of the relationship between angina pectoris and coronary atherosclerosis. Amer. Heart J. 58:539–542 (Oct.) 1959.

36. Levine, S. A.: Carotid sinus massage: new diagnostic test for angina pectoris. J.A.M.A. 182:1332–1334 (Dec. 29) 1962.

37. Mann, F. C., Herrick, J. F., Essex, H. E., and Baldes, E. J.: Effect on blood flow of decreasing lumen of blood vessel. Surgery 4:249–252 (Aug.) 1938.

38. Mason, D. T., Zelis, R., and Amsterdam, E. A.: Action of the nitrites on the peripheral circulation and myocardial oxygen consumption: Significance in the relief of angina pectoris. Chest 59:296–305 (March) 1971.

39. Mitchel, B. F., Adam, M., Lambert, C. J., et al.: Ascending aorta-to-coronary artery saphenous vein bypass grafts. J. Thorac. Cardiovasc. Surg. 60:457–468 (Oct.) 1970.

40. Mosher, P., Ross, J., Jr., McFate, P. A., et al.: Control of coronary blood flow by an autoregulatory mechanism. Circ. Res. 14:250–259 (March) 1964.

41. Mounsey, P.: Prodromal symptoms in myocardial infarction. Brit. Heart J. 13:215–226 (April) 1951.

42. Müller, O., and Rørvik, K.: Haemodynamic consequences of coronary heart disease with observations during anginal pain and on the effect of nitroglycerin. Brit. Heart J. 20:302–310 (July) 1958.

43. Nowlin, J. B., Troyer, W. G., Jr., Collins, W. S., et al.: Association of nocturnal angina pectoris with dreaming. Ann. Intern. Med. 63:1040–1046 (Dec.) 1965.

44. Opie, L. H.: Cardiac metabolism. The effect of some physiologic, pharmacologic and pathologic influences. Amer. Heart J. 69:401–409 (March) 1965.

45. Parker, J. O., West, R. O., and DiGiorgi, S.: The effect of nitroglycerin on coronary blood flow and the hemodynamic response to exercise in coronary artery disease. Amer. J. Cardiol. 27:59–65 (Jan.) 1971.

46. Proudfit, W. L., Shirey, E. K., and Sones, F. M., Jr.: Selective coronary cinearteriography in angina pectoris and myocardial infarction: distribution of obstructive lesions (P). Circulation 32 (Suppl. 2):173–174 (Oct.) 1965.

47. Rees, G., Bristow, J. D., Kremkau, E. L., et al.: Influence of aortocoronary bypass surgery on left ventricular performance. New Eng. J. Med. 284:1116–1120 (May 20) 1971.

48. Resnik, W. H.: Preinfarction angina. II. An interpretation. Mod. Concepts Cardiovasc. Dis. 31:757–761 (Nov.) 1962.

49. Rodriguez, F. L., and Robbins, S. L.: Postmortem angiographic studies on the coronary arterial circulation; intercoronary arterial anastomoses in adult human hearts. Amer. Heart J. 70:348–364 (Sept.) 1965.

50. Rothchild, M. A., and Kissin, M.: Production of the anginal syndrome by induced general anoxemia. Amer. Heart J. 8:729–754 (Aug.) 1933.

51. Russek, H. I.: Intractable angina pectoris. Med. Clin. N. Amer. 54:333–348 (March) 1970.

52. Sampson, J. J., and Eliaser, M., Jr.: Diagnosis of impending acute coronary artery occlusion. Amer. Heart J. 13:675–686 (June) 1937.

53. Sarnoff, S. J., Braunwald, E., Welch, G. H., Jr., et al.: Hemodynamic determinants of oxygen consumption of the heart with special reference to the tension-time index. Amer. J. Physiol. 192:148–156 (Jan.) 1958.

54. Schelling, J. L., and Lasagna, L.: A study of cross-tolerance to circulatory effects of organic nitrates. Clin. Pharmacol. Ther. 8:256–260 (March-April) 1967.

55. Sonnenblick, E. H., Ross, J., Jr., and Braunwald, E.: Oxygen consumption of the heart. Newer concepts of its multifactorial determination. Amer. J. Cardiol. 22:328–336 (Sept.) 1968.

56. Sonnenblick, E. H., Ross, J., Jr., Covell, J. W., et al.: Velocity of contraction as a determinant of myocardial oxygen consumption. Amer. J. Physiol. 209:919–927 (Nov.) 1965.

57. Sowton, E., and Hamer, J.: Hemodynamic changes after beta-adrenergic blockade. Amer. J. Cardiol. 18:317–320 (Sept.) 1966.

58. Spain, D. M., and Bradess, V. A.: Sudden death from coronary heart disease. Survival time, frequency of thrombi and cigarette smoking. Chest 58:107–110 (Aug.) 1970.

59. Spodick, D. H.: Revascularization of the heart—numerators in search of denominators. Amer. Heart J. 81:149–157 (Feb.) 1971.

60. Sutton, D. C., and Lueth, H. C.: Pain. Arch. Intern. Med. 45:827–867 (June) 1930.

61. Vakil, R. J.: Preinfarction syndromes—management and follow-up. Amer. J. Cardiol. 14:55–63 (July) 1964.

62. Vineberg, A. M.: Development of anastomosis between coronary vessels and transplanted internal mammary artery. Canad. Med. Assoc. J. 55:117–119 (Aug.) 1946.

63. Vineberg, A., and Walker, J.: Six months to six years' experience with coronary artery in-
    sufficiency treated by internal mammary artery implantation. Amer. Heart J.
    54:851–862 (Dec.) 1957.
64. Wasserman, S.: Die Angina pectoris ihre Pathogenese und Pathophysiologie. Wien Klin.
    Wochenschr. 41:1514–1518 and 1560–1563 (Nov. 1 and 8) 1928.
65. Wiener, L., Dwyer, E. M., Jr., and Cox, J. W.: Left ventricular hemodynamics in exercise-
    induced angina pectoris. Circulation 38:240–249 (Aug.) 1968.
66. Williams, J. F., Glick, G., and Braunwald, E.: Studies on cardiac dimensions in intact
    unanesthetized man. V. Effects of nitroglycerin. Circulation 32:767–771 (Nov.) 1965.
67. Wolfson, S., Heinle, R. A., Herman, M. V., et al.: Propranolol and angina pectoris. Amer. J.
    Cardiol. 18:345–353 (Sept.) 1966.
68. Wood, P.: Therapeutic application of anticoagulants. Trans. Med. Soc. Lond. 66:80, 1948.
69. Zelis, R., and Mason, D. T.: Demonstration of nitrite tolerance: Attenuation of the vasodi-
    lator response to nitroglycerin by the chronic administration of isosorbide dinitrate. Ab-
    stract. Circulation 40 (Suppl. 3):221 (Nov.) 1969.
70. Zelis, R., Mason, D. T., Spann, J. F., et al.: The mechanism of action of nitroglycerin in the
    relief of angina pectoris: Reduction of myocardial oxygen requirements by ex-
    tracoronary vasodilatation and its attenuation by the chronic administration of isosor-
    bide dinitrate. Abstract. Ann. Intern. Med. 72:779 (May) 1970.
71. Zoll, P. M., Wessler, S., and Blumgart, H. L.: Angina pectoris; clinical and pathologic corre-
    lation. Amer. J. Med. 11:331–357 (Sept.) 1951.

605 Commonwealth Avenue
Boston, Massachusetts 02215

The Management of Paroxysmal Atrial Fibrillation

David I. Rutledge, M.D.

Paroxysmal atrial fibrillation is one of the commonest arrhythmias to plague mankind. It is essentially a benign arrhythmia which responds satisfactorily to treatment.

DIAGNOSIS

If one is fortunate enough to obtain an electrocardiogram during an episode of cardiac irregularity, diagnosis is easy. Too often, however, this is not the case, and one has to depend on the patient's description of the attack for the diagnosis. In contradistinction to chronic atrial fibrillation, which sometimes goes unnoticed by the patient, paroxysmal atrial fibrillation produces unpleasant symptoms. The patient is aware of the tumultuous action in the chest. He may not be able to tell you the pulse rate, but he usually is aware of an irregularity of the pulse. If he has a wife or friend who is a nurse and can take the pulse, this is often a great help in the diagnosis. Usually the rate of the ventricle is not as rapid in paroxysmal atrial fibrillation as it is in the commoner paroxysmal atrial tachycardia. The rate is usually around 100 beats per minute.

The episode tends to last longer than an episode of paroxysmal atrial tachycardia, which is frequently only a matter of a few minutes. The patient is unable to revert the attack by holding the breath, using other methods of straining, or by belching. He may find that if he is able to get to sleep the rhythm will have reverted to normal by morning.

Generally speaking, a cardiac irregularity, with onset in an adult, which is grossly irregular and lasts several hours, should be considered atrial fibrillation, even without an electrocardiogram to confirm the diagnosis.

MECHANISM

The mechanism of atrial fibrillation has long been controversial. For many years the circus movement described by McKenzie was generally held to be the abnormal physiologic state responsible for the arrhythmia. Studies of transmembrane electrical potential have thrown new light on the mechanism of atrial fibrillation.[4] It is now known that other areas beside the sinus node contain cells capable of initiating atrial activity. At times these cells show spontaneous depolarization. They may be automatic, and they may compete with each other for control of the atrium. Such cells are located along the venous tissue sulcus terminalis, along the extent of the junction of the great veins with the right atrium, around the orifice of the coronary sinus, and around the right atrioventricular ring.[2] It can easily be seen that if the activity of the sinus node is depressed, by limitation of its blood supply, the previously mentioned areas may complete for control of the atrial action. By the same token, stimulants to these areas may induce the same process.

There is no uniformity of opinion as to whether a single focus is the cause of atrial fibrillation or whether arrhythmia represents multiple foci. According to Hurst,[3] the weight of evidence supports the unifocal theory. Evidence of Scherf et al.[7] and Prinzmetal et al.[6] tend to support that. As Hurst[3] so aptly put it, "there is no reason why any one mechanism should invariably account for every instance of a given dysrhythmia." Finally it should be emphasized that paroxysmal atrial fibrillation frequently occurs in young adults when no demonstrable evidence of organic heart disease exists, and when there does not appear to be any toxic influence. This is called the idiopathic variety and has also been termed "lone fibrillation."[1]

ETIOLOGY

As I have indicated, paroxysmal atrial fibrillation often occurs in healthy young adults without demonstrable heart disease. However, organic conditions may be present to contribute to the development of arrhythmia, and it is well known that toxic substances are a frequent cause of the disturbance. Causes are listed in Table 1.

MANAGEMENT

If there is underlying disease or toxic influences, attention should first be directed to improving these conditions.

SEDATION. This is of particular value in the idiopathic type. Often a mild sedative and a good night's sleep will result in sinus rhythm by morning.

DIGITALIS. It is not claimed that digitalis has a specific effect in reverting atrial fibrillation. It does tend to slow the ventricular response, and practical experience shows it frequently results in reversion of the rhythm to the sinus variety. If the patient has not been taking digitalis, this is the treatment of choice. In patients who have frequent recurrences of atrial fibrillation, digitalis on a prolonged basis seems to have some beneficial effect in reducing the frequency of attacks. When a non critical situation is present, I prefer to use the oral route for digitalization. Digitoxin or digoxin may be used, depending on the preference of the physician and his familiarity with the use of the drug. If there is any question whether or not the patient has been taking digitalis, I would

Table 1. *Causes of Paroxysmal Atrial Fibrillation*

Organic causes

   Atherosclerotic conditions involving the myocardium and particularly the circulation
      to the sinoatrial node
   Valvular heart disease, most frequently in mitral stenosis; episodes of transient atrial
      fibrillation may be frequent before the arrhythmia becomes fixed
   Atrial septal defects
   Hypermetabolism—once a common cause of atrial fibrillation, either transient or fixed,
      now less frequently seen
   Myocardial infarction, especially if the artery to the sinus node is involved.
   Pulmonary embolus
   Chronic lung disease
   After surgical procedures
      Involving the heart directly
      Involving the thoracic cavity
      Involving the abdomen, particularly upper area

Toxic conditions

   Alcohol excess—one of the commonest causes of the paroxysmal variety of atrial
      fibrillation
   Emotional stress, probably the result of the release of catecholamines into the circulation
   Digitalis intoxication—should always be suspected when the patient taking digitalis
      suddenly begins to fibrillate without other obvious causes[5]
   Excesses of coffee or tea
   Smoking
   Toxic effects from bee stings or spider bites
   Acute pericarditis
   Acute rheumatic fever

Idiopathic variety
   Occurring in healthy young adults without demonstrable evidence of heart disease

prefer to use digoxin because of its more prompt elimination. My preference would be to give digoxin, 0.5 mg., repeating the dose twice in the first 24 hours. This is not a full digitalizing dose, but it is usually sufficient to revert the arrhythmias. If it is necessary to digitalize the patient rapidly, my preference would be crystalline digitalis glycoside (Cedilanid) administered intravenously in an initial dose of 0.8 mg., repeating the dose in a half hour.

QUINIDINE.   This has long been a useful drug in the management of paroxysmal atrial fibrillation ever since a missionary reported to Wenkebach that he was free of atrial fibrillation while taking quinine to offset malaria. Quinidine sometimes tends to increase the ventricular rate. If this might cause a critical situation, then it would be wise to digitalize the patient first. It is always wise to use a trial dose of quinidine, as rarely a person is sensitive to it. Quinidine should be built up rapidly in the bloodstream. My preference is to use 400 mg. at the onset and repeat with 200 mg. every hour until the arrhythmia stops, with the maximum of 12 doses being given within 24 hours.

INDERAL.   More recently, propranolol hydrochloride (Inderal) has proved to be a useful drug in the management of paroxysmal atrial fibrillation. It is a beta-adrenergic blocking agent and for all practical purposes is without side-effects, with the exception of the patient with bronchial asthma. A dose of 20 mg. repeated in half an hour will often revert an episode of atrial fibrillation to sinus rhythm.

CARDIOVERSION. Cardioversion by the direct current introduced by Lown is often a satisfactory way to revert atrial fibrillation to normal sinus rhythm. It is particularly useful when a temporary state exists that cannot be reverted by the drug treatment mentioned previously. If atrial fibrillation has existed for some time, it may be difficult to convert, and it may equally be difficult to maintain sinus rhythm. Maintenance might require the prolonged use of quinidine sulfate with all the problems this therapy presents.

A word should be said about the danger of embolus formation. Generally speaking, patients with brief episodes of atrial fibrillation are not likely to discharge emboli from the atrium unless they existed beforehand because of an organic lesion, such as mitral stenosis. On one occasion, I have seen a patient who had atrial fibrillation of the paroxysmal variety for a period of 24 hours, in whom a large embolism developed at the time of reversion. If the atrial fibrillation has persisted for several days, it is probably wise to use anticoagulants before cardioversion.

SUMMARY

Attention should first be directed to probable cause, and this should be eliminated or controlled when possible. Sedation will control many episodes of paroxysmal atrial fibrillation. Digitalis should be considered first when confronted with atrial fibrillation which is of recent onset. This is particularly true of the postoperative attacks. For the patient known to have paroxysmal atrial fibrillation, propranolol (Inderal), which the patient can take himself, is a very useful drug. Quinidine is useful in the management of the arrhythmia. It requires a little more skill in handling. If an emergency situation exists, cardioversion with the direct current cardioverter should be considered.

REFERENCES

1. Evans, W.: The management of paroxysmal atrial fibrillation. Progr. Cardiovasc. Dis. 2:480–484 (March) 1960.
2. Hoffman, B. F., and Cranefield, P. F.: The physiological basis of cardiac arrhythmias. Amer. J. Med. 37:670–684 (Nov.) 1964.
3. Hurst, J. W., and Logue, R. B.: The Heart, Arteries, and Veins. New York, McGraw-Hill, 1970, p. 507.
4. Hurst, J. W., Paulk, E. A., Jr., Proctor, H. D., et al.: Management of patients with atrial fibrillation. Amer. J. Med. 37:728–741 (Nov.) 1964.
5. Irons, G. V., Jr., and Orgain, E. S.: Digitalis-induced arrhythmias and their management. Progr. Cardiovasc. Dis. 8:539–569 (May) 1966.
6. Prinzmetal, M., Corday, E., Brill, I. C., et al.: Quoted by Hurst, J. W., and Logue, R. B. (ref. 3).
7. Scherf, D., Romano, F. J., and Terranova, R.: Quoted by Hurst, J. W., and Logue, R. B. (ref. 3).

605 Commonwealth Avenue
Boston, Massachusetts 02215

Treatment of Ventricular Arrhythmias in Ambulatory Patients

Robert A. England, M.D.

With the widespread utilization of coronary care units, plans for management of ventricular arrhythmias have evolved. These regimens have come to apply to hospitalized patients who are suspected of having acute cardiac ischemia. The patients are treated when (1) there are more than 5 ventricular ectopic beats per minute, (2) ventricular ectopic beats occur with 2 or more beats in succession, (3) multiform ventricular ectopic beats occur, and (4) ventricular ectopic beats interrupt the T-wave of the preceding beat.

The ambulatory patient presents a situation for which it is much more difficult to establish rules. Ventricular arrhythmias are frequently seen in patients who have no serious disease. The timing of treatment, if any, is rarely clear cut. When a decision is made to suppress the ventricular instability, the choice of therapy is a vexing one.

This paper outlines an approach to ventricular arrhythmias in ambulatory patients who are not suspected of having acute coronary ischemia.

VENTRICULAR ECTOPIC BEATS

Prevalence

Ventricular ectopic beats are frequently seen. Of a group of 122,043 healthy men being screened for flight training by the Air Force, 0.7 per cent had this arrhythmia.[15] Each man had 48 seconds of rhythm recorded.

Of the 12,000 outpatient electrocardiograms that have been reviewed at the Lahey Clinic Foundation,[1] 4.2 per cent of these tracings show ventricular ectopic beats. Of those electrocardiograms showing this arrhythmia, (1) 18 per cent were in patients with "arteriosclerotic heart disease" manifested by old infarctions and angina or congestive failure or both, (2) 25 per cent of the tracings were obtained from patients with hypertension, (3) 10 per cent were obtained from patients with lung disease, (4) 8 per cent were performed on diabetic patients, and (5) 39 per cent were performed on patients with no definite evidence of any disease. This survey of outpatient electrocardiograms shows that ventricular ectopic beats frequently occur in a variety of clinical settings.

Cause of Ectopic Beats

It is likely that spontaneous electrical activity from the ventricle comes from the terminal branches of the Purkinje system.[16] These fibers are composed of cells that have the characteristics of "pacemaker" cells. That is, these cells can depolarize spontaneously. Once the cells fire, a dormant muscle cell will be stimulated to contract (Fig. 1). Factors that tend to cause arrhythmias affect the depolarization process primarily in phase 4. However, stimulants of other segments of the depolarization wave can also play a role (Fig. 2).

Diagnosis

Differentiation from aberrant ventricular conduction can occasionally cause confusion. Aberrant beats may be seen following a long R-R interval between the preceding two beats. They are usually triphasic, with the same initial forces as the normal beats in lead V_1 (Fig. 3).[31]

Ventricular Ectopic Beats and Coronary Artery Disease

The clinical significance of ventricular ectopic beats in ambulatory patients is not certain. In one study,[10] ventricular ectopic beats on routine

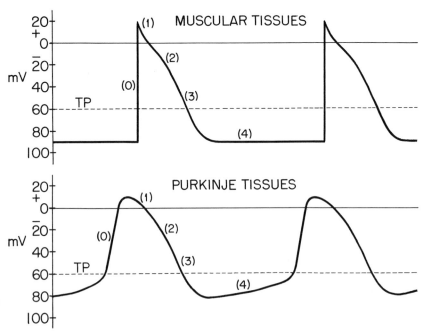

Figure 1.   A Purkinje fiber can reach threshold potential (TP) by its inherent activity. After the TP is reached, the Purkinje fiber is activated. Adjacent muscle fibers are then stimulated to reach their TP. This enables them to depolarize and contract.

FACTORS AFFECTING THE PHASES OF ELECTRICITY
(PURKINJE TISSUES)

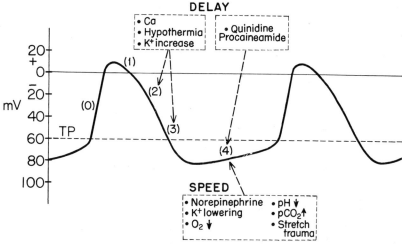

Figure 2. A variety of factors can increase or decrease the tempo of Purkinje fiber activity.

electrocardiograms were not found to be associated with a higher mortality rate. This was determined by making comparisons with patients who had similar heart rates but without any ectopic activity. Ectopic beats were no more significant in their prognosis than was the rate when it was considered by itself. The exception to this observation concerned "multifocal" premature beats. They were thought always to be accompanied by myocardial involvement. ("Multifocal" was not defined but it probably indicated beats that had different electrocardiographic configurations.)

Since these observations of Esler and White[10] in 1929, other efforts

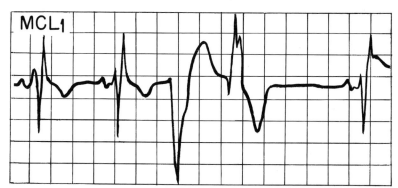

Figure 3. Modified lead V_1 with the third beat conducted normally. Beats 1, 2, and 5 are considered to be conducted aberrantly by virtue of being triphasic and having the same initial force as the normal beat. Beat number 4 is a ventricular premature beat with different initial forces. In addition, the form of QRS is diphasic. (*From* Marriott, H. J. L., and Fogg, E.: Mod. Conc. Cardiovasc. Dis. 39:104, June, 1970, reproduced with permission.)

have been made to continue to clarify the significance of ventricular ectopic beats. In an analysis of some 20,000 "fit air crew men," multifocal beats and those that interrupted T-waves were seen only in subjects who were judged to have some clinical heart disease. Paired ventricular ectopic beats, more specifically, were present only in patients who had coronary artery disease.[25] Hinkle et al.,[14] using long periods of tape monitoring, found that these paired beats were associated with the same risk of sudden death as if the patients had 10 isolated ventricular ectopic beats per 1000 complexes on a recording. These recordings were made during 6 hours of normal activity. Though very extensive, these studies only partially answer the question as to which ectopic beats can be definitely associated with heart disease in an individual patient.

Ventricular Ectopic Beats and Sudden Death

The problem as to whether ventricular ectopic beats are associated with myocardial disease is not the only one that remains unresolved. The overriding issue to be clarified is whether the ventricular ectopic beats are harbingers of sudden death.

Chiang and associates[4] found that a high proportion of patients who died suddenly would have had arrhythmias on routine electrocardiograms. However, these conduction abnormalities were so frequently associated with other risk factors, including hypertensive heart disease, symptomatic coronary artery disease, and diabetes mellitus, that their significance alone remains conjectural.

Hinkle et al.[14] indicated that persons with 10 ventricular ectopic beats per 1000 cardiac cycles had a tenfold increase in the incidence of sudden cardiac death. Lown and Ruberman[24] indicated that an isolated ventricular ectopic beat on an electrocardiogram gave that patient twice the risk of sudden death when compared to a person who had no ventricular ectopic activity on his electrocardiogram.

Thus, these studies implicate ventricular instability with sudden cardiac death. However, it has not been shown how to determine which persons with these ectopic beats will succumb. Nor has it been determined that, once detected, the suppression of this activity will prevent cardiac arrest. Until prophylactic treatment can be shown to be lifesaving, widespread use of antiarrhythmic therapy should not be instituted. These drugs are not invariably successful against ventricular irritability — even when used in high doses — and the side-effects may be difficult to deal with.

Treatment of Ventricular Ectopic Beats

Until studies are completed to indicate the manner in which sudden death can be forestalled in persons with ventricular ectopic beats, treatment should be reserved for those persons whose ectopic beats cause symptoms. Most often, a sensation of chest pounding or "palpitation" is noted. Occasionally, symptomatic ectopic activity can be suppressed simply by correcting electrolyte imbalance. In isolated cases digitalization may work.[23] The younger patient's anxiety can be allayed with a tranquilizer. Sometimes tincture of belladonna will serve to produce relaxation and perhaps to increase the heart rate enough to "overdrive" the ectopic activity.

The vast majority of patients who require therapy for ventricular ectopic beats will need treatment with procainamide, quinidine, or propranolol hydrochloride (Inderal), singly or in combination. The proper regimen can be determined only by trial. Dosage is limited by side-effects in the individual patient.

Use of drugs that have been shown to cause ventricular arrhythmias should be avoided.[17] The common ones are the phenothiazine derivatives, possibly by their effect on the QT interval of repolarization.[2] Catecholamines increase ventricular irritability by themselves, and also may be implicated in ventricular ectopic beats seen with L-Dopa therapy.[28] The role of quinidine in causing syncope and unexpected death has been clinically observed.[32]

James relates the death-dealing properties of quinidine to the prolongation of the QT interval.[17] Procainamide also lengthens the QT interval. Propranolol hydrochloride[7] and diphenylhydantoin[9] both shorten the ventricular refractory period, and thus shorten the QT interval. These latter two drugs, however, are probably less effective than procainamide and quinidine in suppressing most ventricular ectopic beats. Thus, the treatment frequently has the theoretical disadvantage of prolonging the QT interval.

An approach to treating ventricular ectopic beats for symptomatic relief might be outlined as follows: (1) correction of metabolic abnormalities, curtailing stimulants, and avoiding drugs that cause ectopic beats, (2) increasing the slow heart rate with anticholinergic drugs such as tincture of belladonna, (3) digitalization, remembering the role of excess digitalis in causing ventricular arrhythmias,[3] (4) procainamide in doses of 2 gm. a day, (5) propranolol hydrochloride in a dose of 80 mg. a day — this drug has been successful in some cases of L-Dopa-induced ventricular ectopic beats,[22] (6) diphenylhydantoin in a dose of 300 mg. a day, and (7) quinidine in a dose of 800 mg. a day.

Any one or all of these steps can be used to treat patients with symptomatic ventricular ectopic beats. However, treatment should not be undertaken with the idea that suppression of ventricular ectopic beats, when they occur outside a coronary care unit, will prolong life. Studies to evaluate this possibility are now under way.

VENTRICULAR TACHYCARDIA

Ventricular tachycardia is defined as three or more successive ventricular ectopic beats.

Diagnosis

The problem is very much different when dealing with ventricular tachycardia as compared to ventricular ectopic beats. Diagnosis is an illustration of this difference. Massumi and his associates,[27] outlining the difficulty in diagnosing ventricular tachycardia, pointed out that no predictable relationship of atrial activity to ventricular activity exists. In addition, analysis of the first heart sound and jugular venous pulse were shown to be of little help. These findings had been considered as standard criteria in separating nonventricular from ventricular pacemakers[27] (Fig. 4). It has been shown clearly that supraventricular tachycardia with aberrant ventricular conduction can mimic ventricular tachycardia. Marriott[26] has illustrated how this confusion can sometimes be avoided (Fig. 5). Another diagnostic clue is abnormal ventricular conduction interrupted by normal beats for that patient (Fig. 6).

In contrast to ventricular ectopic beats, the diagnosis of ventricular tachycardia means that treatment should be instituted. Ventricular ectopic beats are much easier to diagnose but present a more difficult decision as to when therapy must be instituted. Conversely, ventricular tachycardia is much more difficult to diagnose under certain circumstances, but the decision to treat is straightforward. Two or more episodes of ventricular tachycardia in an ambulatory patient require that steps be taken to prevent recurrent episodes. Paroxysmal ventricular tachycardia is two or more episodes of ventricular tachycardia occurring in ambulatory patients and not during the throes of acute myocardial infarction.

Significance

Not infrequently, paroxysmal ventricular tachycardia will recur in the absence of any definite detectable heart disorders.[21] Ventricular tachycardia in the ambulatory patient must be considered a life-threatening arrhythmia, since it is impossible to tell when any particular episode of ventricular tachycardia will degenerate into ventricular fibrillation. Also, ventricular tachycardia can continue for an indefinite period, and hypotension may ensue as a result of the poor hemodynamics caused by this arrhythmia. When an episode of ventricular tachycardia is noted

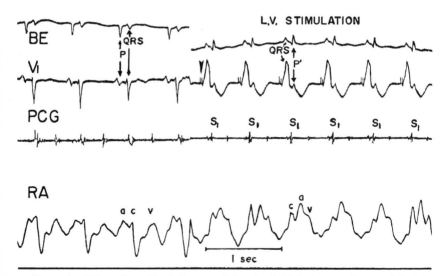

Figure 4.   BE, esophageal lead; V_1, normal chest lead; PCG, phonocardiogram; RA, right atrial pulse tracing. The four first beats are normal. Left ventricular pacing was begun at the fifth beat. This contraction and all the subsequent ones are ventricular in origin (ventricular tachycardia). The atrial activity (P') and the first heart sound (S_1) are constant in relationship to the ventricular contraction (QRS). These characteristics had been used to rule against ventricular tachycardia in the past. This clearly shows that atrial activity and its timing cannot be used to differentiate atrial from ventricular rhythms.

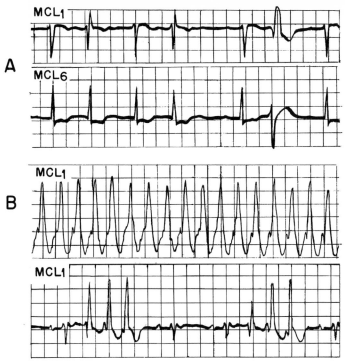

Figure 5. A, The second and fourth beats in both strips are conducted with RBBB-type aberration and show typical aberrant contours (rSR' in MCL₁, qRs in MCL₆); the sixth beat in both strips shows a contour typical of left ventricular ectopy (qR in MCL₁). B, The top strip of MCL₁ shows an anomalous pattern at a rate of 200 that might be either ectopic ventricular or RBBB-type aberration. Aberrancy is confirmed in the bottom strip of MCL₁ where the beat initiating each run of anomalous beats is clearly triphasic (rsR'). (From Marriott, H. J. L., and Fogg, E.: Mod. Conc. Cardiovasc. Dis. 39:106, June, 1970; reproduced with permission.)

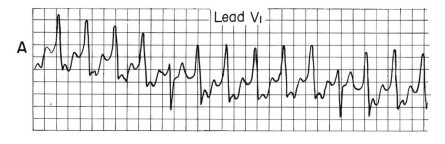

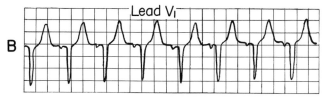

Figure 6. Abnormal ventricular contractions (A) are interrupted by beats (numbers 5 and 11) which are very similar to the patient's usual beats in the precordial leads (B). These beats are not delayed but, rather, are slightly early. If the rhythm was one of aberrant conduction, these early ventricular beats would be more aberrant. Thus, the other beats must be ventricular in origin.

in any ambulatory patient, it is mandatory to observe this patient carefully for any recurrences. Should a recurrence take place, prophylactic
treatment must be undertaken. Before resorting to antiarrhythmic
agents, the effects of hypokalemia[16] and digitalis[23] need to be considered.
Both can cause recurrent ventricular tachycardia as can the phenothiazine derivatives.[20]

Drug Treatment

Procainamide has become the conventional treatment for paroxysmal ventricular tachycardia. Occasionally, doses of more than 10 gm. a
day have been used.[8, 29] However, its use frequently must be stopped
either because it fails to work or because of side-effects, which usually
consist of manifestations of the lupus syndrome.[6] These untoward effects
rarely persist after the drug has been stopped.[33]

Despite an occasional report of the successful use of diphenylhydantoin,[36] it is believed that this drug is not effective in most cases of
ventricular tachycardia.[34]

Quinidine and propranolol hydrochloride have frequently been used
individually. Propranolol hydrochloride has been described as being effective against an unusual type of exercise-induced paroxysmal ventricular tachycardia.[35] Electrocardiographic monitoring during and after exercise has revealed many undetected rhythm disorders.[19] Whether propranolol hydrochloride will be the drug of choice for these is not yet known.

When L-Dopa is necessary for patient care, any ventricular arrhythmias that occur may be suppressed and subsequently prevented with
the use of propranolol hydrochloride.[22]

Perhaps the best drug treatment for paroxysmal ventricular tachycardia has been the combination of quinidine and propranolol hydrochloride. These drugs must be used cautiously in patients with severe
valvular disease or myocardial disease secondary to coronary artery problems. In addition, propranolol hydrochloride has the distinct possibility
of causing distress to patients with obstructive airway disease. The
recommended daily doses range up to 160 mg. of propranolol hydrochloride and 2.6 gm. of quinidine sulfate.[12] However, quinidine doses of more
than 1.2 gm. a day have been shown to cause a 20 per cent incidence of
toxic effects.[30] Diarrhea has frequently been noted when quinidine and
propranolol hydrochloride are combined. However, this frequently responds to mild antidiarrhea therapy.[12]

Nondrug Treatment

Sympathectomy has been used in isolated cases for relief of troublesome recurrent paroxysmal ventricular tachycardia.[11, 19, 37] The use of
intracardiac pacing to control paroxysmal ventricular tachycardia has
met with considerable success.[13, 37] This can be used alone or in combination with drug treatment.[5] The pacing electrode can be implanted
either in the ventricle or in the atrium with good results.[5] Resection of a
ventricular aneurysm has proved successful in an occasional patient
whose condition has been refractory to drug treatment.[18]

SUMMARY

The treatment of ventricular arrhythmias in ambulatory patients must be individualized.

In patients with ventricular ectopic beats the goal is symptomatic relief. If ongoing studies show that ventricular ectopic beats presage sudden cardiac death, then another challenge will lie in selecting the potentially fatal ectopic beats from the benign ones. The different treatment modalities as outlined in this paper will probably still apply.

Paroxysmal ventricular tachycardia in the ambulatory patient presents problems in both diagnosis and treatment. Suggestions to aid in the diagnosis have been presented, and the various choices for treatment have been outlined.

REFERENCES

1. Alexander, S. A., Desai, D., and Hershberg, P.: Unpublished data.
2. Ban, T. A., and St. Jean, A.: The effect of phenothiazines on the electrocardiogram. Can. Med. Assoc. J. *91*:537–540 (Sept. 5) 1964.
3. Beller, G. A., Smith, T. W., Abelmann, W. H., et al.: Digitalis intoxication: Clinical correlations with serum levels. New Eng. J. Med. *284*:989–997 (May 6) 1971.
4. Chiang, B. N., Perlman, L. V., Fulton, M., et al.: Predisposing factors in sudden cardiac death in Tecumseh, Michigan. A prospective study. Circulation *41*:31–37 (Jan.) 1970.
5. Cohen, L. S., Buccino, R. A., Morrow, A. G., et al.: Recurrent ventricular tachycardia and fibrillation treated with a combination of beta-adrenergic blockade and electrical pacing. Ann. Intern. Med. *66*:945–949 (May) 1967.
6. Condemi, J. J., Blomgren, S. E., and Vaughan, J. H.: The procainamide-induced lupus syndrome. Bull. Rheum. Dis. *20*:604–608 (May) 1970.
7. Davis, L. D., and Temte, J. V.: Effects of propranolol on the transmembrane potentials of ventricular muscle and Purkinje fibers of the dog. Circ. Res. *22*:661–677 (May) 1968.
8. Douglas, A. H.: Procainamide prophylaxis in recurrent ventricular tachycardia due to ischemic heart disease. N.Y. State J. Med. *65*:2476–2478 (Oct. 1) 1965.
9. Dreifus, L. S., and Watanabe, Y.: Current status of diphenylhydantoin. Amer. Heart J. *80*:709–713 (Nov.) 1970.
10. Esler, J. W., and White, P. D.: Clinical significance of premature beats with particular reference to heart rate. Arch. Intern. Med. *43*:606–614 (May) 1929.
11. Estes, E. H., Jr., and Izlar, H. L., Jr.: Recurrent ventricular tachycardia: A case successfully treated by bilateral cardiac sympathectomy. Amer. J. Med. *31*:493–497 (Sept.) 1961.
12. Fors, W. J., Jr., Vanderark, C. R., and Reynolds, E. W., Jr.: Evaluation of propranolol and quinidine in the treatment of quinidine-resistant arrhythmias. Amer. J. Cardiol. *27*:190–194 (Feb.) 1971.
13. Greenfield, J. C., Jr., and Orgain, E. S.: The control of ventricular tachyarrhythmias by internal cardiac pacing. Ann. Intern. Med. *66*:1017–1019 (May) 1967.
14. Hinkle, L. E., Jr., Carver, S. T., and Stevens, M.: The frequency of asymptomatic disturbances of cardiac rhythm and conduction in middle-aged men. Amer. J. Cardiol. *24*:629–650 (Nov.) 1969.
15. Hiss, R. G., and Lamb, L. E.: Electrocardiographic findings in 122,043 individuals. Circulation *25*:947–961 (June) 1962.
16. Hoffman, B. F., and Cranefield, P. F.: The physiological basis of cardiac arrhythmias. Amer. J. Med. *37*:670–684 (Nov.) 1964.
17. James, T. N.: QT prolongation and sudden death. Mod. Concepts Cardiovasc. Dis. *38*:35–37 (July) 1969.
18. Kastor, J. A., DeSanctis, R. W., Harthorne, J. W., et al.: Transvenous atrial pacing in the treatment of refractory ventricular irritability. Ann. Intern. Med. *66*:939–945 (May) 1967.
19. Kosowsky, B., et al.: Occurrence of ventricular arrhythmias with exercise as compared to monitoring (in press).
20. Kott, S.: Personal communication.

21. Lesch, M., Lewis, E., Humphries, J. O., et al.: Paroxysmal ventricular tachycardia in the absence of organic heart disease. Report of a case and review of the literature. Ann. Intern. Med. 66:950–960 (May) 1967.
22. Levodopa for parkinsonism. Brit. Med. J. 1:244–245 (Jan. 30) 1971.
23. Lown, B., and Levine, S. A.: Medical progress: Current concepts of digitalis therapy. New Eng. J. Med. 250:771–778, 819–832, and 866–874 (May 6, 13, and 20) 1954.
24. Lown, B., and Ruberman, W.: The concept of precoronary care. Cardiovasc. Dis. 39:97–102 (May) 1970.
25. Manning, G. W., Ahuja, S. P., and Gutierrez, M. R.: Electrocardiographic differentiation between ventricular ectopic beats from subjects with normal and diseased hearts. Acta Cardiol. 23:462–470, 1968.
26. Marriott, H. L.: Constant monitoring for cardiac dysrhythmias and blocks. Mod. Concepts Cardiovasc. Dis. 39:103–108 (June) 1970.
27. Massumi, R. A., Tawakkol, A. A., and Kistin, A. D.: Reevaluation of electrocardiographic and bedside criteria for diagnosis of ventricular tachycardia. Circulation 36:628–636 (Nov.) 1967.
28. Parks, L. C., Watanabe, A. M., and Kopin, I. J.: Prevention or reversal of levodopa-induced cardiac arrhythmias by decarboxylase inhibitors. Lancet 2:1014–1015 (Nov. 14) 1970.
29. Paul, O., and Leigh, C. G.: Ventricular tachycardia: treatment with very large doses of procaine amide. MED. CLIN. N. AMER. 50:271–278 (Jan.) 1966.
30. Rossi, M., and Lown, B.: The use of quinidine in cardioversion. Amer. J. Cardiol. 19:234–238 (Feb.) 1967.
31. Sandler, I. A., and Marriott, H. J.: Differential morphology of anomalous ventricular complexes of RRRB-type in lead V; ventricular ectopy versus aberration. Circulation 31:551–556 (April) 1965.
32. Selzer, A., and Wray, H. W.: Quinidine syncope. Paroxysmal ventricular fibrillation occurring during treatment of chronic atrial arrhythmias. Circulation 30:17–26 (July) 1964.
33. Singson, C. R., Beetham, W. P., Jr., and Alexander, S.: Procainamide-induced lupus syndromes: Review with report of four cases. Lahey Clin. Found. Bull. 19:133–140 (Oct.-Dec.) 1970.
34. Stone, N., Klein, M. D., and Lown, B.: Diphenylhydantoin in the prevention of recurring ventricular tachycardia. Circulation 43:420–427 (March) 1971.
35. Taylor, R. R., and Halliday, E. J.: Beta-adrenergic blockade in the treatment of exercise-induced paroxysmal ventricular tachycardia. Circulation 32:778–781 (Nov.) 1965.
36. Zipes, D. P., and Orgain, E. S.: Refractory paroxysmal ventricular tachycardia. Ann. Intern. Med. 67:1251–1257 (Dec.) 1967.
37. Zipes, D. P., Festoff, B., Schaal, S. F., et al.: Treatment of ventricular arrhythmia by permanent atrial pacemaker and cardiac sympathectomy. Ann. Intern. Med. 68:591–597 (March) 1968.

605 Commonwealth Avenue
Boston, Massachusetts 02215

Prevention and Treatment of Sudden Cardiac Death

Philip I. Hershberg, M.D., and Sidney Alexander, M.D.

In 1969 approximately 800,000 Americans died of coronary heart disease.[3] This figure represented almost half the total deaths in the United States during that year and substantially more than half of those dying before the age of 65.[15, 24] A majority of these deaths were the result of acute myocardial infarction.

Many patients who might have been treated effectively died before they reached the hospital. Bainton and Peterson,[2] for example, reported that 77 per cent of patients who died from acute myocardial infarction did not survive long enough to be seen by a physician while still alive. Among patients who died below the age of 45, Luke and Helpern[20] noted that only 9 of the 78 victims of acute coronary attacks, who died within 24 hours of the onset of symptoms, lived long enough to be admitted to the hospital while still alive.

The logical starting point in the treatment of myocardial infarction lies in the prevention of coronary atherosclerosis and the possible reversal of any such coronary disease which might exist at the initiation of therapy. While little is really known about the basic etiology of acute myocardial infarction, substantial data have been accumulated identifying those factors which render a given individual prone to myocardial infarction. These include heredity, elevated serum lipid levels, heavy cigarette smoking, excessive weight, lack of exercise, psychological stress, diabetes mellitus, and elevated blood pressure.[4, 6, 7, 27] Using these and other factors, such as the electrocardiographic response to exercise, it is possible to predict the probability of future myocardial infarction in a given individual with a relatively high degree of accuracy.[8, 23]

While it may be impractical for the individual physician to apply elaborate predictive cardiologic procedures in his daily practice, in theory at least he may be able to do much to lower the incidence of coronary heart disease. His enthusiasm may be contagious, and the number of patients influenced may be substantial.[11] It must be the physician's responsibility

This investigation was supported in part by grants from the National Aeronautics and Space Administration (NGR 22-007-203) and the U.S. Public Health Service (IR18 HS-00307-01 HCS).

to advise his patients to do those things which might minimize susceptibility to clinical coronary disease.

MORTALITY

A precise estimate of total mortality from all acute myocardial infarctions is difficult. Some patients with mild symptoms never consult a
physician. Others die suddenly and the exact cause of death may not be
apparent. However, a reasonable approximation can be made using data
obtained from several excellent studies.

Gordon and Kannel[9] have noted that two thirds of coronary heart
disease deaths in patients under the age of 65 occurred outside the hospital. In most patients the final episode is sudden, occurring within 1 hour
of onset of symptoms. Spain et al.[26] studied causes of sudden death and
found that a witnessed fatal episode, lasting less than an hour, was the
result of coronary heart disease in more than 90 per cent of all cases.
Since the introduction of coronary care units,[13, 16–19] fewer patients who
reach the hospital alive are dying. Such units, no matter how effective,
obviously have little direct influence on the treatment of patients who die
before they reach the hospital. However, lessons learned from continuous electrocardiographic monitoring and treatment of patients in coronary care units may be applicable to the first aid treatment of sudden
death in the prehospital phase of acute myocardial infarction.

Grace[10] has divided his hospitalized patients into three groups. Those
designated as having "coronoid" disease had typical symptoms but no
positive electrocardiographic or laboratory evidence of acute myocardial
ischemia. In a second group of patients, called the "coronette" group,
subendocardial infarction occurred, manifested chiefly by T wave in-
version. None of the patients in these two groups died acutely from
coronary heart disease. In the third or "coronary" group, acute transmural
myocardial infarction was present. Among these patients a 25 per cent
in-hospital mortality rate was noted.

Shapiro and associates[25] studied coronary deaths among patients in
the 110,000 member Health Insurance Plan in New York City. They
concluded that about 60 per cent of all witnessed deaths from myocardial
infarction occurred within the first half hour after the onset of symptoms. This agrees well with the data of others.[2, 22] Since death in these patients is so rapid, only rarely will a patient survive to reach the hospital.
The overall mortality rate in such patients appears to be considerably in
excess of the average in-hospital mortality rate of about 25 per cent. We
suspect that the overall mortality rate for transmural myocardial infarction is approximately 45 per cent.

DIAGNOSIS AND TREATMENT

Standard medical texts discuss the diagnosis of myocardial infarction by listing the characteristic symptoms, physical findings, and laboratory and electrocardiographic data, producing an authoritative discussion

of the patient who has survived long enough to be seen in the hospital and physician's office. However, little attention is given to the subject of first aid therapy for myocardial infarction. No account is mentioned of the measures which should be taken by the patient's spouse, friend, or business associate before the physician arrives, and rarely is any comment made, however brief, on the immediate treatment by the physician in the patient's home. Not surprisingly, assistance provided by the layman is often ineffective. For practical purposes, the present discussion of the prevention of sudden death will emphasize first aid therapy. Treatment by ambulance personnel and within the hospital will be mentioned only briefly.

First Aid in Myocardial Infarction

First aid training has been applied chiefly to those patients in whom cardiac or respiratory arrest has already developed. Effective external cardiac massage[14] requires fairly comprehensive training, immediate action, and vigorous exertion by a number of well-motivated individuals. Unfortunately, all too often it is unsuccessful. Among hospitalized patients the survival rate is low even when external cardiac massage is applied immediately by a trained staff within a few moments of cardiac arrest.[21] Its application as a first aid measure outside the hospital is obviously limited. Therefore, in those patients in whom cardiac arrest occurs simultaneously with the onset of symptoms, first aid techniques will largely be ineffective. Any decrease in the mortality rate of such individuals must come from proper application of preventive measures. Immediate death is fortunately rare; so-called sudden death usually occurs between 5 minutes and 1 hour after the onset of symptoms, thus allowing some time for the application of appropriate first aid therapy.

Much evidence exists to suggest that the mechanism of death in these patients is either ventricular fibrillation or asystole. Data from patients carefully monitored in coronary care units show that these lethal arrhythmias rarely occur without warning, and that most deaths early in the course of myocardial infarction are potentially preventable by proper drug therapy.

Ventricular premature beats and ventricular tachycardia usually occur before the onset of ventricular fibrillation, the mechanism present in most cases of sudden death. These arrhythmias can be effectively treated by antiarrhythmic drugs, thereby preventing the development of ventricular fibrillation. In selecting an appropriate antiarrhythmic agent for emergency treatment, we therefore must choose an agent with prompt onset of action and little cardiodepressive action. Quinidine and procainamide, two commonly used antiarrhythmic agents, particularly when given intravenously, depress cardiac function and reduce peripheral resistance and blood pressure. Such effects rarely follow the use of intravenously administered lidocaine or intramuscularly administered lidocaine or procainamide.

In the coronary unit, asystole most commonly occurs as a terminal event in patients who die relatively late in the course of myocardial infarction because of intractable heart failure or cardiogenic shock. It occurs infrequently in the absence of massive myocardial infarction.

Asystole may be more common in patients who die suddenly outside the hospital. Adgey et al.[1] studied almost 800 patients with definite coronary episodes by means of electrocardiographic monitoring in a mobile coronary care unit. They were able to perform resuscitative measures within 4 minutes of cardiac arrest in 55 patients. In 7 of these, asystole appeared to be the mechanism of sudden death.

When asystole does occur in hospitalized patients, it rarely develops suddenly. Slowing of the sinus rhythm may first occur, often followed by some degree of heart block. These so-called bradyarrhythmias have in common a slow ventricular rate and predisposition to ectopic ventricular beats. The therapeutic objective should be cardiac acceleration. A period of sinus bradycardia, however, occurs in about 25 per cent of patients with acute myocardial infarction who are monitored in a coronary care unit.[18] Most of these patients do very well without any drug therapy, so that it is difficult to predict in which patients with sinus bradycardia more threatening bradyarrhythmias or asystole will eventually develop. Present evidence suggests that it is perhaps reasonable to apply first aid therapy to those patients with sinus bradycardia who have frequent ventricular ectopic beats or who manifest marked bradycardia (less than 50 per minute). Cardiac rates of less than 50 per minute may reduce cardiac output and coronary flow. Acceleration of the heart rate can usually be achieved with atropine sulfate given subcutaneously or intravenously. Isoproterenol may also be used to accelerate the heart rate, but this drug, which may itself predispose to other arrhythmias, is perhaps best used only in the hospital setting.

The following strategy for prehospital emergency treatment of patients with suspected acute myocardial infarction is offered for consideration. No data are yet available to prove its effectiveness.

1. Pain should be treated promptly with parenterally administered morphine or meperidine.

2. If the heart rate is more than 70 and premature beats are present, lidocaine, 50 to 100 mg., should be given intravenously, followed by 200 mg. intramuscularly. An alternative approach would be the administration of procainamide, 0.5 to 1.0 gm., intramuscularly. However, the onset of action of this latter drug is slower, and treatment with lidocaine is preferred.

3. If the heart rate is less than 50, or between 50 and 70 with frequent premature beats, atropine should be used. It may be administered intravenously or intramuscularly in a dose of 0.6 to 1.0 mg.

Unfortunately physicians are usually not available during the critical few minutes between the onset of symptoms and sudden death. Is it reasonable to suggest that patients who are highly susceptible to acute myocardial infarction or their relatives or close associates be supplied with drugs such as lidocaine or atropine for emergency treatment? Hitherto, such an approach was not feasible because there was no appropriate way of safely administering these medications intramuscularly. Recently, a safe, effective self-injectable syringe has been designed[12] which may alleviate this problem. While we do not necessarily advocate the immediate implementation of such an approach, nonetheless the epidemiology of sudden death suggests that such radical measures may be necessary if we are to lower the high mortality rate. We would strongly urge that research funds be directed toward the study of such an approach.

Generally a lapse of several hours occurs between the onset of symptoms and the arrival of the patient at the hospital. Most of this delay is the result of patient indecision. The well known psychologic mechanism of denial plays a major role in this delay, often abetted by a lack of patient awareness of what constitutes serious symptoms. Surprisingly, once the decision to go to the hospital has been made, the journey itself takes relatively little time. The solution to this problem must be more effective education, urging patients to seek immediate medical assistance at the onset of symptoms.

Treatment By Ambulance Personnel

Recently Pantridge and Geddes[22] described a mobile coronary care unit, housed in a van, and equipped with many of the monitoring and therapeutic devices found useful in its well equipped hospital counterpart. This mobile unit carried a physician and transported 312 patients with myocardial infarction to the hospital without a fatality. Others have reported similarly gratifying results without a physician in attendance and have shown that ambulance personnel can adequately be trained in the prevention and treatment of cardiac arrest. Such an approach may be useful particularly in densely populated areas, but it too will have only limited application to the problem of sudden cardiac death until the major delay in the institution of effective therapy, patient indecision, is overcome.

Treatment in the Coronary Care Unit

General concepts concerning treatment in the coronary care unit have been discussed elsewhere.[5, 16-19] A well equipped and well staffed coronary care unit can reduce in-hospital mortality by 20 to 50 per cent, but since most deaths occur outside the hospital the effect on overall mortality will be considerably less. This decreased mortality has been achieved chiefly by the prompt, aggressive treatment of potentially fatal cardiac arrhythmias. Unlike patients who die suddenly outside the hospital, those who succumb within the coronary unit are more likely to die from cardiogenic shock or severe intractable heart failure. The mortality resulting from both of these conditions, usually associated with massive infarction, has been little altered by the concept of coronary care.

Most physicians in community hospitals are well versed in the proper use of effective antiarrhythmic drugs such as lidocaine, procainamide, quinidine, diphenylhydantoin, propranolol, atropine, and the various catecholamines. There has been justifiable reluctance to attempt pacemaker therapy in patients whose major problem is one of the various bradyarrhythmias or heart block. No longer, however, is it necessary to have mastered the skill of passing a pacing catheter under fluoroscopic control into the right ventricle. Flow-directed pacing catheters, easily passed into the right ventricle, are now available and can effectively control arrhythmias which do not respond to drug therapy. Only a little practice is necessary to accomplish this maneuver successfully. We urge all physicians responsible for treating patients with acute myocardial infarction in the hospital to master this technique.

CONCLUSIONS

The majority of deaths from acute myocardial infarction occur outside the hospital. If we are to lower significantly this mortality rate, a major effort must be made in several areas.

The best treatment is obviously prevention; no longer can the conscientious physician be content with treatment of clinical coronary disease alone. He must play a major role in prevention and patient education. Proper diet, avoidance of smoking, maintenance of a reasonable level of physical activity, and the early treatment of elevated blood pressure and abnormalities of lipid metabolism must be emphasized.

Those patients who have a high risk for the development of acute myocardial infarction must also be instructed properly so that the time between the onset of symptoms and arrival at the hospital is reduced. We have proposed that drug therapy, of proved effectiveness in coronary units, may be useful in the treatment of potentially lethal arrhythmias in patients before they reach the hospital. We urge that studies be instituted to test the effectiveness of this concept.

REFERENCES

1. Adgey, A. A., Scott, M. E., Allen, J. D., et al.: Management of ventricular fibrillation outside hospital. Lancet 1:1169–1171 (June 14) 1969.
2. Bainton, C. R., and Peterson, D. R.: Deaths from coronary heart disease in persons fifty years of age and younger. New Eng. J. Med. 268:569–575 (March 14) 1963.
3. Bethesda Conference Report: Early care for the acute coronary suspect. Amer. J. Cardiol. 23:603–618 (April) 1969.
4. Blakeslee, A. L., and Stamler, J.: Your Heart Has Nine Lives. New York, Simon and Schuster 1963, 269 pp.
5. Brown, K. W., MacMillan, R. L., Forbath, N., et al.: Coronary unit: an intensive-care centre for acute myocardial infarction. Lancet 2:349–352 (Aug. 17) 1963.
6. Frank, C. W., Weinblatt, E., Shapiro, S., et al.: Physical inactivity as a lethal factor in myocardial infarction among men. Circulation 34:1022–1033 (Dec.) 1966.
7. Frank, C. W., Weinblatt, E., Shapiro, S., et al: Myocardial infarction in men. Role of physical activity and smoking in incidence and mortality. J.A.M.A. 198:1241–1245 (Dec. 19) 1966.
8. Gertler, M. M., White, P. D., Cady, L., et al.: Coronary heart disease. Amer. J. Med. Sci. 248:377–398 (Oct.) 1964.
9. Gordon, T., and Kannel, W. B.: Premature mortality from coronary heart disease. The Framingham study. J.A.M.A. 215:1617–1625 (March 8) 1971.
10. Grace, W. J.: Mortality rate from acute myocardial infarction – what are we talking about? Amer. J. Cardiol. 20:301–303 (Sept.) 1967.
11. Harris, W. E., Bowerman, W., McFadden, R. B., et al.: Jogging. An adult exercise program. J.A.M.A. 201:759–761 (Sept. 4) 1967.
12. Hershberg, P. I.: First aid therapy: a new concept in the treatment of myocardial infarction. Med. Times 96:575–591 (June) 1968.
13. Hershberg, P. I.: Angina or no angina: what difference does it make? Amer. Heart J. 81:571–572 (April) 1971.
14. Jude, J. R., Kouwenhoven, W. B., and Knickerbocker, G. G.: Cardiac arrest. Report on the application of external cardiac massage on 118 patients. J.A.M.A. 178:1063–1070 (Dec. 16) 1971.
15. Keys, A. (ed.): Coronary heart disease in seven countries. Circulation (suppl.) 41:1.1–1.211 (April) 1970.

16. Langhorne, W. H.: The coronary care unit. A year's experience in a community hospital. J.A.M.A. *201*:662–665 (Aug. 28) 1967.
17. Likoff, W.: Coronary care conference. Amer. J. Cardiol. *20*:439–440 (Sept.) 1967.
18. Lown, B., Klein, M. D., and Hershberg, P. I.: Coronary and precoronary care. Amer. J. Med. *46*:705–724 (May) 1969.
19. Lown, B., Fakhro, A. M., Hood, W. B., Jr., et al.: The coronary care unit. New perspectives and directions. J.A.M.A. *199*:188–198 (Jan. 16) 1967.
20. Luke, J. L., and Helpern, M.: Sudden unexpected death from natural causes in young adults. A review of 275 consecutive autopsied cases. Arch. Path. *85*:10–17 (Jan.) 1968.
21. Nachlas, M. M., and Miller, D. I.: Closed-chest cardiac resuscitation in patients with acute myocardial infarction. Amer. Heart J. *69*:448–459 (April) 1965.
22. Pantridge, J. F., and Geddes, J. S.: A mobile intensive-care unit in the management of myocardial infarction. Lancet *2*:271–273 (Aug. 5) 1967.
23. Robb, G. P., and Marks, H. H.: Postexercise electrocardiogram in arteriosclerotic heart disease. J.A.M.A. *200*:918–926 (June 12) 1967.
24. Schorr, S. S., Elsom, K. A., Elsom, K. O., et al.: An evaluation of the periodic health examination: a study of factors discriminating between survival and death from coronary heart disease. Ann. Intern, Med. *61*:1006–1014 (Dec.) 1964.
25. Shapiro, S., Weinblatt, E., Frank, C. W., et al.: The H.I.P. study of incidence and prognosis of coronary heart disease, preliminary findings on incidence of myocardial infarction and angina. J. Chron. Dis. *18*:527–558 (June) 1965.
26. Spain, D. M., Bradess, V. A., and Mohr, C.: Coronary atherosclerosis as a cause of unexpected and unexplained death. An autopsy study from 1949–1959. J.A.M.A. *174*:384–388 (Sept. 24) 1960.
27. Walker, W. J., and Gregoratos, G.: Myocardial infarction in young men. Amer. J. Cardiol. *19*:339–343 (March) 1967.

605 Commonwealth Avenue
Boston, Massachusetts 02215

Therapy of Complicated Arterial Hypertension

Donald J. Breslin M.D., and Neil W. Swinton, Jr., M.D.

Effective treatment of the hypertensive patient depends on a comprehensive initial evaluation. Questions which must be answered include:

1. Is the patient's blood pressure consistently elevated or does it fluctuate? An estimate of the mean blood pressure must be made to determine the need for antihypertensive drugs and the response of therapy.

2. What is the patient's emotional status? Many antihypertensive drugs have psychic effects; a few may seriously aggravate a preexisting depression. Can the patient accept the rationale for chronic antihypertensive treatment even though he may be entirely asymptomatic?

3. Is the hypertension the result of some underlying surgically remediable disorder of the kidneys or adrenal glands? Primary (essential) hypertension is an exclusion diagnosis.

4. What is the degree of arteriosclerosis and functional status of the kidneys, brain, heart, and peripheral circulation? Medications which decrease glomerular filtration, produce orthostatic hypotension, or increase cardiac work must sometimes be avoided when abnormal organ function is present.

5. Are there underlying systemic disorders which may be aggravated by antihypertensive medication? Examples of conditions which may influence the choice of medication include diabetes mellitus, gout, peptic ulcer, various conditions causing diarrhea, collagen disorders (particularly systemic lupus erythematosus), and disease of the liver.

6. Is the patient scheduled for elective surgery? Antihypertensive medications must be used judiciously in the preoperative period because of the effect of some antihypertensive drugs during anesthesia and in the postoperative period. Often it is safest to stop drug therapy preoperatively in the mildly or moderately hypertensive patient.

7. Has a surgically remediable lesion of the central nervous system been excluded in the patient presenting with malignant hypertension or encephalopathy? If so, knowledge of several parenteral antihypertensive drugs is important for such emergencies.

LABILE HYPERTENSION

Often the patient with labile hypertension will demonstrate considerable variation in blood pressure during a single examination. Repeating blood pressure determinations after the patient has rested for 5 minutes or after he has taken several deep inspirations may result in a marked fall of blood pressure. At times it is helpful to recheck the blood pressure while the patient is receiving a sedative or tranquilizer. We sometimes teach a relative to take home blood pressures and keep a record of them when labile elevation is suspected.

We desire at least three blood pressure readings before therapy is started for uncomplicated hypertension.[41] If the blood pressure is labile, it should not be ignored, as persistent hypertension eventually develops in many of these hyperreactive individuals. We encourage modest dietary salt restriction, to 5 gm. or less, and for obese hyperreactive persons, a weight-loss diet. Sedatives or tranquilizers are prescribed if the patient is overtly anxious. If the patient is intolerant of dietary salt restriction, diuretic drugs in small dosage may be employed. Occasionally a particular form of hyperreactivity may be observed in which tachycardia is associated with labile hypertension (excess beta-adrenergic syndrome).[17] This may sometimes be related to postural change, with an increase in heart rate and blood pressure occurring on assumption of the erect position or with mild exercise. Such patients who respond best to propranolol hydrochloride (Inderal) may also benefit from reserpine. Most patients with a history of labile hypertension require a urinary vanillic mandelic acid (VMA) or metanephrine measurement to exclude a pheochromocytoma.

EMOTIONAL STATUS OF THE PATIENT

Occasionally a patient will describe unusual intolerance to various antihypertensive medications he has received in the past. While some of these complaints may constitute well-known undesirable side-effects of specific antihypertensive medications, some individuals protest that almost all medications they have received have rendered them relatively incapacitated. If the individual seems depressed, treatment may be started with an antidepressant agent, utilizing their mild antihypertensive effect. In addition, small doses of a diuretic preparation may be begun. Subsequently, with frequent reassurance, the patient can be encouraged to increase gradually the doses of antihypertensive drugs. If a history of depression is present, or if the patient is a compulsive, hard-driving individual, the rauwolfia derivatives and large doses of alpha-methyldopa (Aldomet) may lead to disastrous depression and should be avoided. Many antidepressant agents diminish or block the effectiveness of guanethedine sulfate (Ismelin), so therapy with the latter should be avoided in this combination.

Many anxious hypertensive subjects respond well to alpha-methyldopa (Aldomet). However, if they are already receiving a tranquilizer or sedative agent, the additive effect of the two drugs may produce oversedation. Although the side-effect of sleepiness with alpha-methyldopa tends to decrease after the first few weeks of therapy, the patient should be warned of the possibility of the need to take less of the tranquilizing drug as the dose of alpha-methyldopa is increased.

One of the problems in the ambulatory hypertensive patient is the tendency of the patient to stop taking medication once a relatively normal blood pressure is achieved. A few such patients will remain normotensive without treatment,[14] and some will not become hypertensive again for several months after cessation of therapy. Considerable evidence now exists that control of hypertension improves life expectancy.[42, 43] The patient who understands this, without being unduly frightened by the disease, can be convinced of the need to take adequate antihypertensive medication. Most hypertensive patients have no symptoms related directly to their hypertension. Only careful education by the physician will induce them to take their necessary medication for an indefinite period.

SECONDARY HYPERTENSION

Investigation to exclude underlying disorders of the kidneys or adrenal glands, which may cause hypertension, is usually indicated before initiation of therapy. This is particularly important in younger patients (less than 30 years old) and in those with severe, recent onset, or recent change in level of hypertension. Basic laboratory investigation to detect secondary hypertension should include an intravenous pyelogram with early sequence films, serum potassium, urinalysis, blood urea nitrogen or serum creatinine or both, and often a urine collection for one of the catecholamine degradation products (metanephrines or vanillic mandelic acid). Occasionally a urine culture is also indicated, especially if pyuria is present, or a past history of hematuria, urinary tract infection, or instrumentation is known.

A history of episodes consisting of vascular headaches, blanching, profuse sweating, palpitations, tremor, unexplained anxiety, and chest or abdominal discomfort can be elicited in most patients with pheochromocytoma.[18] A history of labile hypertension, wide blood pressure fluctuations during anesthesia, or of a paradoxical response to antihypertensive agents also suggests a pheochromocytoma. Once the diagnosis is confirmed biochemically (urinary vanillic mandelic acid or metanephrine), we believe visualization of the tumor by contrast aortography is indicated,[35] especially if a flank thoracoabdominal surgical resection is contemplated. Administration of phenoxybenzamine hydrochloride (Dibenzyline) and propranolol hydrochloride (Inderal) before operation results in less blood pressure fluctuation and cardiac arrhythmias during anesthesia.[11, 34] Careful blood volume replacement is important in preventing hypotension following removal of the tumor.[39]

The history is not often helpful in identifying patients with renovascular hypertension. The presence of a renal artery bruit or disparity in size or function between the kidneys on early sequence intravenous pyelogram films detects more than 90 per cent of patients with significant renovascular lesions.[26] Stenoses should be visualized by renal arteriography to determine their operability for excision or bypass graft. Prediction of hypertension benefit from such surgery can only be made with confidence if the renal artery stenosis has been shown to be hemo-dynamically significant by split-function kidney studies (Stamey technique)[15, 33] or bilateral renal vein renin assays[23] or both.

The patient with renovascular hypertension, especially if he is elderly with widespread arteriosclerosis, is not necessarily best treated by renal surgery.[46] If the distal intrarenal arteries are significantly involved, surgery should usually not be attempted. Sacrifice of functioning renal tissue is rarely justified solely for the relief of hypertension which frequently can be controlled with antihypertensive drugs despite renal ischemia. Furthermore, fibromuscular dysplasia which preferentially involves the renal arteries may not progress after the age of 40 years.[28] Azotemia and evidence of renal arteriolar disease are not contraindications to renal artery surgery when a significant main renal artery obstruction is present. In fact, preservation of renal function rather than improvement of blood pressure is increasingly the indication for revascularization surgery in our patients with early azotemia.

Primary aldosteronism resulting from a tumor is usually an indication for adrenal surgery, although the adenoma is rarely malignant and the associated hypertension is usually mild. Hypokalemia is the most undesirable manifestation, sometimes causing neuromuscular symptoms[9] and possible renal tubular damage. Adrenal venography[10] and adrenal vein plasma aldosterone determinations are helpful in distinguishing an aldosterone-producing tumor from primary aldosteronism resulting from adrenal hyperplasia. The characteristic renin suppression and elevation of plasma aldosterone seen in primary aldosteronism tends to be more striking in the tumor group. Study of these variables and of electrolyte levels with the aid of multidimensional computer assisted analysis may be a helpful tool in the future in identifying the nontumor group.[16] Nevertheless, differentiating an adrenal adenoma from adrenal hyperplasia is not always possible before operation.

Good response to a therapeutic trial of adrenal corticosteroids will detect some rare forms of nonsurgical primary aldosteronism[31, 40] but does not always exclude a tumor. If hyperplasia is thought to be present, medical therapy with spironolactone (Aldactone) and potassium supplements may be preferable to bilateral adrenal surgical exploration, especially if surgically induced adrenal insufficiency is the outcome.

Hypertension in young women taking oral contraceptive agents may be associated with elevated renin and aldosterone production. This effect, which may persist for as long as 3 months after cessation of contraceptive therapy, must be considered when seeking causes and appropriate treatment for the new appearance of hypertension in women of childbearing age.[12, 44]

DECREASED FUNCTION OF KIDNEY, BRAIN, OR HEART

Diminished renal function is a common accompaniment of hypertension. Drugs which diminish renal blood flow and glomerular filtration rate (because of diminished effective blood volume, impaired renal vaso-dilatation in the face of generalized vasodilatation, or because of an unforeseen marked drop in systemic blood pressure) must be used with caution to prevent increasing azotemia. In the presence of impaired renal function, alpha-methyldopa (Aldomet) and hydralazine (Apresoline) are the drugs of choice. Thiazide diuretic drugs tend to aggravate azotemia; small doses of furosemide (Lasix) and ethacrynic acid (Edecrin), when given without severe dietary salt restriction, tend not to decrease glomerular filtration rates significantly[25] and yet have an antihypertensive effect. At times an apparent resistance to the antihypertensive properties of alpha-methyldopa (Aldomet) can be avoided by the addition of a small dose of a diuretic agent. Any drug which decreases the blood pressure in the hypertensive patient may decrease the efficiency of renal excretory function if there is significant parenchymal disease. Thus, serum electrolytes and blood urea nitrogen or creatinine or both must be followed closely, titrating the blood pressure response against renal function. Despite the theoretical danger, we usually see improved renal function following control (90 to 100 mm. Hg diastolic pressure) of moderate to severe hypertension in azotemic patients. One should not be overly cautious giving antihypertensive drugs in such situations.[47]

In the presence of ischemic disease of the brain or heart, the drugs which may induce orthostatic hypotension should generally be avoided—ganglionic blocking agents, guanethidine sulfate (Ismelin), and large doses of pargyline hydrochloride (Eutonyl). Hydralazine (Apresoline) increases cardiac work[1] and should not be given to the patient with coronary insufficiency or borderline cardiac compensation. Propranolol hydrochloride (Inderal) and the rauwolfia compounds are also contraindicated in the patient with cardiac decompensation. When diuretic drugs are used with digitalis, we always give supplemental potassium chloride or spironolactone (Aldactone) to prevent hypokalemia and the cardiac arrhythmias of digitalis toxicity.

A diuretic drug, with the subsequent addition of increasing doses of alpha-methyldopa (Aldomet) as needed, is usually chosen when ischemic disease of the brain or heart is present. If this does not prove adequate and the diastolic blood pressure remains significantly elevated, guanethidine can then be added cautiously. When guanethidine sulfate is to be given to such a patient, or when it is to be used in doses greater than 25 mg. daily in any hypertensive patient, it is usually wise to teach the patient to take his own blood pressure both sitting and standing in the morning on arising. In this way, he can be warned of impending symptomatic orthostatic hypotension and decrease the dose of guanethedine sulfate when the standing blood pressure falls too low.

We have not encountered any greater apprehension on the part of patients taking their own blood pressures than one would find in the diabetic patient taking insulin and testing his urine for glycosuria. Much depends on an adequate explanation to the patient of the long-term goals of antihypertensive treatment and reassurance regarding the day-to-day fluctuations in blood pressure he may expect. The patient with controlled hypertension is probably more at ease and more aware of the importance of his taking his own blood pressure than the patient who does not. In addition, we usually exercise such patients (within the limits of their capacities) before measuring their standing blood pressure in the office, since this enhances any orthostatic effect and provides a warning against unsuitable increases in the dose of guanethedine sulfate.

The presence of uncontrolled hypertension in a patient with ischemic heart disease is certainly more detrimental to him than the theoretical risks imposed by a drug which may induce orthostatic hypotension. Control of hypertension is an important part of the therapy of angina pectoris and is mandatory in the treatment of left ventricular heart failure. There is now convincing evidence that control of hypertension may prevent cerebral vascular accidents,[5] increase the longevity of persons who have had a cerebrovascular accident, and also lessen symptoms in patients with cerebrovascular insufficiency.

SYSTOLIC HYPERTENSION

The group most commonly encountered with elevation of systolic blood pressure and normal diastolic pressure is the elderly. Systolic hypertension does alert us to exclude aortic insufficiency, hyperkinetic heart syndromes, anemia, arteriovenous shunting, and hyperthyroidism. Tense, hyperreactive individuals may demonstrate a relative rise in systolic blood pressure alone, but the majority of those with systolic hypertension are over the age of 65. Evidence exists that systolic hypertension is accompanied by an increased mortality rate resulting from cardiovascular disease compared to the general population of similar age.[7, 21, 22] The effectiveness of treatment of systolic hypertension in decreasing the mortality rate requires further assessment. However, the presence of systolic hypertension is now regarded as an indication for antihypertensive therapy.

It has been our experience that patients over the age of 70 often respond relatively poorly to antihypertensive therapy in terms of their general feeling of well-being, mental acuity, and tendency to orthostatic hypotension. Since systolic hypertension in the elderly is also often refractory to mild antihypertensive therapy, it has been our practice not to treat these patients unless they have evidence of cerebral or cardiac decompensation. When we do treat such elderly individuals, it is only when we can be sure that their course will be followed closely by a physician.

SYSTEMIC DISORDERS WHICH MAY BE AFFECTED ADVERSELY BY ANTIHYPERTENSIVE THERAPY

Before initiating antihypertensive therapy, it is important to know if the patient has hyperglycemia or hyperuricemia. Many of the diuretic preparations may modestly elevate the blood sugar[4] and serum uric acid levels[20] which, if borderline high, should be rechecked within a month after beginning diuretic drugs. Diuretic-induced hyperglycemia is not usually a problem in the nondiabetic patient.[24] Moderate elevations in the serum uric acid level, without a history of gout or renal calculi, can probably be ignored. We arbitrarily prescribe probenecid (Benemid) or allopurinol (Zyloprim), both of which counteract the hyperuricemic effect of diuretic agents in the asymptomatic patient with a serum uric acid level above 10 mg. per 100 ml. If renal function is abnormal, allopurinol is given to prevent hyperuricemic nephropathy. If a patient with diabetes mellitus requires diuretic therapy, this can be accomplished by giving an appropriate hypoglycemic drug or insulin when required, but this is not usually necessary. Alpha-methyldopa (Aldomet) may be given initially to individuals with diabetes mellitus or gout, and a diuretic added to the regimen later if necessary.

Spironolactone (Aldactone) is a diuretic which has mild antihypertensive effects and moderate capacity for potentiating the action of other antihypertensive agents. Its advantage lies in its lack of any tendency to aggravate hyperglycemia or hyperuricemia. When it is used, the serum potassium level should be checked periodically since the drug tends to increase potassium retention. However, in the absence of renal dysfunction, hyperkalemia does not usually occur with small doses of spironolactone (50 mg. or less daily).

A variety of other conditions present specific contraindications to antihypertensive drugs. Patients with peptic ulcer or chronic forms of diarrhea should not be given rauwolfia compounds. Hydralazine (Apresoline) and alpha-methyldopa (Aldomet) should not be given to patients with collagen disorders. Hydralazine[8] may produce a lupus-like syndrome when given in doses over 300 mg. daily, and alpha-methyldopa has rarely produced positive lupus erythematosus tests.[38] Individuals with liver disease should not be given alpha-methyldopa (Aldomet).

THE PREOPERATIVE PATIENT

Moderate elevation of blood pressure before surgery should not cause undue concern.[3] Hospitalization, bed rest, and surgery itself tend to lower blood pressure temporarily in the hypertensive patient. The heart, brain, and kidneys should be evaluated carefully before operation since these organs may be affected adversely by prolonged hypotension. In addition, pheochromocytoma presents a special hazard during anesthesia when it may cause marked lability of blood pressure and cardiac arrhythmias. All preoperative patients should be screened to exclude pheochromocytoma with a 24-hour urine for metanephrine or vanillic mandelic acid.

Some antihypertensive agents cause undesirable side-effects for the patient who needs surgery. One of the most important of these is hypokalemia. The serum potassium level should be checked in all patients having taken diuretic drugs, and potassium replacement in the form of liquid potassium chloride must be given before operation to those who are hypokalemic.

Rauwolfia alkaloids (Serpasil, Raudixin) and guanethedine sulfate (Ismelin) may deplete tissue catecholamines that require days or weeks for replacement. This produces an increased tendency for hypotension to develop in response to hypovolemia[13] or anesthesia. When the body's stores of catecholamines are depleted, indirect acting pressor amines, such as methamphetamine hydrochloride (Methedrine, Desoxyn, Desoxyephedrine) and mephentermine (Wyamine), are relatively ineffective. However, the direct acting pressor amines, such as norepinephrine (Levophed), metaraminol (Aramine), phenylephrine (Neo-synephrine) and methoxamine hydrochloride (Vasoxyl), have a potentiated effect in these circumstances. In the past it has been recommended that drugs which deplete tissue catecholamines be discontinued approximately two weeks before operation, when possible. However, anesthesia may usually be performed safely if the anesthesiologist has been warned of their use and avoids the problems of catecholamine depletion by prompt correction of fluid loss and use of direct acting vasopressor agents.

Monoamine oxidase inhibitors such as pargyline hydrochloride (Eutonyl) are used relatively infrequently as antihypertensive agents. These drugs inhibit the inactivation of catecholamines in tissues and may be hazardous to the patient undergoing anesthesia and surgery. They potentiate the effects of many pressor agents, some anesthetic agents, morphine, and insulin.[19] Whenever possible, monoamine oxidase inhibitors should be discontinued at least 2 weeks before operation.

In the patient with a history of mild to moderate hypertension, antihypertensive medication can usually be discontinued several days before surgery. If hypertension is severe or there is significant cardiovascular disease, antihypertensive medication can be continued through the immediate preoperative period. Drugs having effects of short duration and which do not deplete the level of body potassium or cause significant loss of catecholamines are most desirable. Alpha-methyldopa (Aldomet) and hydralazine (Apresoline) fulfill these criteria best.

HYPERTENSIVE CRISIS

Hypertensive emergencies, such as intracerebral hemorrhage and dissecting hematomas of the aorta, require prompt knowledgeable management.[2] Headache, nausea, lethargy, confusion, and other transient neurologic abnormalities, which can progress to coma and death unless treated rapidly, may develop in the patient with severe hypertension. The neurologic abnormalities associated with severe hypertension (hypertensive encephalopathy) are histologically related to findings in the brain of hyaline degeneration in the wall of arterioles, diffusely scattered microinfarctions, perivascular hemorrhages, and diffuse or localized cerebral edema.[37] Such conditions as subarachnoid hemorrhage, traumatic intracranial bleeding, and brain tumor must be excluded. One must be particularly suspicious of an underlying primary neurologic problem when the pretreatment levels of diastolic blood pressure are relatively low (less than 120 mm. Hg in the adult) or when hypertensive retinopathy is not present. Persistence or progression of neurologic abnormalities despite successful antihypertensive therapy must also suggest the possibility of a primary neurologic disorder. It should be noted that xanthochromia and elevated protein content in the spinal fluid are not uncommon in hypertensive encephalopathy.

Treatment of the hypertensive emergency requires familiarity with only a few parenterally administered hypotensive drugs. Reserpine (Sandril, Serpasil) and pentolinium (Ansolysen) should provide adequate therapy for most acute hypertensive crises. Hydralazine (Apresoline) and alpha-methyldopa (Aldomet) are occasionally useful. Infrequently, one needs a rapid-acting antihypertensive drug with transitory effect, such as trimethaphan camphorsulfonate (Arfonad). Intravenous diazoxide holds great promise as a useful drug for such emergencies but is not yet generally available.

Reserpine has many undesirable side-effects, particularly its sedating and depressing properties. This is particularly undesirable when assessing the course of intracranial bleeding or head injury. In addition, reserpine causes relative increased parasympathetic activity—bradycardia, slowed atrioventricular cardiac conduction, activation of a peptic ulcer, and increased bronchial constriction. Reserpine depletes tissue catecholamines, which may decrease cardiac output.[6] If it is given in large doses for several days, temporary parkinsonism may result. Despite these disadvantages, intramuscularly administered reserpine is useful. Since its maximum effect occurs in 2 to 5 hours, intervals between doses should not be less than 3 hours, with an initial dose of 1.25 to 2.5 mg. and a total dose not exceeding 20 mg. in 24 hours.

Since pentolinium (Ansolysen) is a ganglionic blocking agent, it produces parasympathetic as well as sympathetic blockade. Consequently, it may cause paralytic ileus, urinary retention, aggravation of glaucoma, and undesirable effects in the fetus during pregnancy. It decreases venous return to the heart, which is an advantage in the presence of congestive heart failure but may be a disadvantage when renal function is impaired. Pentolinium is free of sedating effects and more rapid in action than reserpine. Its maximum effect appears within 30 to 60 minutes after administration. Although it may be used by either intravenous or intramuscular routes, we prefer the intramuscular route because of an increased risk of inducing an excessive drop in blood pressure when it is given intravenously. It may be given in initial intramuscular doses of 2 to 5 mg., gradually increasing the dose as needed to a maximum of 50 mg. The initial interval between doses is 30 minutes and is increased to intervals of 6 to 8 hours once a satisfactory hypotensive effect is achieved.

Alpha-methyldopa[32] (Aldomet) and hydralazine[27] (Apresoline) cause relatively little decrease in glomerular filtration rate and are therefore helpful when renal function is impaired. Both drugs, given parenterally, have a less reliable hypotensive effect than reserpine or pentolinium. Alpha-methyldopa also has a relatively slow onset of action. It may have some effect in 2 to 5 hours, but its maximum hypotensive effect may not occur for 10 to 20 hours after administration. It may cause drowsiness and rarely hepatotoxicity. It is given intravenously in doses of 250 to 500 mg. in 100 ml. of 5 per cent dextrose in water over a period of 30 minutes at intervals of 6 to 8 hours.

Hydralazine, which increases cardiac output, should be avoided when angina pectoris or congestive heart failure is present. It is most commonly used in treating the acute hypertension of glomerulonephritis or the toxemia of pregnancy. It may be given by the intravenous or intramuscular route. Intramuscular doses are usually 10 to 40 mg. given at intervals of 4 to 6 hours. A slow intravenous infusion containing 40 to 100 mg. in 1 liter of 5 per cent glucose and water may be used.

A rapidly active drug with transient effect such as trimethaphan camphorsulfonate (Arfonad) is rarely needed. Its use requires continual monitoring of the patient's blood pressure. It is sometimes employed for treating a dissecting hematoma of the aorta[45] or severe hypertension associated with intracranial bleeding. Arfonad is also excellent in the treatment of systemic hypertension causing left ventricular failure and pulmonary edema.[36]

The effect of any of these parenteral antihypertensive agents may be potentiated by administration of a diuretic such as furosemide (Lasix) administered in an initial dose of approximately 40 mg. intravenously. The use of such a diuretic is particularly important with intravenously administered diazoxide which may become the drug of choice for hypertensive emergencies but is not yet commercially available for this purpose.[29]

REFERENCES

1. Ablad, B.: A study of the mechanism of the hemodynamic effects of hydralazine in man. Acta Pharmacol., 20(Suppl. 1):1–53, 1963.
2. Breslin, D. J.: Hypertensive crisis. MED. CLIN. N. AMER., 53:351–360 (March) 1969.
3. Breslin, D. J., and Swinton, N. W., Jr.: Elective surgery in hypertensive patients – preoperative consideration. Surg. Clin. N. Amer., 50:585–593 (June) 1970.
4. Carliner, N. H., Schelling, J. L., Russel, R. P., Okun, R., and Davis, M.: Thiazide- and phthalimidine-induced hyperglycemia in hypertensive patients. J.A.M.A., 191:535–540 (Feb. 15) 1965.
5. Carter, A. B.: Hypotensive therapy in stroke survivors. Lancet, 1:485–489 (March 7) 1970.
6. Cohen, S. I., Young, M. W., Lau, S. H., et al.: Effects of reserpine therapy on cardiac output and atrioventricular conduction during rest and controlled heart rates in patients with essential hypertension. Circulation, 37:738–746 (May) 1968.
7. Colandrea, M. A., Friedman, G. D., Nichaman, M. Z., and Lynd, C. N.: Systolic hypertension in the elderly. An epidemiologic assessment. Circulation, 41:239–245 (Feb.) 1970.
8. Condemi, J. J., Moore-Jones, D., Vaughan, J. H., and Perry, H. M.: Antinuclear antibodies following hydralazine toxicity. New Eng. J. Med., 276:486–491 (March 2) 1967.
9. Conn, J. W., Knopf, R. F., and Nesbit, R. M.: Clinical characteristics of primary aldosteronism from an analysis of 145 cases. Amer. J. Surg., 107:159–172 (Jan.) 1964.
10. Conn, J. W., Rovner, D. R., Cohen, E. L., et al.: Preoperative diagnosis of primary aldosteronism. Including a comparison of operative findings and preoperative tumor localization by adrenal phlebography. Arch. Intern. Med., 123:113–123 (Feb.) 1969.
11. Cooperman, L. H., Engleman, K., and Mann, P. E. G.: Anesthetic management of pheochromocytoma employing halothane and beta adrenergic blockade. Anesthesiology, 28:575–582 (May-June) 1967.
12. Crane, M. G., Harris, J. J., and Winsor, W., III: Hypertension, oral contraceptive agents, and conjugated estrogens. Ann. Intern. Med., 74:13–21 (Jan.) 1971.
13. Dingle, H. R.: Antihypertensive drugs and anaesthesia. Anaesthesia, 21:151–172, 1966.
14. Dustan, H. P., Page, I. H., Tarazi, R. C., and Frohlich, E. D.: Arterial pressure responses to discontinuing antihypertensive drugs. Circulation, 37:370–379 (March) 1968.
15. Fair, W. R., and Stamey, T. A.: Differential renal function studies in segmental renal ischemia. J.A.M.A., 217:790–793 (Aug. 9) 1971.
16. Ferriss, J. B., Neville, A. M., Brown, J. J., et al.: Hypertension with aldosterone excess and low plasma-renin: preoperative distinction between patients with and without adrenocortical tumour. Lancet, 2:995–1000 (Nov. 14) 1970.
17. Frohlich, E. D.: Beta adrenergic blockade in the circulatory regulation of hyperkinetic states. Amer. J. Cardiol., 27:195–199 (Feb.) 1971.

18. Gifford, R. W., Jr., Kvale, W. F., Maher, F. T., et al.: Clinical features, diagnosis and treatment of pheochromocytoma: a review of 76 cases. Mayo Clin. Proc., *39*:281–302 (April) 1964.
19. Goldberg, L. I.: Monoamine oxidase inhibitors: adverse reactions and possible mechanisms. J.A.M.A., *190*:456–462 (Nov. 2) 1964.
20. Healey, L. A., Magid, G. J., and Decker, J. L.: Uric acid retention due to hydrochlorothiazide. New Eng. J. Med., *261*:1358–1362 (Dec. 31) 1959.
21. Kannel, W. B., Gordon, T., and Schwartz, M. J.: Systolic versus diastolic blood pressure and risk of coronary heart disease. The Framingham study. Amer. J. Cardiol., 27:335–346 (April) 1971.
22. Kannel, W. B., Wolf, P. A., Verter, J., and McNamara, P. M.: Epidemiologic assessment of the role of blood pressure in stroke. The Framingham study. J.A.M.A., *214*:301–310 (Oct. 12) 1970.
23. Kirkendall, W. M., Fitz, A. E., and Lawrence, M. S.: Renal hypertension. Diagnosis and surgical management. New Eng. J. Med., 276:479–485 (March 2) 1967.
24. Kohner, E. M., Dollery, C. T., Lowy, C., and Schumer, B.: Effect of diuretic therapy on glucose tolerance in hypertensive patients. Lancet, *1*:986–990 (May 15) 1971.
25. Laragh, J. H.: The proper use of newer diuretics. Ann. Intern. Med., 67:606–613 (Sept.) 1967.
26. Maxwell, M. H., Gonick, H. C., Wiita, R., and Kaufman, J. J.: Use of the rapid-sequence intravenous pyelogram in the diagnosis of renovascular hypertension. New Eng. J. Med., 270:213–220 (Jan. 30) 1964.
27. Moyer, J. H.: Comparative clinical pharmacology on antihypertensive drugs. *In* Milliez, P., and Tcherdakoff, P. (eds.): International Club on Arterial Hypertension. Paris, L'Expansion Scientifique Française, 1965, pp. 479–490.
28. Meaney, T. F., Dustan, H. P., and McCormack, L. J.: Natural history of renal arterial disease. Radiology, *91*:881–887 (Nov.) 1968.
29. Miller, W. E., Gifford, R. W., Jr., Humphrey, D. C., and Vidt, D. G.: Management of severe hypertension with intravenous injections of diazoxide. Amer. J. Cardiol., 24:870–875 (Dec.) 1969.
30. Mroczek, W. J., Davidov, M., Gavrilovich, L., and Finnerty, F. A., Jr.: The value of aggressive therapy in the hypertensive patient with azotemia. Circulation, *40*:893–904 (Dec.) 1969.
31. Newton, M. A., and Laragh, J. H.: Manipulation by corticotropin and cortisol of aldosterone secretion in primary aldosteronism. Arch. Intern. Med., *123*:147–151 (Feb.) 1969.
32. Onesti, G., Brest, A. M., Novack, P., et al.: Pharmacodynamic effects of alpha-methyl dopa in hypertensive subjects. Amer. Heart J., 67:32–38 (Jan.) 1964.
33. Palmer, J. M.: Prognostic value of contralateral renal plasma flow in renovascular hypertension. Analysis of 55 surgically treated patients with proved unilateral lesions. J.A.M.A., *217*:794–802 (Aug. 9) 1971.
34. Prichard, B. M. C., and Ross, E. J.: Use of propranolol in conjunction with alpha receptor blocking drugs in pheochromocytoma. Amer. J. Cardiol., *18*:394–398 (Sept.) 1966.
35. Rossi, P., Young, I. S., and Panke, W. F.: Techniques, usefulness, and hazards of arteriography of pheochromocytoma. Review of 99 cases. J.A.M.A., *205*:547–553 (Aug. 19) 1968.
36. Sarnoff, S. J., Goodale, W. T., and Sarnoff, L. C.: Graded reduction of arterial pressure in man by means of a thiophanium derivative (Ro 2-2222). Preliminary observations on its effect in acute pulmonary edema. Circulation, 6:63–73 (July) 1952.
37. Scheinker, I. M.: Hypertensive disease of the brain. Arch. Path., *36*:289–296, 1943.
38. Sherman, J. D., Love, D. E., and Harrington, J. F.: Anemia, positive lupus and rheumatoid factors with methyldopa: a report of three cases. Arch. Intern. Med., *120*:321–326 (Sept.) 1967.
39. Sjoerdsma, A., Engelman, K., Waldmann, T. A., Cooperman, L. H., and Hammond, W. G.: Pheochromocytoma: current concepts of diagnosis and treatment. Combined clinical staff conference of the National Institutes of Health. Ann. Intern. Med., 65:1302–1326 (Dec.) 1966.
40. Sutherland, D. J. A., Ruse, J. L., and Laidlaw, J. C.: Hypertension, increased aldosterone secretion and low plasma renin activity relieved by dexamethasone. J. Canad. Med. Assoc., *95*:1109–1119 (Nov. 26) 1966.
41. Swinton, N. W., Jr., and Breslin, D. J.: The clinical evaluation of arterial hypertension. Lahey Clin. Found. Bull., *18*:143–153 (Oct.–Dec.) 1969.
42. Veterans Administration Cooperative Study Group on Antihypertensive Agents: Effects of treatment on morbidity in hypertension. Results in patients with diastolic blood pressures averaging 115 through 129 mm. Hg. J.A.M.A., *202*:1028–1034 (Dec. 11) 1967.
43. Veterans Administration Cooperative Study Group on Antihypertensive Agents: Effects of treatment on morbidity in hypertension. II. Results in patients with diastolic blood pressure averaging 90 through 114 mm Hg. J.A.M.A., *213*:1143–1152 (Aug. 17) 1970.

44. Weinberger, M. H., Collins, R. D., Dowdy, A. J., Nokes, G. W., and Luetscher, J. A.: Hypertension induced by oral contraceptives containing estrogen and gestagen. Ann. Intern. Med., 71:891–902 (Nov.) 1969.

45. Wheat, M. W., Jr., Palmer, R. F., Bartley, T. D., and Seelman, R. C.: Treatment of dissecting aneurysms of the aorta without surgery. J. Thorac. Cardiovas. Surg., 50:364–373 (Sept.) 1965.

46. Wollenweber, J., Sheps, S. G., and Davis, G. B.: Clinical course of atherosclerotic renovascular disease. Amer. J. Cardiol., 21:60–71 (Jan.) 1968.

47. Woods, J. W., and Blythe, W. B.: Management of malignant hypertension complicated by renal insufficiency. New Eng. J. Med., 277:57–62 (July 13) 1967.

605 Commonwealth Avenue
Boston, Massachusetts 02215

Hyponatremia

Richard M. Finkel, M.D.

Hyponatremia is a common electrolyte disturbance that occurs in a variety of clinical situations (Table 1). Rational therapy requires determination of whether the patient has water overload or sodium depletion, or whether he has hyponatremia on some other basis.

PSEUDOHYPONATREMIA

Normally the water content of serum is about 93 per cent. The concentration of sodium in the serum water is about 154 mEq. per liter, whereas the concentration of sodium in total serum, which is what we determine in the clinical laboratory, is lower owing to the volume occupied by the 7 per cent nonaqueous material. Thus, the normal serum sodium concentration is 144 mEq. per liter, not 154 mEq. per liter.

In patients with hyperlipidemia and hyperproteinemia a further lowering of serum sodium can be seen as a result of the increase in volume occupied by these materials. The concentration of sodium in water and the concentration of other solutes remains normal, and thus the serum osmolality is also normal. Any patient with hyponatremia and normal serum osmolality should have a determination of serum lipids and serum proteins, and any patient with hyponatremia with known hyperlipidemia or hyperproteinemia should be suspected of having pseudohyponatremia. The concentration of lipids or proteins must be quite high, however, to produce a significant depression in serum sodium. For example, total lipids of 6 gm. per 100 ml. or total proteins of 14 gm. per 100 ml. would account for a drop in serum sodium of about 5 per cent.[12] These patients with pseudohyponatremia have no symptoms, since the concentration of solutes in intracellular and extracellular fluid is within normal limits. The only appropriate treatment is that directed at the underlying protein or lipid disorder.

SOLUTE ACCUMULATION

Hyponatremia is also seen whenever an accumulation of solute in extracellular fluid is present. The solute raises the serum osmolality, draws

Table 1. *Causes of Hyponatremia*

Pseudohyponatremia
    Hyperlipidemia
    Hyperproteinemia

Solute accumulation
    Hyperglycemia
    Mannitol

Water overload
    Compulsive water drinking
    Endocrinopathies
    Postoperative, postanesthetic
    Oxytocin
    Inappropriate antidiuretic hormone syndrome
    Chlorpropamide
    Edematous states

Sodium depletion

Essential hyponatremia

fluid out of the cells into the extracellular fluid, and dilutes the serum sodium. As in pseudohyponatremia, the serum osmolality is not low. This is a useful observation in the differential diagnosis of hyponatremia since in all other types serum osmolality is low. Solute accumulation occurs most commonly with hyperglycemia, but it can also be seen in the patient who has been given large doses of mannitol and in whom a diuresis has not developed. One can expect a fall in the level of serum sodium of 3 mEq. per liter for every 100 mg. per 100 ml. elevation in blood glucose. Of course, the patient with diabetes mellitus may well have additional factors influencing the level of serum sodium, including deficits in sodium and water and perhaps hyperlipidemia as well. However, it is helpful to calculate what component of the hyponatremia is attributable to hyperglycemia and a consequent water shift, since otherwise water needs may be underestimated and sodium needs overestimated.

WATER OVERLOAD

Normally the kidney is adept at promptly excreting whatever water loads are presented to it. This capacity to form dilute urine is of critical importance in maintaining the normal concentration or tonicity of body fluids. Rarely, a patient may take or be given such massive amounts of fluid that he cannot excrete water fast enough to prevent positive water balance although renal diluting capacity is normal. The patient's level of total body water increases, and he becomes hyponatremic. This is seen in the compulsive water drinker who may drink as many as 20 liters a day and dilute his serum osmolality from a normal of about 285 to as low as 240.[1] Serum sodium concentrations are commonly between 130 to 140, but they may be even lower. A nearly lethal water overloading has been reported in a patient with polydipsia who, in addition, had a compromise in diluting capacity from the use of a thiazide diuretic.[4]

Most patients with clinically significant water overloading have a defect in water excretion. This occurs with a wide variety of clinical situations[5] including endocrinopathies such as hypopituitarism, myxedema, and Addison's disease, following surgery and anesthesia, following the use of oxytocin, with sodium-retaining states such as cardiac failure, cirrhosis, and nephrotic syndrome, and with the inappropriate antidiuretic hormone syndrome.[9]

If the water excess is profound or rapid in onset, the syndrome of water intoxication may develop. The symptoms are anorexia, headache, blurred vision, muscle cramps, and ultimately stupor, convulsions, and death. This syndrome is seen if a large fluid intake is provided for patients who have an unrecognized defect in water excretion. Certainly any patient whose fluid intake is large, or whose intake and output record suggests positive fluid balance, should have the serum sodium measured periodically.

The inappropriate antidiuretic hormone syndrome occurs in patients with pulmonary disease, including pneumonia, tuberculosis, lung abscess, and fungal infections, with central nervous system disease such as neoplasm, trauma, hemorrhage, and inflammatory processes, with porphyria, with the Guillain-Barré syndrome, and with certain tumors, including those of the lung, pancreas, thymus, and duodenum, and lymphoma. Direct isolation of antidiuretic materials from tumor[10] and tuberculous lung[11] has been achieved. Recently the syndrome has been described in patients receiving chlorpropamide (Diabinese), perhaps through a potentiation of the action of antidiuretic hormone,[3, 13] and in a patient with leukemia following vincristine sulfate (Oncovin) therapy.[2]

Patients with the inappropriate antidiuretic hormone syndrome have low levels of serum sodium and serum osmolality but fail to form a dilute urine in response to this. Thus, the urine osmolality is inappropriately high. It need not be hypertonic in this syndrome since even osmolalities as low as 200 in the urine may be inappropriately high for the degree of dilution of body water. With a normal water excretory mechanism, for example, it should be possible to reduce the urine osmolality below 100 in order to excrete excessive water loads. The level of urinary sodium is often high in patients with the inappropriate antidiuretic hormone syndrome, and this often leads to the erroneous conclusion that the patient is a "salt waster" and has the hyponatremia on the basis of salt depletion. An important differential point is that the blood urea nitrogen and serum creatinine levels are normal or even low as a result of increased renal plasma flow. This is against salt depletion. Physical examination reveals no evidence of salt depletion, nor does it show edema, but weight gain may be noted. Although pure water excess is likely the major factor accounting for the hyponatremia, it has been shown recently that this alone cannot account for the degree of hyponatremia observed. It is likely that other factors, as yet unidentified, are involved.[8]

The treatment for water intoxication is fluid restriction. If the hyponatremia is very severe and the patient has major symptoms of water intoxication, hypertonic saline can be given. However, this is hazardous if the patient has sodium overload, as occurs in cirrhosis, nephrotic syndrome, and congestive heart failure. In the inappropriate antidiuretic hormone syndrome the benefit of hypertonic saline is transient, since the administered sodium is promptly excreted. Hypertonic saline is administered at a rate of less than 100 mEq. per hour, and the patient is monitored carefully for signs of congestive failure and for hypernatremia. Hyponatremic patients who are also edematous are treated with both water restriction and with diuretic therapy to remove the excessive salt. It is not necessary to restore serum sodium to normal levels in many patients as long as the level of serum sodium is greater than 130, and they are asymptomatic and are cautioned about the risks of increased fluid intake. Patients with severe congestive heart failure who are treated with water restriction may complain bitterly of thirst despite their state of dilution, and may suffer more morbidity from the water restriction than from the hyponatremia itself. In these patients and in those with cirrhosis, the tendency to hyponatremia will persist and treatment will be difficult unless the underlying cardiac or hepatic disease can be improved.

SODIUM DEPLETION

Since sodium has a critical role in determining plasma volume, sodium depletion produces plasma volume contraction. The usual response to sodium depletion is retention of water, which serves to reexpand the plasma volume, and thus hyponatremia develops.[6] The patient sacrifices the tonicity of body fluids in order to help defend himself against circulatory collapse. If the patient does not have access to water, however, the serum sodium level may remain normal.

Sodium depletion may occur from urinary losses because of renal disease, Addison's disease, or diuretic therapy, from gastrointestinal losses or less commonly from losses in sweat. The findings on physical examination are quite important to the diagnosis of sodium depletion and include postural hypotension, flat neck veins, tachycardia, and diminished skin turgor. Patients will exhibit weight loss, and laboratory studies usually reveal an increase in blood urea nitrogen or creatinine due to reduced renal perfusion. This is in striking contrast to the findings in patients with the inappropriate antidiuretic hormone syndrome. In the salt-depleted patient there is also commonly an increase in hematocrit and serum proteins due to the plasma volume contraction; urinary sodium concentration is low if the losses have been extrarenal in origin.

The treatment of hyponatremia due to sodium depletion is, of course, the administration of sodium. For mild sodium depletion in which the major finding is decreased skin turgor, the deficit of sodium is usually in the range of 500 mEq. per liter. This can be treated with 2 to 3 liters of normal saline. For more severe losses with hypotension and oliguria, the administration of hypertonic saline is warranted at a rate of about 50 mEq. per hour, especially if the patient has severe hyponatremia. Such patients may have a sodium depletion amounting to 1000 mEq.

ESSENTIAL HYPONATREMIA

Rarely the regulatory mechanisms that control tonicity of body fluids undergo a change that allows dilution to occur and persist.[7] Water loads are handled normally in these patients, and no evidence of sodium depletion exists. If water is restricted, the state of dilution is improved but on resumption of normal intake the osmolality and serum sodium levels drop back to the original level. This has been appropriately called "resetting of the osmostat." No treatment is practical other than that for any underlying systemic disease.

SUMMARY

Difficulties in treatment of patients with hyponatremia usually arise because consideration has not been given to the underlying pathophysiology. It is usually possible on the basis of simple clinical and laboratory observations to distinguish whether the hyponatremia is the result of depressed serum water content, solute accumulation in extracellular fluid, water overload, sodium depletion, or to "resetting of the osmostat." When the cause is determined, appropriate treatment can be given.

REFERENCES

1. Barlow, E. D., and De Wardener, H. E.: Compulsive water drinking. Quart. J. Med. 28:235–258 (April) 1959.
2. Cutting, H. O.: Inappropriate secretion of antidiuretic hormone secondary to vincristine therapy. Amer. J. Med. 51:269–271 (Aug.) 1971.
3. Fine, D., and Shedrovilzky, H.: Hyponatremia due to chlorpropamide. A syndrome resembling inappropriate secretion of antidiuretic hormone. Ann. Intern. Med. 72:83–87 (Jan.) 1970.
4. Kennedy, R. M., and Earley, L. E.: Profound hyponatremia resulting from a thiazide-induced decrease in urine diluting capacity in a patient with primary polydipsia. New Eng. J. Med. 282:1185–1186 (May 21) 1970.
5. Kleeman, C. R., and Fichman, M. P.: The clinical physiology of water metabolism. New Eng. J. Med. 277:1300–1307 (Dec. 14) 1967.
6. Leaf, A.: The clinical and physiologic significance of the serum sodium concentration. New Eng. J. Med. 267:77–83 (July 12) 1962.
7. Miles, A. I., and Needle, M. A.: Fixed hyponatremia with normal responses to varying salt and water intakes. New Eng. J. Med. 284:26–28 (Jan. 7) 1971.
8. Nolph, K. D., and Schrier, R. W.: Sodium, potassium, and water metabolism in the syndrome of inappropriate antidiuretic hormone secretion. Amer. J. Med. 49:534–545 (Oct.) 1970.
9. Schwartz, W. B., Bennett, W., Curelop, S., and Bartter, F. C.: A syndrome of renal sodium loss and hyponatremia probably resulting from inappropriate secretion of antidiuretic hormone. Amer. J. Med. 23:529–542 (Oct.) 1957.
10. Vorherr, H., Massry, S. G., Utiger, R. D., et al.: Antidiuretic principle in malignant tumor extracts from patients with inappropriate ADH syndrome. J. Clin. Endocrin. 28:162–168 (Feb.) 1968.
11. Vorherr, H., Massry, S. G., Fallet, R., et al.: Antidiuretic principle in tuberculous lung tissue of a patient with pulmonary tuberculosis and hyponatremia. Ann. Int. Med. 72:383–387 (March) 1970.
12. Waugh, W. H.: Utility of expressing serum sodium per unit of water in assessing hyponatremia. Metabolism 18:706–712 (Aug.) 1969.
13. Weissman, P. N., Shenkman, L., and Gregerman, R. I.: Chlorpropamide hyponatremia: drug-induced inappropriate antidiuretic-hormone activity. New Eng. J. Med. 284:65–71 (Jan. 14) 1971.

605 Commonwealth Avenue
Boston, Massachusetts 02215

A Multidisciplined Approach for the Management of Metastatic Breast Cancer

Richard A. Oberfield, M.D., Blake Cady, M.D.,
Artemis G. Pazianos, M.D., and Ferdinand A. Salzman, M.D.

Extremely complex and difficult diagnostic and therapeutic problems frequently arise in patients with metastatic or recurrent breast cancer. A multidisciplined panel of specialists has been established to analyze and manage these patients. The panel consists of a chemotherapist, a general surgeon, an endocrinologist, and a radiotherapist. The patterns of therapy instituted have been based on the following concepts:

1. Therapy is palliative, not curative, and therefore significant symptoms or the potential for them must be present before instituting therapy.

2. Only one treatment modality must be utilized at a time, to simplify management and gain maximum predictive information for future therapeutic judgments.

3. The hormonal status of each patient must be ascertained as early as possible in the course of the disease as a basis for most future management.

4. Objective measurable disease must remain after diagnosis so that the effect of treatment can be quantitated.

5. Menstrual status at the time of recurrence must be clearly established as premenopausal, menopausal, or postmenopausal for aid in classification of therapy.

6. Localized disease is treated by localized therapy; systemic disease is treated by systemic therapy.

7. Progressive disease is treated; stable disease is observed.

8. All patients with metastatic breast cancer must receive some form of systemic therapy before terminal stages are reached, as only 20 per cent of patients are completely unresponsive to all attempts at treatment.

9. Multiple attempts at systemic control by a succession of systemic approaches are usually justified before death, because palliation can be achieved in a large majority of patients.

10. "Response" means 6 months of subjective cessation of symp-

toms and objective decrease in disease without appearance of new lesions.

With these guidelines in mind, general concepts about therapy can be outlined.

1. Radiation therapy is used at all stages for localized symptomatic disease, particularly for palliation of bone pain, but it is also used to prevent fractures in weight-bearing bones or progression of disease in the central nervous system.

2. Premenopausal patients are subjected to oophorectomy (Fig. 1).

a. If response occurs, further relapse warrants adrenalectomy or hypophysectomy.

b. If oophorectomy response does not occur, or when all hormonal responses end, androgens, chemotherapy, and adrenal steroids are used.

3. Postmenopausal patients are given estrogens (Fig. 2).

a. If response occurs, further relapse warrants adrenalectomy or hypophysectomy.

b. If estrogen response does not occur, chemotherapy, adrenal steroids, or androgens are used.

4. Menopausal patients (defined as patients over 45 years of age with irregular periods, or with menopausal symptoms, or patients within 5 years of spontaneous cessation of menses, or menstruating patients over 50 years who do not respond to oophorectomy) are given androgens *or* are subjected to adrenalectomy with oophorectomy, or hypophysectomy (Fig. 3).

a. If hormonal response occurs, further hormonal measures are used for relapses before the eventual use of chemotherapy.

b. If hormonal response fails to occur, chemotherapy is used.

5. Corticosteroids can frequently produce subjective palliation for a brief period of 2 to 3 months. Response to corticosteroids is *not* classified as a hormonal response.

6. Life-threatening situations not amenable to x-ray therapy and for which the 6 weeks' observation period for judgment of hormonal

METHOD OF SEQUENTIAL TREATMENT IN PREMENOPAUSAL WOMEN

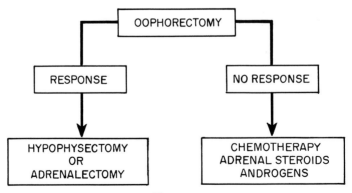

Figure 1.

METHOD OF SEQUENTIAL TREATMENT IN POSTMENOPAUSAL WOMEN

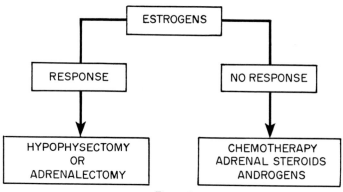

Figure 2.

response is too long would receive chemotherapy as the primary treatment of choice.

SPECIAL SURGICAL CONSIDERATIONS IN LOCALLY ADVANCED OR METASTATIC BREAST CANCER

Mastectomy

Mastectomy is occasionally necessary to prevent or control local fungation and ulceration when disease can no longer be controlled by radiation or other measures. Significant palliation can be achieved by removing painful ulcers or unsightly masses. Care must be taken, however, to view this in a strictly palliative light, and to modify the traditional

METHOD OF SEQUENTIAL TREATMENT IN MENOPAUSAL WOMEN

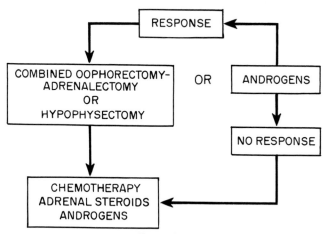

Figure 3.

mastectomy to avoid opening too many tissue planes that have no pertinence to a noncurative operative procedure. Carcinoma en cuirasse can be the penalty of too vigorous dissection for advanced lesions.

Radiation necrosis of chest wall recurrences after several courses of radiotherapy occasionally causes ulceration and extreme pain. Occasionally such ulcers are free of tumor but some may also be recurrent disease. Full-thickness excision of the chest wall with underlying ribs or sternum may be necessary with the ensuing defect covered by a large pedicle flap from nearby chest wall or the opposite breast. Such problems occur significantly less often after total (simple) mastectomy or modified radical mastectomy because of the thicker bulk of tissue overlying the ribs and the ability to mobilize local skin flaps more easily.

Pathologic fractures or impending pathologic fractures are best handled by internal rod fixation and radiation therapy if symptomatic. If no symptoms are present, there is usually enough time to give x-ray therapy alone and allow judicious motion while awaiting healing. However, femoral or humeral shafts or femoral necks lend themselves to stabilization, which prevents fracture site motion, relieves pain, and allows activity while radiation therapy is completed.

Biopsy

The simplest possible biopsy techniques should always be used. Needle aspiration biopsy of a supraclavicular lymph node is faster, cheaper, and less disturbing to the patient than open excision biopsy. Dermal punch biopsy of a small portion of a chest wall nodule with local anesthesia is nearly always more satisfactory than excision of such a nodule. These biopsy techniques are particularly noteworthy because visible or palpable disease is left in place for evaluation of therapeutic response. Our most perplexing problems arise from patients referred after total excision of isolated chest wall nodules and subsequent oophorectomy. The most valuable indicator of response (the chest wall nodule) is gone and frequently there is little else that can be measured objectively. How much more rational management can be achieved when a small dermal punch biopsy of such a lesion has been done before the hormonal manipulation or oophorectomy! Then clear objective data are obtained about response. Six or 9 months later, when further disease appears, a clear recommendation for adrenalectomy or hypophysectomy can be made with the assurance of response rates that exceed 50 per cent.

On occasion, needle aspiration biopsy of a concomitant breast mass will allow intelligent assessment of a lytic bone lesion in patients presenting initially with bone pain. At least two such cases each year present to our orthopedic service. Seldom is it necessary to do open bone biopsy or even open breast biopsy. Such aspiration biopsy techniques are inexpensive and rapid and are associated with no morbidity.

THE ROLE OF RADIOTHERAPY IN THE MANAGEMENT OF METASTATIC BREAST CANCER

Almost every woman with breast cancer in whom metastases develop will at some time receive radiation therapy for its palliative value. That it is palliative should not imply that it is an indifferent or necessarily slack form of treatment, for palliative radiotherapy can be every bit as difficult and demanding, and often more so, than is curative radiotherapy. Palliative radiotherapy in this disease is most useful and rationally used when the radiotherapist is fully aware of the patient's total clinical condition. This implies that he be aware of what curative and palliative measures have been used in the past, what others are available, and where the patient stands, at that moment, in the total spectrum of sequential palliative therapy (hormonal, chemotherapeutic, and ablative).

Modern radiotherapeutic techniques, even in palliative situations, imply the use of megavoltage radiations for optimal results. Although kilovoltage radiations have had an honorable past in this disease and are quite adequate in some situations, megavolt radiations are preferred because of their skin-sparing quality, their improved depth dose, and lessened side scatter, and because they permit a more accurate estimation of the actual delivered dose of radiation. They are more likely to permit attainment of the major goal in palliation: the most effective relief in the shortest time with the least morbidity.

Whenever possible, our aim is to deliver the desired dose of radiation within a 2 week period. This is usually attainable, although exceptions exist, particularly when large volumes of tissue must be included and the daily dose of radiation must be lowered in order to lessen radiation morbidity.

Bone Metastases

Irradiation is the treatment of choice for a local bone lesion causing pain. Solitary lesions in nonweight-bearing bones that can be encompassed in fields up to 10 cm.^{2} respond to single doses of 800 or 1400 rads delivered in 1 week. Such situations however are uncommon. Usually treatment fields have to be larger, and we prefer to extend the treatment to 2 weeks and administer doses in the range of 2000 to 3000 rads. Vertebral metastases, for example, are rarely solitary, and it is generally unwise to restrict the radiation only to the one or two obviously involved vertebrae. Usually several bodies are included and at least 2000 rads, preferably 2500 rads, are given in 10 fractions through a single direct posterior field. Whenever there seems to be a discrepancy between the roentgenologic findings of vertebral involvement and the clinical pattern of pain we do not hesitate to extend the treatment fields to satisfy both criteria; thus, fields may be 30 cm. long, for example, to include the entire lumbar spine and sacrum or several segments of both dorsal and lumbar spine. Similar diagnostic-therapeutic problems may arise in the neck and shoulder region. When the obvious cervical vertebral lesion does not clinically agree with the brachial plexus distribution of pain and there is no palpable disease either in the supraclavicular or high axillary regions, we will irradiate, using appropriately shaped fields, both regions to a minimum dose of 3000 rads.

It may be appropriate to irradiate a particularly painful bone lesion even in the presence of multiple progressive bone lesions for which the main treatment is hormonal or chemotherapeutic. The painful nonweight-bearing bone lesions usually respond rapidly with relief evident within 1 week. Osteolytic lesions respond better than osteoblastic lesions in general.

Not all osseous lesions cause pain. Osseous metastatic lesions that are not particularly painful may be better managed by other measures (hormonal, and so forth) particularly if they are progressive. The single exception is the osteolytic lesion in a weight-bearing long bone, usually the femur. It is our rule that such a lesion in the femoral shaft that is eroding one cortical margin and is over 2 cm. in diameter heralds an impending pathologic fracture and should be irradiated whether symptomatic or not. These lesions usually respond to tumor doses of 2500 to 3000 rads given in 2 to 2½ weeks. Where a pathologic fracture has already occurred or is about to occur, we recommend internal fixation followed by irradiation.

Soft Tissue Metastases

This category of breast metastases includes a wide variety of lesions, the majority of which are less painful than bone lesions. However, certain frequently recurring types have special significance to the patient.

Intracranial Metastases

Headache and nausea are the usual indicators, although ocular and gait disturbances in various combinations are not uncommon. Corticosteroids are usually administered the moment the diagnosis is made or suspected. We believe whole brain irradiation should be given if one or more intracranial metastatic sites are identified. A dose of 2500 to 3000 rads in 2 weeks is administered by opposing right and left lateral fields. Corticosteroids are discontinued as soon as feasible. Metastases localized to the orbit, retro-orbital space, or gasserian ganglion do occur. In this situation where small fields are feasible, we administer 2000 rads in 1 week.

Intrathoracic Metastases

Mediastinal lymph node disease may cause esophageal obstruction or a superior vena cava syndrome or cause distressing cough, either singly or in combination. Appropriately shaped opposed anterior and posterior megavoltage fields irradiated to 4000 rads in 3 weeks give effective relief. Only on rare occasions is higher dosage necessary. Problems arise only when the patient has had previous radiotherapy to the dorsal spine, as this would cause further irradiation of the spinal cord at this level. Here the judgment and experience of the radiotherapist are stressed the most. Special rotational and oblique techniques may help to circumvent partially the implied dangers of high dosage to the cord, or it may be necessary to combine chemotherapy with smaller doses of radiation. Such problems increase in frequency in any large group of patients with metastatic cancer and demand close coordination between the various specialists involved in the care of these patients.

Intra-Abdominal Metastases

Large intra-abdominal masses may or may not be symptomatic. They may threaten intestinal obstruction, ulceration, and hemorrhage. Nodal enlargement in the choledochoduodenal area can be distressing. Liver involvement can be the sole evidence of breast metastases. Cul-de-sac metastases in the pelvis can ulcerate through the vagina and cause bleeding. Radiation may be helpful in these situations alone or in conjunction with surgical, hormonal, or chemotherapeutic manipulation. Soft tissue metastases respond less readily to radiation in the palliative sense than do bony metastases. Some shrinkage of the mass can always be obtained, but doses in the range of 4000 rads are required. This is easily administered to the pelvis with little morbidity, but irradiation of the intestine outside the pelvis is more likely to cause varying degrees of anorexia, nausea, and vomiting. Thus, large abdominal fields are rarely employed or efficacious for breast metastases.

Often, more localized radiotherapy is combined with other measures if the age and general condition of the patient warrant distressing treatment regimens. On rare occasions we have irradiated localized metastases at the porta hepatis. Doses up to 2500 rads can be given with moderate morbidity. It is difficult to generalize on the efficacy of this type of treatment; response, when it does occur, is brief.

Chest Wall Metastases

Isolated chest wall recurrences, if few in number, can easily be irradiated with good results. Multinodular recurrences in the mastectomy scar usually herald more widespread disease in the chest wall than is apparent at the time. Whether in fact radiotherapy or hormonal alteration or chemotherapy is chosen will depend on several factors, mainly the hormonal status, age, previous response to endocrine alteration if such was accomplished for other recurrence, and whether the patient had previous chest wall irradiation as, for example, following mastectomy. If radiation is indicated and permissible, chest wall irradiation must be carried to at least 3500 rads and usually to 4500 rads in 2 to 4 weeks, depending on field size, in order to obtain satisfactory regression. Again megavolt irradiation is preferred. At our institution low megavolt electron irradiation at 3 to 3.5 million volts is used, or if a large area and nodes are involved, a special sector scanning technique using 2 million volt x-rays is used.

HORMONAL AND ABLATIVE CONSIDERATIONS IN METASTATIC MAMMARY CANCER

Extensive studies in man and in experimental animals have established that estrogens play an important role in the growth of some breast cancers. The concept of hormonal dependence has evolved with the observation that certain women respond to alterations in their hormonal environment whereas other patients fail to respond at all. Initial therapy in individuals with metastatic disease, therefore, is directed at abolishing endogenous estrogen or in some way blocking its effect.

Oophorectomy

Castration remains the treatment of choice in the young, menstruating woman. Unfortunately, no practical means for selecting patients for oophorectomy has been found. Since it is relatively innocuous, this should be selected as the primary treatment in the premenopausal patient. Approximately 40 to 50 per cent of patients will respond, presumably because of removal of the primary source of estrogen, with remissions averaging 9 months.[8, 12] Castration should also be performed in the patient who has had a previous hysterectomy and is still in the premenopausal age group.

In the late premenopausal patient an oophorectomy can be performed, bearing in mind that lack of response does not necessarily imply lack of hormonal dependence, since the ovaries in these patients may not be the major source of estrogens. Failure of these individuals to respond would not, therefore, contraindicate further ablative therapy, such as adrenalectomy or hypophysectomy.

Menopausal patients are subjected to androgen therapy or adrenalectomy with oophorectomy or hypophysectomy.

Castration alone should not be considered in the older patient who is clearly postmenopausal since the yield of beneficial results is too small.

Our group favors surgical castration unless the patient's condition is too poor to tolerate anesthesia. Radiation castration can be offered such a patient with the knowledge that it may take 6 weeks to achieve ablation of function.

Hormonal Therapy

Sex hormones continue to have a role in the palliation of mammary cancer. The disasters which have been reported[9] have been related to exacerbation of the disease and the ensuing hypercalcemia. For this reason hospitalization for close observation and daily serum calcium measurements are strongly urged, particularly in the patient with bone metastases.

Androgen Therapy

This mode of therapy should be considered in the younger patient who has had castration with or without a response and in the early menopausal patient. Approximately 30 per cent of patients in these age groups will respond, with an average duration of response of 8 months. Androgen therapy is occasionally elected in the patient who is more than 5 years postmenopausal if she looks physiologically younger. Some groups have recommended androgen therapy in the older population, but the results are not quite as good as those achieved with estrogen therapy. Approximately 20 per cent of the postmenopausal patients will respond.

The mechanism by which androgen therapy induces remission is not known but it may in some way neutralize or block endogenous estrogen. It apparently can also exert a direct tumor effect, since some short remissions have been obtained even after hypophysectomy.

The obvious side-effects are the only major drawback and may be unacceptable to some patients.

Estrogen Therapy

Objective remissions can be obtained with estrogens in 40 to 45 per cent of postmenopausal patients. The average duration of response is comparable to that of androgen therapy, that is, 8 months. Here again the mechanism by which remissions are induced is not known. The effect may be mediated through the pituitary with suppression of function, or estrogens may in some way block the endogenous hormones.

The side-effects of nausea and fluid retention can be controlled in most patients.

Corticosteroid Therapy

Cortisone and its analogues play a useful role in breast cancer. With large doses of prednisone, 30 to 60 mg. daily, or cortisone, 200 to 400 mg., short objective remissions can be obtained in 30 per cent of patients. This approach is generally reserved for patients too ill to undergo ablative therapy. It is also useful in patients with hepatic or pulmonary disease. Sufficient improvement may be obtained in a few weeks so that surgery may be feasible. Ablative therapy is of course preferable because the marked side-effects of long-term corticosteroid therapy can be avoided.

Corticosteroids often provide considerable subjective improvement and may be useful even in the patient with terminal disease because of the euphoria and sense of well being which they produce.

Bilateral Adrenalectomy or Hypophysectomy

Depending on the surgical talent available, either bilateral adrenalectomy or hypophysectomy can be offered, since these procedures yield approximately the same results. Forty to 45 per cent of unselected patients will obtain an objective remission averaging 18 months.[2, 11] Either of these should be considered in the patient who has had a previous castration response or is late premenopausal or clearly menopausal. Failure to respond to castration in a premenopausal patient is a general contraindication to further ablative therapy. If adrenalectomy is selected rather than hypophysectomy, a simultaneous castration should be performed if the ovaries have not been removed previously. Hypophysectomy should not be considered in a patient who has had a previous beneficial adrenalectomy. Less than 20 per cent of such patients will obtain an additional remission, and most of these are too brief to be worthwhile.[2]

Age is not necessarily a contraindication to surgery. A decision must be based on the patient's clinical condition and willingness to follow a program of substitution therapy. The latter is not a major consideration since replacement is relatively simple, and patients with malignancy are accustomed to some program of therapy.

Unfortunately there is no absolute way to predict which patients will definitely respond to such procedures. On the basis of previous experience, however, certain guidelines can be followed. The most consistent index has been the previous response to castration in premenopausal women. The great majority of these patients will obtain a second remission from either hypophysectomy or adrenalectomy.

If the disease is in any way altered by hormonal therapy, that is, ameliorated or exacerbated by either androgens or estrogens, a more favorable response may be anticipated. The previous response to corticosteroids is less predictable.

A long "disease-free" interval from the time of mastectomy to the first appearance of metastases also favors a response. This is consistent with the observation that more slowly growing tumors in general respond better to various modalities of therapy. A disease-free interval from mastectomy to onset of metastases of less than 1 year precludes a high response rate to hormonal manipulation.

Once again it should be emphasized that age is not a contraindication but actually an indication for ablative therapy. A high percentage (60 to 65 per cent) of women more than 60 years of age can be expected to benefit. There is no reasonable explanation for this since estrogen production in this age group is minimal. This, too, may be related to the fact that the disease is often less aggressive in the older patient.

The optimum time to recommend ablative therapy is often difficult. It is usually deferred until the disease is fairly widespread and yet the patient must be a reasonable operative risk and have a life expectancy of several months in order to assess any possible benefit. Even in the best of clinics with close supervision the opportunity may be missed in a patient whose tumor suddenly escapes control and any surgical procedure becomes extremely hazardous. Ablative surgery is clearly not a heroic procedure and should be performed early enough in the course of the disease to be of possible long-term benefit rather than in a life-threatening situation.

INDICATIONS FOR CHEMOTHERAPY IN METASTATIC BREAST CANCER

Cancer chemotherapeutic agents, nonhormonal in nature, can be effective in the treatment of advanced breast cancer and are reserved for patients no longer responsive to hormones or surgical ablative procedures, such as hypophysectomy or adrenalectomy, or whose disease is rapidly progressive. Unlike hormone therapy or ablative surgical procedures, chemotherapeutic agents produce toxic reactions involving the bone marrow, gastrointestinal tract, and other sites depending on the specific drug involved. Hence, they should only be given by physicians experienced in their use and familiar with their toxic reactions.

The main indications for chemotherapy are: (1) progressive cancer with demonstrated unresponsiveness to hormones and in which x-ray therapy provides no practical benefit, and (2) rapid progression involving vital organs, such as liver, lungs, central nervous system, and so forth, in which the length of expected survival precludes the usual 6 week observation period for maximum effectiveness of hormones for surgical ablative procedures.

Special indications for chemotherapy have been: (1) Hypercalcemia. Hypercalcemia secondary to progressive breast cancer has responded dramatically to the antibiotic mithramycin. This appears to be more useful than the usual treatment with steroids. Generally, 0.25 mcg. per kilogram of body weight per day for 1 to 3 days by single intravenous injection is an adequate dose to lower the serum calcium of most patients. (2) Adjuvant chemotherapy. Chemotherapy has *also* been valuable as an adjuvant treatment with x-ray therapy. When used in combination with x-ray therapy, enhanced antitumor responses have been seen, in part related to increased sensitivity to the ionizing radiation. This has been helpful in difficult situations, such as liver and brain metastases. Chemotherapy has also been used in combination with surgical ablative procedures although no controlled studies have been employed. It has also been suggested that they be employed in patients who have undergone remission with hormonal therapy or surgical ablative procedures in the hope of prolonging survival or remissions. This approach is currently being studied by various cooperative study groups.

Patients with significant bone marrow involvement, when treated with chemotherapeutic drugs, may show enhanced toxicity, and treatment must be used cautiously. Patients with a survival of less than 1 month can also be treated, but this will be at the discretion of the physician. As long as these drugs do not cure breast cancer, palliation should be our aim. This might preclude asymptomatic patients, but if it can be shown that survival will be prolonged, this group of patients should also be treated.

Table 1. *Drug Doses of Chemotherapeutic Agents in Metastatic Breast Cancer*

DRUG	ROUTE OF ADMINISTRATION	DOSAGE
Triethylene thiophosphoramide (Thio-tepa)	Intravenous or intramuscular	0.2 mg./kg. × 5
Cyclophosphamide	Orally Intravenously	3.5 to 5.0 mg./kg./day × 10 8 mg./kg. × 5; 15 mg./kg./ week; 40 mg./kg. × 1
Melphalan[13]	Orally	0.3 mg./kg. × 4 days (4 to 6 week intervals)
5-Fluorouracil (5-FU)	Intravenously	12 mg./kg./day × 4 to 5 and 6 to 12 mg./kg. every other day × 5 or until toxicity
Methotrexate (Mtx)	Orally	1.25 mg. orally four times a day

COMBINATION TREATMENT

5-FU — 12 mg./kg./day I.V. × 4
then 500 mg./week
Methotrexate — 25 to 50 mg./week I.V.
Cytoxan — 2.5 mg./kg./day orally
Vincristine — 35 mcg./kg./week I.V. 4 to 10 doses
Prednisone — 0.75 mg./kg./day × 4 to 5; then
reduced to 25 mg./day for 8 weeks,
then decreased to zero. Maintenance
is carried out with reduced doses
of all drugs except for Vincristine
and prednisone which is decreased
after 8 to 12 weeks

Methods and Drugs Used in Chemotherapy

Chemotherapeutic drugs can be given either systemically, orally, intravenously, intramuscularly, or regionally, either by perfusion, infusion, topical intratumor, or direct instillation into a serous cavity. Systemic chemotherapy is most often used and in Table 1 are listed the agents most commonly used. For most of these agents, the drug toxicity has been well described in the literature. Physicians should be familiar with one or two agents and use them in an intelligent manner.

Recently, combinations of chemotherapeutic drugs have been used and response rates have varied from 50 to 80 per cent in various reports (Table 2). It is becoming evident that response rates are markedly enhanced in comparison to single agent chemotherapy. Previous studies in combination chemotherapy in acute leukemia and Hodgkin's disease have shown the superiority of this approach over single drug administration, but in breast cancer such controlled studies have not been reported to date.

We have recently been exploring the five drug combination of 5-FU, methotrexate, Cytoxan, Vincristine, and prednisone as originally reported by Cooper.[5] In our own clinic, 42 patients with advanced breast cancer either resistant to hormonal therapy or in relapse following remission

Table 2. *Results of Chemotherapeutic Agents in Metastatic Breast Cancer*

	NUMBER OF PATIENTS	OBJECTIVE RESPONSE	
		Number	Per cent
Alkylating Agents			
Collected Series[4]			
Nitrogen mustard, thio-tepa, cyclophosphamide	724	188	26
Melphalan[13]	52	12	23
Antimetabolites			
Fluorinated Pyrimidine			
5-Fluorouracil[16]	251	91	36
5-Fluorouracil[1]	158	52	33
5-Fluoro-2'-deoxyuridine[1] (FUDR)	46	22	48
Folic Acid Antagonists			
Methotrexate (Mtx)[15]	37	16	43
Vinca Alkaloids			
Vinblastine (VLB)[6]	40	10	25
Vincristine (VCR)[3]	35	12	34
Combined Chemotherapy			
Thio-tepa and Mtx[7]	40	24	60
5-FU, Mtx, Cytoxan, Vincristine, prednisone[5]	60	54	90
5-FU, Mtx, Cytoxan, Vincristine, prednisone[10]	43	27	63

with ablative surgical procedures were treated. Of these, 27 have shown complete objective responses (63 per cent response rate) and this is far superior to our previous experience with single agents. Because of the enthusiasm for this form of chemotherapy, further controlled studies are in order.

In addition, because of our previous studies involving regional infusion chemotherapy of the liver, we have adapted this in the treatment of occasional instances of breast cancer.[14] Twelve patients have been treated by regional infusion, with a 50 per cent response rate using the fluorinated pyrimidines.

Thoracentesis or Paracentesis

The early and vigorous treatment of pleural effusion may prevent lung trapping and maintain maximum pulmonary volume. This can best be accomplished by removal of fluid and obliteration of the pleural space at the earliest stage possible. Many agents have been described for this – talcum powder, chloroquine, nitrogen mustard, thio-tepa, P32, and radioactive colloidal gold.

Our practice is to withdraw as much fluid as can be obtained *easily* by use of a needle or, preferably, the largest bore intracath tubing placed through its needle, followed by the instillation of 0.4 mg. per kilogram of HN_2 (not to exceed 20 mg.) followed by rapid changes in patient position after removal of the needle or catheter to attempt better mixing of the drug with residual pleural fluid and contact with the entire pleural surface. Leukopenia is occasionally seen in 7 to 10 days, in addition to nausea and vomiting in the immediate 12 hour period. Careful check of the pleural fluid should be made over the next several days and attempts made to keep the space fairly dry so that pleural adhesions can occur easily.

CONCLUSIONS

Intelligent therapeutic management in patients with advanced breast cancer offers useful control and prolongation of a comfortable life. A more aggressive approach is justified in this form of cancer with an appropriate sequential long-range therapeutic plan designed for each patient. A multidisciplined approach involving surgeons, radiotherapists, endocrinologists, and medical oncologists can be of significant value for these difficult management problems.

REFERENCES

1. Ansfield, R. J., and Curreri, A. R.: Further clinical comparison between 5-fluorouracil (5-FU) and 5-fluoro-2 -deoxy-uridine (5-FUDR). Cancer Chemother. Rep., 32:101–105 (Oct.) 1963.
2. Byron, R. L., Jr., Yonemoto, R. H., Bashore, R., Bierman, H. R., et al.: Bilateral adrenalectomy in advanced breast cancer. Surgery, 52:725–732 (Nov.) 1962.
3. Clinical Staff Conference. Breast cancer. Combined clinical staff conference at the National Institutes of Health. Ann. Intern Med., 63:321–341 (Aug.) 1965.

4. Comparative clinical and biological effects of alkylating agents. Ann. N.Y. Acad. Sci., 68:245–657 (Oct. 21) 1958.
5. Cooper, R.: Report on data presented at special meeting held at NCI (New Jersey) to discuss therapy of advanced breast cancer. September 11, 1969. Eastern Cooperative Oncology Group Minutes, p. 53.
6. Frei, E., III, Carbone, P., and Shnider, B., et al.: Quoted by Clinical Staff Conference (Ref. 3).
7. Greenspan, E. M., Fieber, M., Lesnick, G., and Edelman, S.: Response of advanced breast carcinoma to the combination of the antimetabolite, methotrexate, and alkylating agent, thio-TEPA. J. Mount Sinai Hosp. N.Y., 30:246–267 (May-June) 1963.
8. Kennedy, B. J., and Fortuny, I. E.: Therapeutic castration in the treatment of advanced breast cancer. Caner, 17:1197–1202 (Sept.) 1964.
9. Moore, F. D., Woodrow, S. I., Aliapoulios, M. A., et al.: Carcinoma of the breast. A decade of new results with old concepts. New Eng. J. Med., 277:292–296, 343–350, 411–416, and 460–468 (Aug. 10, 17, 24, and 31) 1967.
10. Oberfield, R.: Unpublished data.
11. Pearson, O. H., and Ray, B. S.: Hypophysectomy in the treatment of metastatic mammary cancer. Amer. J. Surg., 99:544–552 (April) 1960.
12. Pearson, O. H., and others: Scientific exhibits; endocrine therapy of metastatic breast cancer. Arch. Intern. Med., 95:357–364 (Feb.) 1955.
13. Sears, M. E.: Chemotherapy for advanced breast cancer. In Breast cancer: Early and late. 13th Annual Clinical Conf. on Cancer, 1968, University of Texas M.D. Anderson Hospital and Tumor Institute at Houston, Houston, Texas. Chicago, Year Book Medical Publishers, Inc., 1970, pp. 387–393.
14. Sullivan, R. D., Watkins, E., Jr., Oberfield, R. A., and Khazei, A. M.: Current status of protracted arterial infusion cancer chemotherapy for treatment of solid tumors. Surg. Clin. N. Amer., 47:769–784 (June) 1967.
15. Sullivan, R. D., Miller, E., Zurek, W. Z., Oberfield, R. A., and Ojima, Y.: Re-evaluation of methotrexate as an anti-cancer drug. Surg. Gynec. Obstet., 125:819–824 (Oct.) 1967.
16. Zubrod, G. G.: The limited usefulness of 5-fluorouracil (5-FU) and 5-fluorodeoxyuridine (5-FUDR) in the management of patients with adenocarcinoma. In Ingelfinger, F. J., Relman, A. S., and Finland, M. (eds.): Controversy in Internal Medicine. Philadelphia, W. B. Saunders Co., 1966, pp. 591–600.

605 Commonwealth Avenue
Boston, Massachusetts 02215

Practical Aspects of Investigation and Treatment of Colorectal Cancer

Richard A. Oberfield, M.D.

Colorectal cancer ranks in mortality and incidence as the second commonest form of cancer; it is preceded by cancer of the breast in women, and by cancer of the lungs in men.[24] In 1967, 43,513 patients died from cancer of the colorectal region, and approximately 46,000 new cases are expected in 1971.[24] The only known curative approach to date has been surgical removal of the tumor. Although the surgical mortality rate has been reduced, the 5 year recurrence rate remains approximately the same—50 per cent.[15, 24] In this article I will attempt to review three aspects of colorectal cancer. These include basic problems relating to the primary treatment of the disease, the present chemotherapy program for systemic metastatic disease, and management of liver metastasis from colorectal cancer. This involves a regional form of chemotherapy that at our institution has produced increased remission rates and possibly prolonged survival for this most difficult form of metastasis.

PROBLEMS RELATED TO THE PRIMARY TREATMENT OF COLORECTAL CANCER

If we are to improve our results in colorectal cancer, we first must improve the diagnosis of the disease, and an early diagnosis is essential. Swinton,[30] from the Lahey Clinic Foundation, has reviewed a series of 334 patients who presented with various signs and symptoms leading to the diagnosis of colorectal cancer (Table 1). This is very similar to the experience of others.[2, 5] Signs and symptoms will vary depending on whether the tumor arises in the right colon, where unexplained anemia, vague abdominal pain, and palpable masses are often present, or in the left colon, where a change in bowel habit, rectal bleeding, and pain are more frequent. The cardinal signs and symptoms have been bleeding, altered bowel function, and abdominal pain. Classic problems appeared in the majority of patients, although a small percentage of patients were asymptomatic.

After a careful history and physical examination, a proctoscopic

Table 1. *Classical Signs and Symptoms in Colorectal Cancer
(334 Patients)**

	PER CENT
Bleeding	73
Altered bowel function	73
Abdominal pain	63
Weight loss (> 5 lb.)	26
Hemoglobin (< 12 gm.)	24
History of benign polyps	7
History of polyps with carcinoma	24
Classical signs and symptoms	95.5
No signs and symptoms	4.5

*Adapted from Swinton, N. W., Samaan, S., and Rosenthal, D.: Surg. Clin. N. Amer., 47:657–662, 1967.

examination is mandatory. Some rectosigmoid carcinomas are too high for a rectal examination and too low to be detected by barium enema. Certainly, small polypoid carcinomas of the lower sigmoid can be seen on proctoscopic examination and cured in 90 to 95 per cent of cases.[2] A barium enema should also be performed, and if results are negative but symptoms persist, it should be repeated. Air-contrast enemas often are helpful for small polypoid lesions, which can be cured in 9 of 10 cases.

Although much work has been done with the use of tumor-specific antigens, such as the carcinoembryonic antigens (CEA), as yet it has not been useful as a practical method of diagnosis. This was described by Gold[11] in 1965 when tumor-specific antigens were detected in embryonal human epithelium and in colonic cancer and were called carcinoembryonic antigen.

After a diagnosis of colorectal cancer has been established, operation has been the treatment of choice. What has been the experience with the end result in colorectal cancer? It is of interest that over the years, despite sophisticated techniques and improvements in many areas relating to surgery, 5 year survival rates have been approximately 50 per cent.

Swinton has reviewed a vast number of patients with cancer of the colon and rectum from 1941 through 1945 and from 1956 to 1961 (Tables 2 and 3).[29] Over the two periods, the operative mortality rate has decreased from 8.2 to 3.1 per cent. We have increased the degree of resectability, and no significant change has been noted in the two series on the number of patients operated on. However, patients with nodal involvement or nodal and blood vessel involvement still have a similar 5 year survival rate.

The difference in the group with blood vessel invasion is hard to explain. Even in the Dukes A cases, the survival rate has only increased from 56.3 to 67.1 per cent over this 20 year period. Patients with regional nodal involvement alone or combined with blood vessel invasion still have a poor survival rate despite early diagnosis and improvement in surgical techniques. Patients with blood-borne metastasis are found most frequently in the younger age groups when prognosis is poor.

Table 2. *End-Results, Cancer of Colon and Rectum*
*1941–1945 Inclusive**

INVOLVEMENT		TOTAL SERIES		5 YEAR SURVIVAL	
Lymph Node	Blood Vessel	Number	Per cent	Number	Per cent
None	None	355	56.2	200	56.3
Present	None	128	20.3	41	32.1
None	Present	82	13.0	22	26.8
Present	Present	67	10.6	6	9.0
Total with nodal or vessel involvement or both		277	43.8	69	24.9
Total operated on (operability)		732	100.0	338	46.2
Total resected (resectability)		632	86.3	269	42.6
Operative mortality		60	8.2	0	0

*From Swinton, N. W., Sr., and Nahra, K. S.: *In* Sullivan, R. D., ed.: Clinical Cancer Chemotherapy Including Ambulatory Infusion. Springfield, Illinois, Charles C Thomas, 1970.

A large number of cases reviewed by Gabriel at St. Mark's Hospital from 1928 to 1957 showed that a majority of patients still present with Dukes C classification, for which 5 year survival rates are very poor (Table 4).[10] Therefore, despite all that we can do, metastasis will eventually develop in most patients with a tendency to spread that will either be lymphatic or vascular.

As a generalization, one concludes that of 100 per cent of the patients operated on, 50 per cent will be cured, hematogenous spread will develop in 35 per cent, lymphatic involvement will develop in 5 per cent, and local recurrence will develop in 10 per cent. What is the significance of all this? Despite early diagnosis and sophisticated surgical techniques, we can expect little in improvement of resectability and operative mortality and survival rates. What will the future hold? Some of the solutions will be in early diagnosis, surgical improvements, adjuvant therapy involving

Table 3. *End Results, Cancer of Colon and Rectum*
*1956–1961 Inclusive**

INVOLVEMENT		TOTAL SERIES		5 YEAR SURVIVAL	
Lymph Node	Blood Vessel	Number	Per cent	Number	Per cent
None	None	280	45.9	188	67.1
Present	None	128	20.9	46	36.0
None	Present	88	14.4	53	60.2
Present	Present	114	18.7	15	13.0
Total with nodal or vessel involvement or both		330	54.1	114	34.5
Total operated on (operability)		620	100.0	316	50.9
Total resected (resectability)		610	98.4	302	49.5
Operative mortality		19	3.1	0	0

*From Swinton, N. W., Sr., and Nahra, K. S.: *In* Sullivan, R. D., ed.: Clinical Cancer Chemotherapy Including Ambulatory Infusion. Springfield, Illinois, Charles C Thomas, 1970.

Table 4. *Proportions of Dukes A, B, and C Cases in a Series of 2,950 Cases of Carcinoma of the Rectum (St. Mark's Hospital Statistics, 1928–1957)**

GROUP	NUMBER OF CASES	PERCENTAGE
A	436	14.8
B	1,005	34.1
C	1,509	51.1
Total	2,950	

*From Gabriel, W. B.: The Principles and Practice of Rectal Surgery. London, H. K. Lewis, 5th ed., 1963.

chemotherapy, radiotherapy, and, hopefully, immunotherapy involving bacille Calmette Guérin (BCG) or corynebacterium parvum.

Rousselot[22] has described an intraluminal technique using 5-fluorouracil (5-FU) at the time of operation. This involves a two-tape procedure to isolate the bowel segment with the tumor. An injection of 5-FU, 30 mg. per kilogram of body weight, diluted to 50 ml. of saline, is injected into the bowel lumen. After 30 minutes, resection is performed, and on the first and second postoperative day, 5-FU, 10 mg. per kilogram of body weight, is injected intravenously. It was hoped that this method would improve recurrence rates, especially those related to dissemination of tumor cells at the time of operation.

Rousselot[22] reviewed a series of cases randomized between the control group and the 5-FU group. The overall 5 year survival rate has significantly been improved in Stage III groups with a 5 year survival rate of 65 per cent compared with 26 per cent in the control groups. It is of interest that the women in the 5-FU group had significantly better survival rates than the men. The difference in 5 year survival rates between the 5-FU treated group compared with the control group and also the national average group is significant. It is clear from these studies that this appears to offer significant improvement. A prospective randomized study in cooperation with other hospitals is being performed now to substantiate this finding. Other investigators, such as Curreri,[3, 20] have used systemic 5-FU in Dukes B and C cases postoperatively and then at a later date have a second look. They have noted a delay in local recurrence, and this would indicate a need for further work in this area.

At the Lahey Clinic Foundation, we have attempted to develop a protocol for prophylactic regional infusion of liver metastasis in asymptomatic patients in the hope that we could improve this difficult area of treatment. We have attempted to randomize those patients with lymph node and blood vessel involvement who, at the time of surgery, have a poor prognosis and will have liver metastasis and will die from their disease within 2 years. One group will receive regional infusion chemotherapy; the other will not receive any chemotherapy. Other groups have attempted this, but no reports of studies are available to date.

In summary, for the primary treatment of colorectal cancer, we have reached the zenith of early diagnosis and surgery, and we must look toward adjuvant methods for improving our results. A multidisciplined approach is necessary in this area.

SYSTEMIC CHEMOTHERAPY FOR METASTATIC
COLORECTAL CANCER

We have relied primarily on antimetabolites, fluorinated pyrimidines, such as 5-FU, 5-fluoro-2'-deoxyuridine (5-FUDR), and the folic acid antagonist, 4-amino-N[10] methyl pteroylglutamic acid (methotrexate), for the management of this condition. What is the mechanism of action of the fluorinated pyrimidines, 5-FU, since it is the best agent available in the treatment of advanced cancer of the colon? In 1954, Rutman, Cantarow, and Paschkis[23] showed an increase in concentration of uracil in rat liver tumors compared with the normal rat liver. This was not true of orotic acid. Duschinsky et al.,[6] in 1957, in collaboration with Hoffmann-LaRoche, synthesized 5-FU. A substitution of fluorine at position five of uracil had a profound effect. Just by altering molecules, we can produce significant effects such as the changing of acetic acid to 5-fluoroacetic acid, which is the difference between salad dressing and commercial rat poison.[12]

In 1958 Curreri and associates[4] reported clinical results that prompted further studies. The fluorinated pyrimidines, 5-FU and 5-FUDR, inhibit thymidylate synthetase leading to block of deoxyribonucleic acid (DNA) synthesis.[13] Thymidylate synthetase catalyzes the methylation of 2-deoxyuridylic acid to thymidylic acid. This inhibition of thymidylate synthetase is responsible for the antitumor effect of 5-FU and 5-FUDR. This action is related to the degree of phosphorylation. Kessel and Hall[16] are trying to relate the degree of phosphorylation to the sensitivity of tumors to 5-FU and 5-FUDR. Certainly, when 5-FU is given by continuous infusion, the toxicity is decreased, whereas 5-FUDR toxicity is enhanced.[28] This is definitely related to the action of these antimetabolites and how they are metabolized by the tumor cells and normal cells.

A review of many different series using 5-FU has shown response rates on the average of 20 per cent, although they have varied from 8 to 85 per cent, depending on the series.[33] Patients with advanced disease are selected after having a tissue diagnosis and objective measurable disease, and if possible with some degree of palliation to be expected. A patient who is entirely asymptomatic and who is unaware of his disease should not be subjected to systemic chemotherapy, since no cure is to be expected. Some persons believe that it is contraindicated in the more senile, emotionally disturbed patients or after a recent major operation. This is quite variable.

Various dose schedules for intravenous administration are shown in Table 5. In any dose schedule, one should try to obtain slight toxicity or antitumor response. The initial course is preferably given in the hospital, with subsequent courses given on an outpatient basis. Leukocyte counts are obtained every 2 to 3 days during therapy, and hemoglobin and platelet counts twice a week. The second course is given in about 4 to 5 weeks after completion of the last course. If weekly maintenance is considered, therapy is begun in 2 to 3 weeks, starting with 500 mg. intravenously and increasing by increments of 250 mg. weekly, depending on the white blood cell count.

Table 5. *Dosage Regimens (5-FU)*

INDUCTION	FOLLOWED BY
15 mg./kg. × 4 or 5 doses (intravenous push)	7.5 mg. on alternate days for 4 or 5 doses or to toxicity
12 mg./kg. × 4 to 5 doses (intravenous push)*	6 mg. on alternate days for 4 or 5 doses or to toxicity
12 mg./kg. × 5 doses (intravenous push; infusion over 4 hours)*	12 mg./kg. on alternate days for 5 doses or to toxicity
5 mg./kg. × 3 doses (intravenous push)	7.5 mg./kg. on alternate days to toxicity
10 mg./kg. × 5 doses (intravenous push)	At monthly intervals
7.5 to 15.0 mg./kg. weekly (intravenous push)	Weekly
25 to 30 mg./kg. every 3 weeks (intravenous push)	Every 3 weeks

*Maximum daily dose = 1 gm.

Orally administered 5-FU is absorbed by the gastrointestinal tract.[18, 19] It has been used with antitumor effect, and the dose schedules have been essentially similar with the drug being given with juice for breakfast.[18, 19] The dose schedule is 12 mg. per kilogram of body weight in juice for breakfast every day for 4 or 5 days, followed by the same amount every other day to toxicity. Various modifications can be used. The response patterns have been similar to those obtained with prolonged intravenous infusion of 5-FU, but the response rates have been low. Toxic reactions are well recognized and are mainly limited to the gastrointestinal tract and bone marrow depression. Again, the important thing is to be familiar with one dose schedule and know exactly the toxic reactions. It is believed that toxicity is not essential, but should there be no antitumor response, one is not sure whether optimal treatment has been administered.

In summary, systemic chemotherapy using 5-FU has resulted in response rates around 20 per cent, with minimal to moderate toxicity. Although 5-FUDR might be slightly more effective, the results of studies[1, 8, 21] that have been done do not warrant its preference, especially in view of the cost. Other drugs with the same antitumor effect but response rates below that of 5-FU have been methotrexate, BCNU, mitomycin-C, and combinations of drugs. However, their response rates reveal little hope for the future. Because of this, new drugs in addition to other drugs with little previous trial in colon cancer should be tried. The Eastern Cooperative Oncology Group is presently employing a protocol for the continuous evaluation of new therapy in patients with metastatic cancer of the colon and rectum (phase 2).[9] With this protocol, ineffective regimens will be eliminated rapidly and replaced by new agents, including combinations.

PROLONGED REGIONAL ARTERIAL INFUSION IN THE TREATMENT OF METASTATIC LIVER DISEASE

Of the 44,000 patients with cancer of the colon, 22,000 will have recurrence in 5 years. Of these 22,000, 11,000 will die from liver disease, and 8,000 of these will not have dissemination. Systemic chemotherapy, surgery, and radiation therapy have given slight benefit. Since the tumor is limited to the liver, which is supplied by one major artery, a regional form of chemotherapy would be desirable. These tumors are supplied predominantly by the hepatic artery and not the portal vein; therefore, the hepatic artery is preferred.

Approximately 8 or 9 years ago, our oncology group at the Lahey Clinic developed a rational and aggressive approach to the management of these patients, known as prolonged arterial infusion of antimetabolites, using administration of methotrexate, 5-FUDR, and 5-FU to these tumors for clinical benefit. This is not a perfusion technique but a prolonged arterial infusion technique. The rationale for this approach is that we can provide high concentrations of the drug to the tumor site.

Since these solid tumors have doubling times of only 3 months or more, and since we are using antimetabolites that interfere with cell turnover, it is logical to use a prolonged infusion technique because at any given time only a small percentage of tumor cells are dividing. An intermittent approach would destroy only a small percentage of tumor cells. By providing continuous exposure of tumor cell populations as they divide over a prolonged period, a majority of tumor cells would be affected with a greater antitumor effect. This may also result in enhanced toxicity, but drugs such as 5-FUDR and 5-FU are primarily detoxified by the liver, and only a local hepatic toxic effect will be obtained.[17]

In previous reports, we have described our techniques and results of continuous infusion chemotherapy.[25, 27] We have been able to obtain a prolonged infusion technique by the use of a portable pump that allows the patient to be ambulatory while receiving chemotherapy in high concentrations 24 hours a day. Occasionally, a large volume pump is necessary in patients confined to the hospital for whom drugs other than 5-FUDR and 5-FU are used.

Patients with no extrahepatic disease and only liver metastasis are explored after a preoperative arteriogram shows no anomalies. A catheter is inserted into the hepatic artery, and fluorescein is injected to make sure that both lobes of the liver are fluoresced well. Then a Teflon catheter is attached to a portable pump. The patients are discharged from the hospital after about 2 weeks with continuation of the chemotherapy. The pump can be removed manually (Fig. 1).

We have used primarily 5-FUDR and 5-FU (Table 6). 5-FUDR is now available, and although methotrexate could be used, it is not detoxified to the same degree as 5-FUDR and 5-FU, and systemic toxicity develops. These patients receive 5-FUDR for periods of 4 to 6 weeks, at which time a chemical hepatitis or local toxicity develops, as manifested by an increase in the serum glutamic oxaloacetic transaminase (SGOT), alkaline phosphatase, and occasionally bilirubin. Following this, nonmedicated solution containing distilled water is infused for another 4 to 6 weeks, at which time toxicity abates and the liver will improve. Liver scans, which will show improvement in the majority of patients, are performed at 6 week intervals. The catheters are checked by infusion angiography to make sure the catheter is intact. Over a long period cystic

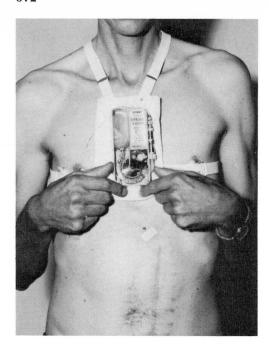

Figure 1. The patient is receiving continuous ambulatory arterial cancer chemotherapy through a treatment catheter, using a low-volume portable pump apparatus. The self-contained pump is worn beneath the clothing like a hearing aid.

areas will develop in the liver in some patients, and calcifications of liver metastasis in others.

In 1965 Sullivan and Zurek[26] reported results of treatment of liver cancer by protracted ambulatory infusion employing predominantly 5-FUDR. In 73 patients, objective response rates were 60 per cent without extrahepatic metastasis and 55 per cent with extrahepatic metastasis for patients with advanced liver metastasis. An average expected survival of 2.1 months was increased to 9.4 months. Analysis of the natural history of hepatic metastases in 390 patients indicated that only 70 per cent of patients live beyond 1 year with an overall median survival time of 75 days.[14] Therefore, any techniques or therapeutic modalities should show a net survival beyond that of untreated patients.

Recently at the Lahey Clinic, an analysis of 82 patients treated by hepatic artery infusion between 1961 and 1967 was compared to an untreated group of 67 patients from 1950 to 1960.[32] The treated group

Table 6. *Effective Drug Dose Schedules for Hepatic Artery Infusion*

DRUG	DOSAGE
5-Fluorouracil (5-FU)	5.0 to 7.5 mg./kg./24 hours; 3 mg./kg./24 hours*
5-Fluoro-2′-deoxyuridine (5-FUDR)	0.1 to 0.3 mg./kg./24 hours**
Methotrexate (Mtx)	5.0 to 10.0 mg./24 hours

*Maximum amount possible via hepatic artery using chronometric infusion pump.
**20 mg./day average dose.

Table 7. *Survival after Onset of Abnormal Liver Function Tests**

SURVIVAL (MONTHS)	TREATED GROUP (82 PATIENTS)		CONTROL GROUP (67 PATIENTS, 1950–1960)	
	Number	Per cent	Number	Per cent
6	54	65.9	12	17.9
12	30	36.6	7	10.4
18	13	15.9	5	7.5
24	3	3.7	2	3.0
36	0	0	1	1.5

*From Swinton, N. W., et al.: Proc. Roy. Soc. Med., 63(Suppl.): 21–23, 1970.

showed a survival of 65.9 per cent at 6 months and 36.6 per cent at 1 year, compared to 17.9 per cent of the untreated group at 1 year (Table 7).[31]

In view of these data a prospective and randomized study was started within the Eastern Cooperative Oncology Group, comparing two modalities of treatment — prolonged arterial infusion with 5-FUDR via the hepatic artery, as performed at the Lahey Clinic over the past 6 to 7 years, and conventional 5-FU chemotherapy (by intravenous administration) as performed throughout the country.[7] No results have been reported yet. 5-FU, by prolonged regional arterial infusion, will not be used in this study because the total dose that can be delivered by this method employing a small chronometric infusion pump (approximately 3.0 to 5.0 mg. per kilogram of body weight) is insufficient to produce comparable hepatic toxicity to 5-FUDR by similar administration. Since 5-FUDR and 5-FU have shown comparable antitumor responses in metastatic adenocarcinoma in liver arising from the colorectal region,[21] 5-FUDR will be the drug used for regional arterial infusion in this study.

For patients with very advanced disease who cannot undergo laparotomy, we have used percutaneous catheters. These catheters can also be attached to our portable pump. We have also used regional infusion for recurrent cancer of the colon and rectum involving the perineum, for which a catheter is inserted into the lower abdominal aorta, attached to a pump, and 5-FU or 5-FUDR is given. Favorable results can be obtained. However, more extensive local toxicity will be seen, primarily involving the skin. As one approaches the larger arteries, the doses producing local toxicity and systemic toxicity are almost identical.

SUMMARY

We have many problems to resolve as to the control of colorectal cancer. It is hoped that new clinical programs will explore new drugs with varying doses and new methods of administration will try to improve our dose-toxicity response ratios. These studies, combined with the recent work in tumor immunology and in conjunction with similar improvements in surgery, radiotherapeutic techniques, biochemical knowledge involving the cancer cell, and cell kinetic patterns, hopefully will improve our results. However, a multi-disciplined approach will have to be instituted. Only this will dispel the gloom that exists concerning the treatment of cancer. The cancer patient is often a much neglected individual, and the challenge he presents can be stimulating and rewarding for the physician.

REFERENCES

1. Ansfield, F. J., and Curreri, A. R.: Further clinical comparison between 5-fluorouracil (5-FU) and 5-fluoro-2'-deoxyuridine (5-FUDR). Cancer Chemother. Rep. 32:101–105 (Oct.) 1963.
2. Colcock, B. P.: Carcinoma of the colon. Surg. Clin. N. Amer. 47:647–655 (June) 1967.
3. Curreri, A. R.: Further clinical studies with 5-fluorouracil. Proc. Amer. Assoc. Cancer Res. 3:14 (March) 1959.
4. Curreri, A. R., Ansfield, F. J., McIver, F. A., et al.: Clinical studies with 5-fluorouracil. Cancer Res. 18:474–484 (May) 1958.
5. dePeyster, F. A., and Gilchrist, R. C.: Pathology and manifestations of cancer of the colon and rectum. In Turell, R. (Ed.): Diseases of the Colon and Anorectum. Philadelphia, W. B. Saunders Co., 1959, vol. 1, pp. 384–409.
6. Duschinsky, R., Pleven, E., and Heidelberger, C.: The synthesis of 5-fluoropyrimidines. J. Amer. Chem. Soc. 79:4559–4560 (Aug. 20) 1957.
7. Eastern Cooperative Oncology Group Protocol, EST 0470.
8. Eastern Cooperative Group in Solid Tumor Chemotherapy. Comparison of antimetabolites in the treatment of breast and colon cancer. J.A.M.A. 200:770–778 (May 29) 1967.
9. Eastern Cooperative Oncology Group Protocol activated December 1970.
10. Gabriel, W. B.: The Principles and Practice of Rectal Surgery. London, H. K. Lewis, 5th ed., 1963, p. 739.
11. Gold, P., and Freedman, S. O.: Specific carcinoembryonic antigens of the human digestive system. J. Exp. Med. 122:467–481 (Sept. 1) 1965.
12. Heidelberger, C.: Chemical carcinogenesis, chemotherapy: cancer's continuing core challenges – G. H. A. Clowes Memorial Lecture. Cancer Res. 30:1549–1569 (June) 1970.
13. Heidelberger, C., Kaldor, G., Murkherjee, K. L., and Danneberg, P. B.: Studies on fluorinated pyrimidines. XI. In vitro studies on tumor resistance. Cancer Res. 20:903–909 (July) 1960.
14. Jaffe, B. M., Donegan, W. L., Watson, F., et al.: Factors influencing survival in patients with untreated hepatic metastases. Surg. Gynec. Obstet. 127:1–11 (July) 1968.
15. James, J. A. G.: Cancer Prognosis Manual. New York, American Cancer Society, Inc., 1966.
16. Kessel, D., and Hall, T. C.: Influence of ribose donors on the action of 5-fluorouracil. Cancer Res. 29:1749–1754 (Oct.) 1969.
17. Khazei, A. M., Morgenthaler, F. R., Patel, D. D., and Watkins, E., Jr.: Liver dysfunction during protracted hepatic artery infusion of massive doses of fluorinated pyrimidine. Surg. Forum 16:72–73, 1965.
18. Khung, C. L., Hall, T. C., Piro, A. J., et al.: A clinical trial of oral 5-fluorouracil. Clin. Pharmacol. Ther. 7:527–533 (July-Aug.) 1966.
19. Lahiri, S. R., Boileau, G., and Hall, T. C.: 5-Fluorouracil (5-FU) by mouth in metastatic colo-rectal carcinoma. Abstract 35. Seventh Annual Scientific Program of the American Society of Clinical Oncology, Chicago, Illinois, April 7, 1971.
20. Machman, S., and Curreri, A. R.: Re-operation in colon carcinoma following 5-FU administration. Abstract. Third Annual Scientific Program of the American Society of Clinical Oncology, Chicago, Illinois, April 12, 1967.
21. Moertel, C. G., Reitemeier, R. J., and Hahn, R. G.: Therapy with the fluorinated pyrimidines. In Moertel, C. G., and Reitemeier, R. J. (Eds.): Advanced Gastrointestinal Cancer; Clinical Management and Chemotherapy. New York, Hoeber Medical Division, Harper & Row, Publishers, 1969, pp. 86–107.
22. Rousselot, L. M., Cole, D. R., Gross, C. E., et al.: A five year intraluminal chemotherapy (5-fluorouracil) adjuvant to surgery for colorectal cancer. Amer. J. Surg. 115:140–147 (Feb.) 1968.
23. Rutman, R. J., Cantarow, A., and Paschkis, K. E.: Studies in 2-acetylaminofluorene carcinogenesis; utilization of uracil-2-C^{14} by preneoplastic rat liver and rat hepatoma. Cancer Res. 14:119–123 (Feb.) 1954.
24. Silverberg, E., and Holleb, A. I.: Cancer Statistics, 1971. 21:13–31 (Jan.-Feb.) 1971.
25. Sullivan, R. D., and Oberfield, R. A.: Chemotherapy of metastatic gastrointestinal cancer. MED. CLIN. N. AMER., 50:427–438 (March) 1966.
26. Sullivan, R. D., and Zurek, W. Z.: Chemotherapy for liver cancer by protracted ambulatory infusion. J.A.M.A. 194:481–486 (Nov. 1) 1965.

27. Sullivan, R. D., Norcross, J. W., and Watkins, E., Jr.: Chemotherapy of metastatic liver cancer by prolonged hepatic artery infusion. New Eng. J. Med. 270:321–327 (Feb. 13) 1964.

28. Sullivan, R. D., Young, C. W., Miller, E., et al.: The clinical effects of continuous administration of fluorinated pyrimidines (5-fluorouracil and 5-fluoro-2'-deoxyuridine). Cancer Chemother. Rep. 8:77–83 (July) 1960.

29. Swinton, N. W., Sr., and Nahra, K. S.: The natural evolution of colorectal cancer. *In* Sullivan, R. D. (Ed.): Clinical Cancer Chemotherapy Including Ambulatory Infusion. Springfield, Illinois, Charles C Thomas, 1970, pp. 37–46.

30. Swinton, N. W., Samaan, S., and Rosenthal, D.: Cancer of the rectum and sigmoid. Surg. Clin. N. Amer. 47:657–662 (June) 1967.

31. Swinton, N. W., Sr., Cady, B., Nahra, K. S., and Watkins, E., Jr.: Arterial infusion chemotherapy of liver metastases arising from rectal and colonic cancer. Proc. Roy. Soc. Med. 63(Suppl.):21–23, 1970.

32. Watkins, E., Jr., Khazei, A. M., and Nahra, K. S.: Surgical basis for arterial infusion chemotherapy of disseminated carcinoma of the liver. Surg. Gynec. Obstet. 130:580–605 (April) 1970.

33. Zubrod, C. G.: The limited usefulness of 5-fluorouracil (5-FU) and 5-fluorodeoxyuridine (5-FUDR) in the management of patients with adenocarcinoma. *In* Ingelfinger, F. J., Relman, A. S., Finland, M. (Eds.): Controversy in Internal Medicine. Philadelphia, W. B. Saunders Co., 1966, pp. 591–600.

605 Commonwealth Avenue
Boston, Massachusetts 02215

The Physician's Responsibility To The Dying Patient

Richard C. Lippincott, M.D.

Traditional medical concepts relying heavily on diagnosis, treatment, cure, and relieving suffering have recently been giving way to an onslaught of humanistic papers suggesting that the physician must take a more active role in the experience of dying. In addition to the traditional issues of patient care, therefore, the concepts of the integrity of the whole person, honesty with the incurably ill, and dignity in the face of death have been exposed. Thus a subspecialty of thantology has given new understanding to human life. Although Bromberg and Schilder[1] in 1933 presented some guarded views of the denial-hostility mechanisms associated with dying, almost all the significant psychologic evaluations have been since 1958 giving the science a span of only 15 years. Wahl,[6] Rhoads,[5] and Weisman and Hackett[7] have added valuable insight into the psychologic process of human death. Finally, two definitive books[3, 4] published in the last three years have added significantly to new understanding of the process of dying, especially the clarification by Kubler-Ross[3] of the five psychologic stages. Our attempt will be to summarize the basic attitudes, crystalize the emotional conflicts, and suggest the relevant interventions that the physician might make.

Death is a frequent component to a busy physician's life and is so frequent that its effect on patient management may be overlooked. Sudden, precipitous death is a problem to the physician and the family, but when the process of dying allows time for human experience and reaction, it is a universal problem for the patient as well.

The patient's and the physician's attitudes about dying greatly influence the quality and compassion of care. Primary is the patient's attitude regarding the appropriateness of his death, that is, "one (an experience) which the patient would choose for himself if he had an option." For example, the young child, the man in the prime of his life, and the patient with cancer are approached as inappropriate death experiences by all. Cancer gives rise not only to general anxiety but also to specific feelings of helplessness, loss of control, and images of deformity and tissue destruction. A patient's attitude about dying is influenced as well, if not determined, by his own life experience and history. Needless to say, so are those of their physicians. Spiritual, cultural, and existential views as well as that difficult to define concept, self-image, are inherently important. For some patients, death is a repugnant intruder into a well-ordered life; for others, it may represent a welcome solution to problems of living. The significance is in understanding which, so that this dynamic process does not perplex or complicate the treatment program to the extent that we lose the precious reality that successful treatment is not necessarily tantamount to total physical recovery. A realistic approach to the understanding of the patient's special needs will lead to more complete relief of suffering, maintenance of human dignity, and a recognition that the meaning of a patient's life must be relevant to treatment consideration.

The psychologic conflicts associated with dying are in three distinct areas. First is the intrapsychic, representing, as we have outlined briefly, the attitudes the patient brings to the experience and the unique anxieties or psychologic mechanisms that are in operation. As the terminal experience approaches, the patient becomes more aware of his relationships, more sensitive, and proceeds through a rather consistent communication pattern. Initially, anxiety predominates either overtly or covertly. There is a need to talk, to express his or her fears, and to attempt to gain some meaning. Impulsivity, hyperactivity, tangentiality, or denial may be present, especially if the verbal process is frustrated. The patient in this stage is very sensitive to the physician's own anxiety or rejection and may manipulate to receive more attention. Intermediately, the anxiety may give way to complicated rationalization and denial. Clearly, dependency needs increase, but these may be masked by hostility at having been failed by his physician; this is projected on to him by the patient.

This then gives way to increased needs for reassurance, especially for the physical presence of the physician, depression, and finally a protective denial spreads on to the physician, who now becomes all knowing and caring. Terminally, the patient's communications become increasingly constricted. Dependency upon physical presence, touching, and reassurance of hope are requested. Many have described the marked sense of isolation and abandonment which occurs at this stage. These later feelings are often accompanied by what has been described as the attitudes of acceptance—a kind of psychologic death preceding the biologic death. Samuel Butler said, "The organism dies when it is too much bewildered and no longer remembers what to do next."

The second area of conflict is within the relationship of the patient and his physician and, by extension, the entire health team. These health personnel are products of their society, history, and personal experience. Anger, guilt, jealousy with the implied death solution, and feelings of failure at not having "cured" the patient are complicating factors. The physician who sees himself as a healer, a restorer of health and life, may set up a conspiracy of silence with his patient, having similar needs to deny the inevitable. The patient's advancing disease is a concrete symbol of the frustrating knowledge that he has been unable to cure the patient and is thus not omnipotent. The physician may begin to call less frequently or rationalize that other patients are more interesting or need his services more. In most hospitals the terminal patient is given a low priority regarding care and often isolated so as "not to upset other pa-

tients." A further conflict complication is the continued diagnostic testing and medical procedures undertaken despite the clear inevitability of
death. Daily blood tests to confirm what is already known, chemotherapeutic agents for terminal cancer patients, and heroic cardiac procedures, all can be greatly rationalized and abused. A clear perspective of
the reasons and the need for procedures will prevent focusing on the
treatment program and not the patient.

Lastly, the patient's family relationships must be considered. There
will be denial, dependency, and depression as seen in the patient. Addi-
tionally, there is the feeling related to loss of relationship, loss of security (financial and emotional), resentment at being left, guilt following
old love-hate dynamics, and most difficult for the physician, the tendency
to project these feelings on to him in the form of accusation or anger.

As stressed earlier, for the physician, death is inappropriate also,
representing a failure of his medical skills, lowered self-esteem, and
some threat to his prestige in the form of judgments from his colleagues
on the hospital staff. Thus guilt, anxiety, anger at the patient not getting
well, and sincere ambivalence push the physician toward a conspiracy of
silence and withdrawal to mechanical techniques and use of drugs. This
occurs at a time when the patient needs most to discuss his concerns and
needs. Providing this requires time, patience, and a well thought out philosophy of life and death so that the physician faces his patient with
honest control and openness. Someone said, "The trouble with dying is,
it's so final." Frankl[2] suggests that this is both the trouble and the joy, for
as he points out, it is the very finiteness of life that gives our activities
meaning. Without an ending, life becomes meaninglessly monotonous,
removed from the creative drive and the need to use time appropriately.
The existential view of finality places the process of dying and death in a
proper and logical position in regard to the patient's life and gives the
physician an honest stand from which he may discuss with the patient
whatever needs to be discussed. Patients with terminal disease often
wish to fulfill obligations, settle family matters, or, specifically, "make
the most" of the time left to them. The physician's insistence on curative
or disease-oriented treatments blocks the patient's needs and increases
isolation. Further, the physician who delegates these responsibilities to
others has lost a unique opportunity to share a basic experience and
meaning of his profession as well as the gratitude of his patients. He has
lost immeasurably the ability to allow his patient to feel in control and to
sense a dignity of life and death in this control and isolates himself from a
real understanding of man.

In summary, there is a basic need for understanding of the patient's
and one's own (physician's) needs, history, and expectations when facing
the terminal experiences of life. A firm philosophy allowing honesty with
oneself and with the patient, the ability to tell the truth but to listen as
well with enough sensitivity so as not to burden him, and a recognition of
the communication and emotional changes taking place are important
features in the care of the dying patient. This is coupled with the maximal use of surgical skills and medical treatment to reduce pain and suffering, to restore optimal functioning, and to allow time to openly discuss

the process of dying. The patient may use control and dignity in the process.

REFERENCES

1. Bromberg, W., and Schilder, P.: Death and dying: A comparative study of the attitudes and mental reactions toward death and dying. Psychoanal. Rev., 20:133–185 (April) 1933.
2. Frankl, V.: Man's Search for Meaning: An Introduction to Logotherapy. New York, Washington Square Press, 1963, 220 pp.
3. Kubler-Ross, E.: On Death and Dying. New York, Macmillan Co., 1969, 260 pp.
4. Pearson, L.: Death and Dying: Current Issues in the Treatment of the Dying Person. Cleveland, Press of Case Western Reserve University, 1969, 132 pp.
5. Rhoads, P. S.: Management of the patient with terminal illness. J.A.M.A., *192*:661–665 (May 24) 1965.
6. Wahl, C. W.: The physician's management of the dying patient. *In* Masserman, J. H. (ed.): Current Psychiatric Therapies. New York, Grune and Stratton, 1962, vol. 2, pp. 127–136.
7. Weisman, A. D., and Hackett, T. P.: Predilection to death. Death and dying as a psychiatric problem. Psychosomat. Med., 23:232–256 (May-June) 1961.

605 Commonwealth Avenue
Boston, Massachusetts 02215

Effectiveness of Lithium Carbonate in the Prevention of Manic and Depressive Episodes

Walter I. Tucker, M.D., and George O. Bell, M.D.

The purpose of this article is to indicate the effectiveness, safety, and practicability of prophylactic lithium carbonate treatment in office and general hospital practice. Many patients with cyclic mood swings may manifest somatic symptoms as well as behavioral changes, which first come to the attention of medical practitioners who are not psychiatrists. Mood swings of less than major degree are often not recognized as such, although they may cause serious disability and maladjustment. The risks and problems of lithium carbonate treatment, such as the effect on thyroid function, have generally been overdrawn in the medical press, resulting in some hesitancy in using this treatment when indicated. It is hoped that this report will help to alert medical practitioners to the prevalence of this disorder and the effectiveness of lithium carbonate when episodes are frequent and disabling. The results reported are based on experience in the treatment of private patients, and no claim is made of a controlled study, but they do corroborate the findings reported in more controlled hospital studies and indicate that effective treatment can be carried out on such a patient population with minimum risk.

Other studies[3, 4, 8] have reported varying results in the prevention of manic and depressive episodes on a long-term basis, although evidence for effectiveness has regularly been reported. Our experience covers 105 patients who have been treated in a general hospital and on an office basis for 1 to 4 years. All patients had had a previous history of cycles of mood swings at least once a year for a number of years previously, and all had had medical examinations in the medical department. All were treated by one psychiatrist during the period.

Patients were selected who had had frequent mood swings, usually with rapid changes over weeks or months. Manic-depressive reactions constituted the largest group, characterized by manic or depressive episodes or both, without precipitants. Other conditions were also included to assess the effectiveness of treatment: recurrent depressive episodes of reactive or involutional type, schizo-affective reactions which appeared to be cyclic, and some patients having cycles of somatic symptoms and personality changes without evident medical or psychiatric cause.

In some patients lithium carbonate was started during a manic episode, in other patients treatment was started after recovery from a treated depressive episode, and in others treatment was started while the patient was in a normal period. The dosage of lithium carbonate was usually 300 mg. three times daily, which was regulated up or down in accordance with a blood level between 0.5 and 1.5 mEq. per liter and the avoidance of side-effects. Blood lithium levels were taken twice within the first 4 weeks or until the dosage was stabilized and thereafter every 6 months or when indicated by medical or psychiatric status. Antidepressive or tranquilizing medication was continued in gradually decreasing doses to zero in patients having no recurrences.

The study includes all patients in whom lithium carbonate was started between August 1967 and August 1970, with the final follow-up in August 1971. Patients were classified as 2+ who had no episodes of manic or depressive reactions during the period of one to four years. Patients were classified as 1+ who had some episodes during the period but much less severe and less frequent than those that had occurred during the years before treatment with lithium carbonate. Patients were classified as 0 who showed no significant improvement during the period of treatment.

RESULTS

Of the 59 manic-depressive patients, 42 had no episodes of depression or manic reaction (2+), 12 were improved compared to the years before lithium carbonate treatment (1+), and 5 showed no improvement (0). All 5 of those unimproved discontinued treatment during the first year. Of the 23 patients with recurrent depression, 7 had no recurrences (2+), 7 were improved (1+), and 9 were unimproved (0). Of the 12 patients with schizo-affective reactions, 4 had no recurrences (2+), 1 was improved (1+), and 7 were unimproved (0). Of the 11 with personality disorders, 2 had no recurrence of symptoms (2+), none were improved (1+), and 9 were unimproved (0).

LITHIUM AND THYROID FUNCTION

The occurrence of goiter or thyroid disorder has not been found to be a serious problem, and no patient had to discontinue lithium on this account. Thyroid problems after lithium carbonate treatment developed in only 5 patients with no finding of goiter or hypothyroidism before starting lithium carbonate. All five had symptoms of mild hypothyroidism confirmed by protein-bound iodine or thyroxine (T-4) and responded promptly to thyroid replacement therapy. Only one had a small goiter. Four patients with pretreatment findings of a small goiter or history of thyroidectomy showed some increase in goiter or decrease in protein-bound iodine, and all responded to thyroid replacement therapy. Seven patients with pretreatment findings of small goiter or history of thyroidectomy showed no change after lithium carbonate therapy.

In 1967 attention was drawn to the possible adverse effects of lithium on thyroid function at a symposium on "Lithium and Goitre" in Sweden. Thyroid enlargement occurred in isolated patients during treatment with lithium.[1, 2]

An excellent review of the effects of lithium on thyroid function has been reported by Shopsin.[5] Thyroid enlargement with normal thyroid function, goiter with myxedema, and myxedema without goiter have been reported. In both man and rat protein-bound iodine levels are reduced and thyroidal uptakes of radioactive iodine are increased following short-term lithium treatment. In lithium-treated ewes, radioactive iodine uptakes have been elevated significantly in the absence of elevated levels of thyroid stimulating hormone. This latter finding tends to cloud the possibility of a thyroid-pituitary feedback mechanism as a cause of elevated radioactive iodine uptake values.

Lithium actively accumulates within the thyroid gland in greater concentrations than in the serum. The possibility of a competitive mechanism between lithium and iodide in goitrogenesis has neither been proved nor disproved. Nor is there definite proof that lithium interferes with the intrathyroidal mechanisms for thyroxine production. The occurrence of antithyroid antibody titers in one subject reported by Shopsin et al.[6, 7] points to the likelihood of a preexisting lymphocytic thyroiditis. Goiter and hypothyroidism developed in this patient while taking lithium. Elevated titers of antithyroid antibody persisted independently of lithium ingestion, and presumably lithium played no role in causing the high antithyroid antibody titers.

The dye used in coloring capsules of lithium is a xanthine derivative containing 57.7 per cent iodine. Thus, ingestion of such colored capsules provides the patient with two or three times the normal optimal daily iodine requirement.[6, 7] The significance of the increased iodine intake in thyroid dysfunction needs further evaluation.

Although evidence is somewhat conflicting and incomplete, available data suggest that lithium interferes with thyroxine production in some manner. Lithium, therefore, is capable of producing goiter or hypothyroidism or both in some patients. The thyroidal disturbances are not frequent or serious. They are readily reversed by stopping lithium or by the administration of thyroid hormone along with lithium.

Before the institution of lithium treatment, examination of the patient for thyroid enlargement and baseline measurements of serum levels of protein-bound iodine, thyroxine, and thyroid antibody titers are advisable. Periodic reevaluation of thyroid function and size should be part of the management of all lithium-treated patients. At the first sign of thyroid enlargement or decrease in level of thyroid function, concomitant administration of thyroid hormone should be initiated and maintained as long as lithium ingestion is continued.

OTHER MEDICAL COMPLICATIONS

Other medical complications necessitating discontinuance of lithium carbonate were rare. Congestive heart failure developed in 2 patients in the older age group, and lithium carbonate was stopped, but in 3 other patients in whom cardiac decompensation of mild degree developed, lithium carbonate was continued without further difficulty. One patient in whom a severe renal infection developed stopped the lithium carbonate. In none of these instances could the cardiac or renal disorders be attributed specifically to lithium carbonate treatment.

SIDE-EFFECTS

The most common side-effects were tremor, nausea, and fluid retention. These symptoms could usually be eliminated or decreased to great degree by reducing the dosage and controlling salt and fluid intake, but 7 patients discontinued lithium carbonate because of these side-effects, in most instances because they were not willing to persist in dosage regulation and the lithium carbonate was not evidently effective in preventing recurrence of symptoms. There were no more serious side-effects as reported with higher doses of lithium carbonate, as the lithium carbonate level was maintained below 1.5 mEq. per liter. The lithium carbonate was discontinued temporarily during periods of intercurrent illness, such as acute infections with fever, excessive sweating, operations, or other conditions involving fluid and electrolyte changes.

REPORTS OF CASES

Case 1

A 44 year old man was first seen in 1961 by the Department of Internal Medicine with what was originally considered by the referring physician to be recurrent relapses of lead poisoning. Subsequent history indicated typical history of mood swings for 17 years and previous history of electroshock therapy on two occasions. In the course of the next 6 years he had episodes of severe disabling manic or depressive episodes at least twice a year, resulting in loss of jobs in manic episodes during which police arrests were necessitated because of threats of violence to his family. Hospital treatment was needed 6 times, and episodes were terminated by electroshock therapy or tranquilizing medication, but depression was usually followed soon by a manic episode and vice versa, and efforts at prevention by medication and preventive electroshock therapy were not successful.

Lithium carbonate treatment was started in 1967, and for 4 years he has been well, with no side-effects and no relapses. Thyroid tests have been within normal limits. He has maintained a steady job and is considered a valuable employee. His family life is stable and happy for the first time since marriage, whereas divorce was imminent when lithium carbonate was started.

Case 2

A 46 year old woman was first seen in 1961 with a past history of menstrual irregularities and alleged "hyperthyroidism" in 1934 treated with iodine. She came with a present status of severe depression and guilt and delusions that people were talking accusingly about her. Medical examination was normal with a protein-bound iodine of 4.3. Emergency hospitalization was soon necessitated when she set fire to herself in a suicidal attempt. She recovered after treatment for severe burns and electroshock therapy and was entirely well with no psychiatric symptoms and was diagnosed as schizoaffective reaction. Relapses tended to occur at least yearly despite antidepressive medication and phenothiazines, but prompt response to electroshock therapy was noted, and for 4 years she had electroshock therapy at intervals for prevention. In 1967 lithium carbonate treatment was started, and she has had no significant relapses since. In 1968 signs of hypothyroidism developed, confirmed by laboratory tests, but no goiter was present. She was given desiccated thyroid, 120 mg. a day, with clearing of signs and symptoms, and laboratory tests returned to normal limits. She has continued lithium carbonate without further complications or relapse of schizoaffective symptoms.

Case 3

A 59 year old man was first seen in the psychiatric department in 1965 but had been seen in various departments since 1954 and treated for gastrointestinal symptoms, anemia, and headaches. A history was obtained of mood swings all his life, usually with depression and somatic symptoms in the winter and excessive energy and ambition in the summer. He had learned to adjust his activities to these changes and had, of his own accord, taken "pep" pills when down and sedatives when up.

The episodes were managed better, with less prolonged and less severe cycles, with antidepressive or tranquilizing medication, but they continued to occur during the next 2 years, and hospitalization was required briefly on one occasion for depression. Two weeks after starting lithium carbonate in 1967 he reported "feeling more on an even keel" than he could ever recall. He has had no mood swings of depression or overactivity in 4 years, has had no significant somatic symptoms, and has taken no medication except lithium carbonate. He has a slight hand tremor from lithium carbonate at times which does not bother him. Thyroid tests and examinations have been within normal limits.

DISCUSSION

In our experience with private patients treated largely on an office basis, we have found lithium carbonate treatment to be quite safe when contact is maintained with the patient and the established guidelines regarding dosage, blood level, and intercurrent illness are followed.

The value of lithium carbonate treatment in manic patients has been established, and our experience supports this, although the use of phenothiazines in conjunction with lithium carbonate is more rapidly effective.

We had undertaken to assess the effectiveness of lithium carbonate in cyclic disorders which could not be classified as strictly manic-depressive illness, and generally the results were poor. However, a few patients in the schizoaffective and other categories did respond well, which suggests that possibly the basic disorder was an atypical manic-depressive disorder. For best results, however, it is necessary to limit lithium carbonate treatment to definite manic-depressive disorders with frequent rapid mood swings.

Patients generally accepted the treatment very well and tended to continue to take the medication much more faithfully than antidepressive medication or tranquilizers previously prescribed for prevention. I would ascribe this cooperation to the relative lack of side-effects as well as the eventual realization of effectiveness. A further factor in promoting faithfulness in taking medication was that failure to take medication could be proved by blood test.

In the practice of psychiatry, we have been able to terminate depressive episodes (with antidepressives and electroshock therapy) and manic episodes (with phenothiazines and lithium carbonate), but lithium carbonate has been found to be quite effective in preventing recurrences of both in cyclic mood disorders. When mood swings tend to be frequent and changes rapid, it has been next to impossible to control them by change of medication and other treatment, particularly in the hypomanic stage when patients tend to ignore all advice. The problem of regulation could be compared to that in the brittle diabetic. With lithium carbonate used prophylactically, these problems can often be eliminated and patients often state spontaneously that they "feel more on an even keel" for the first time.

In medical practice, less severe degrees of mood swings, often manifested by somatic symptoms, are frequently not recognized as manifestations of manic-depressive illness. Exacerbations of gastrointestinal symptoms or headaches are often associated with a depressive episode. One patient whose course was followed for 12 years always had symptoms of sore throat and malaise, and was treated for what she insisted was a virus infection for weeks or months, at the onset of her many depressive episodes. Other patients in hypomanic episodes are likely to cause family disruptions or lose jobs as a result of moral indiscretions or poor judgment. A wider recognition of such episodes as manifestations of a cyclic mood disorder is more likely if the possibility is kept in mind and sometimes can lead to the solution in a problem patient. A realization of the effectiveness and safety of lithium carbonate in prevention of cyclic mood swings in patients whose course can be followed over a period of years could result in the wider use of this treatment not only by psychiatrists but by other medical practitioners who are likely to encounter less severe degrees of manic-depressive illness.

REFERENCES

1. Allgen, L. A., Almgren, S., and Martens, S.: Report at symposium on "Lithium and Goitre" in Risskov, Denmark, 1967.
2. Baastrup, P. C.: Report at Symposium on "Lithium and Goitre" in Risskov, Denmark, 1967.
3. Baastrup, P. C., and Schou, M.: Lithium as a prophylactic agent. Its effect against recurrent depressions and manic-depressive psychosis. Arch. Gen. Psychiat., 16:162–172 (Feb.) 1967.
4. Coopen, A., Noguera, R., Bailey, J., et al.: Prophylactic lithium in affective disorders. Lancet, 2:275–279 (Aug. 7) 1971.
5. Shopsin, B.: Effects of lithium on thyroid function. (A review). Dis. Nerv. System, 31:237–244 (April) 1970.
6. Shopsin, B.: Paper presented at the First Murfreesboro Roundtable on Basic Mechanisms of Lithium. Murfreesboro, Tennessee, April, 1969.
7. Shopsin, B., Blum, M., and Gershon, S.: Lithium-induced thyroid disturbance: case report and review. Compr. Psychiat., 10:215–223 (May) 1969.
8. Van der Velde, C. D.: Effectiveness of lithium carbonate in the treatment of manic-depressive illness. Amer. J. Psychiat., 127:345–351 (Sept.) 1970.

605 Commonwealth Avenue
Boston, Massachusetts 02215

The Role of Hypnotherapy in Clinical Medicine

Andrew E. St. Amand, M.D.

"Nothing should be omitted in an art which interests the whole world, one which may be beneficial to suffering humanity and which does not risk human life or comfort." These words are attributed to Hippocrates. Medical hypnosis is such an art and an important yet virtually neglected therapeutic tool in clinical medicine. Hypnosis can be "prescribed" as a medicine because it is in reality the "art of medicine" based upon the fundamental tenets of faith. No physician will deny that his greatest ally is faith. Voltaire once stated that there is probably more cure in the doctor's words than in many of the drugs he prescribes. Many legitimate drugs exert their therapeutic effect not so much because of their pharmacologic effects per se but as a result of the existing relationship between the patient and the physician prescribing the drug. This *faith* is also known as the "placebo effect" or *suggestion*.

Hypnotic-like techniques have been in use for centuries. The "sacred sleep" of the Egyptian soothsayers apparently was a trance state induced in those followers who came to seek relief from their symptoms. The "laying on of the hands" produced a hypnotic state which was both a religious experience and a therapeutic modality. The Greek oracles, the Hindu priests, the Persian Magi, and the Indian Yogi all induced trance-like states with varying techniques. The references in the Talmud and Bible to the "laying on of the hands" led to the formation of several religions that introduced healing through touch and prayer. Despite the growth of science, faith-healing has persisted and still persists in non-medical cults.

Faith-healing as practiced today differs from the fetish, amulets, and rituals practiced among primitive cultures. So-called civilized cultures practice faith-healing in the guise of Christian Science, miracles, prayer meetings, "secret drugs," and pseudohealing cults referred to as quackery.

Many metaphysicians over the centuries claimed that the magnet had curative powers. In 1773 Franz Anton Mesmer presented his thesis on "The Influence of the Stars and Planets as Curative Powers" to the medical faculty of the University of Vienna. The planets, he believed, affected humans through an invisible force he called "animal magnetism." He claimed that this force could be derived from a magnet. Mesmerism became a byword throughout Europe and thousands of invalids sought his services.

Mesmer accented two important ingredients: *belief* and *expectation*. When a person believed what he heard about mesmerism, he expected a cure. Where suggestion could cure, it did. James Braid, a Scottish physician, became interested in mesmerism in 1843. He recognized the true nature of the trance state. He scoffed at the mysterious and occult and branded as false the "magnetic fluid" of Mesmer. Emphasizing clinical observation and the scientific method, he verified that it was primarily the degree of expectation that increased a subject's susceptibility to suggestion. Braid was responsible for the term used today, hypnosis. James Eisdale (1845), a Scottish surgeon practicing in India, performed over 200 major and thousands of minor surgical procedures using hypnosis as the sole anesthetic.

The acceptance of hypnosis as a therapeutic tool by the medical profession has been slow. It was not until 1958 that the Council on Mental Health of American Medical Association endorsed hypnosis as a useful adjunct to therapy. Hypnosis, today, is utilized in many professional fields for a wide variety of conditions. The news media, however, has dwelt entirely on the spectacular features creating misconceptions about the phenomenon. There is probably no other phenomenon in clinical medicine where reasonable, rational, and intelligent individuals abandon these attitudes when they think or talk about hypnosis. The number of extreme statements we hear or see written for or against the use of hypnosis is large. The reason, in part, is that hypnosis is often associated with quackery, occultism, magic, and charlatanism. The hypnotic trance does exist. Therefore, it seems that we would be better clinicians if we learned to identify this phenomenon and perhaps learn how to use it as an adjunct to therapy.

WHAT IS HYPNOSIS?

Braid was first to call the trance state hypnosis after the Greek word for sleep, *hypnos*. Years later he recognized that the trance was not a sleep state but one of wakefulness characterized by deep concentration and relaxation. He abandoned the term *hypnosis* and substituted the word "monoideism," the concentration on one idea.

Hypnosis may be defined as an altered state of awareness or consciousness whereby the subject becomes more receptive to suggestions be they heterosuggestions or autosuggestions. Hypnosis, therefore, is *not* an unconscious or sleep state but a wakeful or dissociative state often called the *trance*. Normally most persons are suggestible. This is the key premise of the advertising industry. The subject or patient in a hypnotic trance, however, accepts suggestions more readily and uncritically. The trance or hypnotic state, therefore, is a natural, inherent phenomenon that can be experienced by almost everyone. Contrary to popular belief, the more intelligent the subject, as a rule, the more readily the trance state can be induced. The depth of trance varies widely. Patient motivation, confidence in the physician, and the experience of the physician using hypnosis are a few of the factors leading to successful use of the trance state.

The dangers of hypnosis are grossly exaggerated. It is indeed surprising how few complications occur when one considers how many untrained or unsophisticated operators use hypnosis for entertainment or treatment. The trained physician, dentist, or psychologist using hypnosis within the boundaries of his professional competence or specialty will encounter no difficulties. The proper use of hypnosis is not dangerous; it is the misuse that is dangerous.

When using hypnosis several principles should be kept in mind. (1) Hypnosis is *adjunctive* to conventional therapy and, as a rule, not a form of treatment. There are some exceptions to this rule, for example, insomnia and chronic tension states. If no underlying physical or emotional cause can be found to account for these conditions, the use of hypnosis and autohypnosis can alleviate or mitigate these symptoms. Otherwise, the physical or emotional cause must be dealt with first. (2) Nothing can be done in hypnotherapy that cannot be done without hypnosis. The difference is that therapy is greatly facilitated and accelerated with hypnosis. (3) Goal orientation of the trance state between the patient and physician, be it implied or explicit, is imperative. A clear-cut, accepted goal is necessary, and the physician should respect this contract. The physician who treats a patient for intractable pain with hypnosis and who also decides to break the patient's smoking habit without prior discussion with the patient may precipitate an anxiety reaction. (4) Competence in the main application of hypnosis must be assumed. A physician with poor clinical judgment will not become a better physician because hypnosis is used. An error in clinical judgment can be intensified rather than corrected through the use of hypnosis.

HYPNOTHERAPY AND SUGGESTIVE THERAPY

A wide variety of organic and functional conditions are amenable to hypnotherapy and suggestive therapy. Hypnotherapy is dependent on the induction of the hypnotic trance and the acceptance by the patient in trance of structural suggestions dealing with a particular symptom. Suggestive therapy relies on the use of suggestion, direct or indirect, without the use of the trance state.

Direct removal of symptoms through the use of hypnosis and suggestion has been a controversial topic among physicians. Some feel that the removal of a patient's symptom will precipitate a more serious problem, while others regard the symptom as a self-perpetuating vestige of a long forgotten or resolved "triggering incident," such as an emotional or religious conflict. In other words, the cause of the symptom may have long passed into oblivion, but the symptom lingers on. The bulk of medical therapeutics is aimed at alleviating symptoms. Medical and surgical measures are employed, often without benefit. If an analgesic drug is prescribed to relieve pain without criticism, why should the use of hypnosis to relieve this symptom be criticized? Are drugs considered safe and suggestions dangerous? This, of course, is ridiculous. Suggestions dealing with a particular symptom are given to the patient in trance in a permissive manner – not in an authoritative or commanding nature. If the patient has a *strong,* perhaps unrecognized, need for the symptom the suggestions will not be accepted. Medical and surgical procedures usually fail also. Sir William Osler pointed out that doctors are often ignorant of their own faith cures when prescribing medications and are very sensitive about those performed outside their ranks.

Some physicians believe that if a symptom is removed through hypnosis and suggestion, another, perhaps more serious one, will appear or that the patient will have some emotional crisis. This is simply not true. This belief denies years of sound clinical experience by qualified, reputable physicians and dentists who use hypnosis as an adjunct to therapy.

CLINICAL HYPNOTHERAPY

From March 1967 through June 1969 a number of patients were evaluated for hypnotherapy at the Lahey Clinic Foundation. The patients were referred only after appropriate and sometimes extensive studies were performed to determine the cause or causes of their symptoms. During the initial interview a history was taken with particular emphasis on the patient's emotional background. Some symptoms were the result of some organic disease and all conventional modes of therapy failed; other symptoms were thought to be functional. Patients with manifestations of depression, anxiety, suicide, or other emotional or major personality disorders were refused and referred to the psychiatrist. Pain is often a manifestation of depression, and a direct attack on this symptom using hypnosis, drugs, or surgical procedures only results in failure or temporary remissions.

Motivation of the patient to be free of symptoms was also assessed. The smiling patient with *constant* severe pain or the patient with "la belle indifference" toward his symptoms was refused. Patients thought to be using their symptom for some secondary gain, such as monetary compensation or to manipulate a situation, were likewise refused. These patients usually failed to respond to hypnotherapy. If the need of the symptom was no longer present, the patient improved with hypnotherapy. Perhaps this was merely an "honorable way out" or a face-saving method of giving up their symptom.

The patients accepted were given a brief orientation on hypnosis. A plan of therapy was outlined. The patients were seen for two or three sessions. They were also taught self-hypnosis using, when possible, tape recordings as a teaching aid. After three sessions a subjective and objective evaluation of results was made. If the patient was free of symptoms or improving but required more hypnotic sessions, that decision was made. If no improvement or benefit occurred, hypnotherapy was terminated.

Teaching the patient self-hypnosis forces him to take an active role in therapy. It shifts the responsibility of "getting well" to the patient where it properly belongs and reduces the dependency of the patient on the therapist.

RESULTS

A total of 184 patients was accepted for hypnotherapy. Twenty-nine (16 per cent) were seen only once or twice. Perhaps these patients were disillusioned about hypnosis or were free of symptoms. No follow-up was made with this group. The remaining 155 patients were treated through the use of hypnosis.

Excellent results with complete control or removal of symptoms were obtained in 66 of the 155 patients (43 per cent). An example is the case of a 32 year old man who sustained a self-inflicted, *accidental* gunshot wound of the right foot five years earlier. Cosmetically he had a normal-appearing foot, having lost only a portion of the fifth metatarsal bone. However, he complained of pain between the fourth and fifth toes with weight bearing. Over a 5 year period this man had 14 operations on his foot to find the "neuroma" causing his pain. Obtaining no relief, the patient was referred to the Department of Neurosurgery at the Lahey Clinic Foundation. After consultation with the Department of Orthopedic Surgery, a trial of hypnotherapy was suggested. During the course of three sessions the patient became free of symptoms and has remained so. The patient was instructed in self-hypnotic techniques.

Another example of a difficult therapeutic problem successfully treated through hypnosis is the case of an 18 year old single girl with a diagnosis of "scoliosis." She was referred to the neurosurgical department where it was determined that her "scoliosis" of 6 months' duration was due to posture and not a true curvature of the spine. The problem was completely eliminated after two hypnotic sessions. Psychotherapy consultation was advised and refused. A discussion with the patient's parents helped ease the tensions at home between siblings. The patient is currently enthusiastically using hypnosis successfully to manage her obesity.

A more dramatic case was that of a 42 year old religious teacher assigned to the Philippines for 15 years. Paresthesias of the left arm and neck developed. Myelography performed in Manila showed blockage of the dye at the cervical level. Because a spinal cord lesion was suspected, the patient was transferred to the clinic. In transit the patient's condition worsened. He became extremely tense and held all his muscles rigid. He was so disabled that he required assistance, and had to be fed and clothed. When not in bed, he sat in a wheelchair.

A repeat myelogram revealed normal findings, and a diagnosis of "conversion reaction" was made. A consultation for hypnotherapy was suggested and the patient agreed. The consultation was acknowledged 3 days later *deliberately*. This helps by developing a heightened state of expectation in the patient so that when he is finally seen by the therapist suggestions are more readily accepted.

In this situation no hypnotic trance was induced. Direct suggestions that by holding the hands of the therapist he could get up from the wheelchair and walk was all that was necessary. His gait was unsteady at first but improved to normal within four days. After 3 years he remains a normal, physically active member of his religious community. It was learned later through his superior that the patient's symptoms began soon after the patient was informed of his transfer to another school in the Philippines. His superiors did not know that the patient had a long-standing dislike for the new headmaster he was about to serve. His symptoms were an unconscious mechanism for extricating himself from an unpleasant situation since, being bound by the vow of obedience, he had to accept the transfer.

Of the 155 patients, 45 (29 per cent) had partial improvement of symptoms. A woman with widespread metastasis and pain was able to reduce the use of meperidine (Demerol) to a single dose per day. Another patient, a 37 year old woman with severe headaches unrelieved after bilateral temporal arteriectomy, was markedly improved after hypnotherapy. She now requires very little medication.

Outright failure occurred in 44 of the 155 patients (28 per cent). An 18 year old girl with back pain did not obtain relief from lumbar laminectomy and spinal fusion. A trial of hypnotherapy resulted in relief of pain for 1 week only. Subsequent sessions failed. A 42 year old executive with functional dysphonia failed to improve with hypnotherapy.

In the group of patients who obtained good or partial relief, recurrence of symptoms developed in 6; in 2 patients, intensity was decreased. A question of secondary gain has been considered in 3 of the 6 patients.

SUMMARY

Hypnotherapy is not a panacea for all patients. Enthusiasm for the use of hypnosis must not replace good clinical judgment. In the properly selected patient, however, hypnotherapy can be a rapid adjunct to other conventional modes of therapy. Results, at times, can be quite dramatic. The late Arthur Guedel, dean of American anesthesiologists, once remarked regarding hypnosis, "there is something to it, but wait before using it until you are old enough to be laughed at."

REFERENCES

1. Cheek, D. B., and LeCron, L. M.: Clinical Hypnotherapy. New York, Grune and Stratton, 1968, 245 pp.
2. Frank, J. D.: Persuasion and Healing: A Comparative Study of Psychotherapy. Baltimore, Johns Hopkins Press, 1961, 282 pp.
3. Hartland, J.: Medical and Dental Hypnosis and Its Clinical Applications. Baltimore, Williams and Wilkins, 1966, 346 pp.
4. Kroger, W. S.: Clinical and Experimental Hypnosis. Philadelphia, J. B. Lippincott Co., 1963, 361 pp.
5. Marmer, M. J.: Hypnosis in Anesthesiology. Springfield, Illinois, Charles C Thomas, 1959, 168 pp.
6. Meares, A.: A System of Medical Hypnosis. Philadelphia, W. B. Saunders, 1960, 484 pp.
7. Schneck, J. M.: Hypnosis in Modern Medicine. Springfield, Illinois, Charles C Thomas, 1953, 472 pp.
8. Scott, M. J.: Hypnosis in Skin and Allergic Diseases. Springfield, Illinois, Charles C Thomas, 1960, 164 pp.

605 Commonwealth Avenue
Boston, Massachusetts 02215

The Management of Parkinson's Syndrome

Stephen L. Wanger, M.D.

Parkinson's syndrome, estimated to occur in more than 400,000 patients, is one of the most prevalent of the serious neurologic diseases in the United States. Each year more than 37,000 persons are newly afflicted, and the increasing life span of our growing population can be expected to aggravate this problem further.[46]

Although multiple etiologic factors have been recognized, the vast majority of cases are idiopathic. Postencephalitic Parkinson's syndrome occurs with decreasing frequency; very few new cases are reported as a result of the pandemic of von Economo's encephalitis lethargica during the years 1918 to 1926.[16] Arteriosclerotic parkinsonism is more common in older age groups. Other symptomatic cases, following carbon monoxide poisoning, chronic manganese exposure, or hypoxia, are relatively infrequent. Transient Parkinson's syndrome, following the use of rauwolfia, phenothiazine, and related compounds, usually disappears within a few weeks after the drug is discontinued.

CLINICAL FEATURES

With rare exceptions, it is not possible to distinguish the various etiologic types of Parkinson's syndrome on the basis of clinical symptoms.[42] The major features are those of motor dysfunction:[64] *tremor,* resulting from relatively rhythmic alternating contraction of agonist and antagonist muscle groups, usually maximal at rest, diminishing with initiation of movement and absent during sleep; *rigidity,* caused by hypertonicity, which is present simultaneously and equally in agonists and antagonists, and which may assume a characteristic cogwheel quality because of superimposed tremor; *bradykinesia,* with exasperating slowness in initiating movements and marked reduction in both spontaneous movements and associated automatic and auxiliary movements; and *impairment of postural and righting reflexes.* Significant problems in functional self-sufficiency result from these basic symptoms, which combine to produce a characteristic progressive decrease in amplitude in tasks requiring repetitive movements, and affect facial expressiveness, speech, writing, eating, dressing, rising from bed or chair, and walking and turning. Autonomic symptoms of sialorrhea and seborrhea often cause embarrassment. Intellectual functioning is not characteristically impaired, but individual instances of irritability or depression are common, and dementia secondary to pseudobulbar or cortical degenerative lesions may coexist in postencephalitic and arteriosclerotic patients.

The natural history of Parkinson's syndrome is highly variable, with age at onset ranging from the third or fourth decade in cases related to encephalitis, through middle age for idiopathic cases, and often into the seventh or eighth decade in cases associated with arteriosclerosis. Involvement usually is asymmetric, especially for tremor and rigidity, but bilateral functional impairment often overshadows predominant unilateral motor features. The rate of progression of symptoms, while usually totally unpredictable at onset, tends to remain constant for each patient, permitting meaningful prediction of future functional status after the initial year or two of disease.[18, 26] Such long-term uniformity of progression for the individual patient tends to offset the diurnal variability which often reflects transient emotional factors, and enables reproducible evaluation of treatment measures.

MANAGEMENT

Physical, medical, and surgical measures have been developed in the treatment of Parkinson's syndrome. The development of stereotactic neurosurgical procedures during the past two decades has been overshadowed in scientific brilliance and therapeutic triumph by neurochemical discoveries during the 1960's. The medical treatment of Parkinson's syndrome must now be discussed as a series of phases.

Physical Therapy

Physical therapy of some type has probably the longest history of use, although the basic neurologic symptoms of tremor and rigidity are not affected by physical therapy.[52] Bradykinesia, however, both leads to and is increased by diminished range of joint motion in all limbs; thus, active range of motion exercises are vital in maintaining limb function. Reciprocal movements of legs, essential to reestablishing more normal rhythm of gait, can be practiced several times a day on a stationary bicycle against minimal resistance. The complex task of walking is further impaired by paraspinal muscle rigidity which, combined with abnormal postural and righting reflexes, results in progressive forward-shifting of the center of gravity, producing anteropulsive and festinating gait. The simplification of gait retraining into two basic instructions as "lift the foot and bend the knee with each step" and "keep the shoulders back and the head straight forward" frequently produces significant progress in walking, transforming automatic involuntary movements into voluntary ones. An important goal of physical therapy is the preservation, as much as possible, of the mechanical ability to utilize improvements in basic neurologic symptoms produced by medical and surgical treatment.

Medical Treatment—Phase 1

Pathologic findings of dramatic loss of melanin pigment in the substantia nigra and variable degeneration in the basal ganglia and other areas of brain stem and cerebral cortex have been established for 50 years.[24] However, until recently, medical treatment has largely been empirical, based on time-honored observations of the beneficial effects of atropine and scopolamine, and continuing with the synthesis of compounds possessing anticholinergic effects similar to naturally occurring belladonna alkaloids but producing fewer undesirable side-effects.[18] Antihistamines and a nonhalogenated phenothiazine have been of secondary value (Table 1).

Rarely (with the exception of mild, phenothiazine-induced parkinsonian symptoms) is any one of these agents sufficient to control symptoms of Parkinson's syndrome. No significant difference exists among drugs within each category. Side-effects limit their use in large doses. For these reasons, conventional drug treatment consists of combinations of individual drugs from the first two groups, with agents from the second.[18, 67]

Some degree of impairment in acuity of mentation is to be expected with the use of anticholinergic medications, ranging from subtle difficulty in concentration and memory through more dramatic confusion to vivid hallucinations, usually with high doses of group A or B drugs in elderly patients. Other side-effects of anticholinergics are experienced by almost all patients, including dry mouth, blurred vision, constipation, and urinary hesitancy. Urinary retention is a potential hazard in patients with preexisting prostatic hypertrophy. The presence of narrow-angle glaucoma contraindicates the use of anticholinergic drugs. The chief side-effects of the antihistamines are dizziness and drowsiness.

Table 1. *Standard Drugs Employed in Treating*
Parkinson's Syndrome

Group A
Anticholinergics
   Trihexyphenidyl hydrochloride (Artane)
   Biperiden (Akineton)
   Cycrimine (Pagitane)
   Procyclidine (Kemadrin)

Group B
Combined anticholinergic and antihistaminic action
   Benztropine (Cogentin)

Group C
Antihistamines
   Diphenhydramine hydrochloride (Benadryl)
   Chlorphenoxamine (Phenoxene)
   Orphenadrine hydrochloride (Disipal)

Group D
Nonhalogenated phenothiazine
   Ethopropazine (Parsidol)

It has been estimated that, with optimal combinations of these drugs at the best adjusted dose levels, objective improvement is no more than 25 per cent and may be closer to 10 per cent.[18] Characteristic progression of disease continues, unabated by these drugs.

Medical Treatment—Phase 2

The serendipitous observation[54] of marked improvement in parkinsonian symptoms of rigidity, tremor, and bradykinesia, coincident with the administration of amantadine hydrochloride (Symmetrel) as prophylaxis against Asian influenza, type A-2, has led to a number of reports concerning the efficacy of this drug in the treatment of Parkinson's syndrome.[31, 48, 49, 51, 54] Although reports of improvement vary from 20 to 80 per cent of patients, it is generally agreed that the effect is significantly superior to combinations of standard antiparkinsonian drugs listed in phase 1. As in phase 1, the rationale has been empirical.

Amantadine hydrochloride is extremely rapid in speed of onset, producing significant improvement within 2 to 10 days. If no response has occurred by 2 weeks, the drug should be discontinued. In a few patients, however, a second trial after one or more months has been successful.[54] Discontinuation of the drug results in significant deterioration within one or two days. All investigators have noted partial decline in effectiveness after 4 to 8 weeks of use, but observation for 1 year has documented persisting benefit at a slightly reduced level of effectiveness.[47]

Amantadine hydrochloride in usual therapeutic doses of 200 mg. a day may have a mild stimulating effect, with increasing restlessness and insomnia at doses of 300 to 500 mg. a day[49] and convulsive liability at 800 mg. a day.[54] The ingestion of 2.8 gm. of amantadine hydrochloride by a man with postencephalitic parkinsonism in a suicide attempt caused an acute toxic psychosis without decrease in level of consciousness. Convulsions did not occur, possibly because the patient had been receiving diphenylhydantoin (Dilantin) for an unrelated reason. The patient was treated with hydration and recovered within 4 days.[21] No significant increase in therapeutic benefits accrues from daily doses in excess of 300 mg., and the frequency of restlessness at this dose level requires careful supervision.[49]

Anticholinergic side-effects are potentiated when amantadine hydrochloride is added to a regimen of phase 1 drugs, with symptoms ranging from dry mouth through hallucinations. Doses of anticholinergics and antihistamines should be reduced slightly when amantadine hydrochloride is begun, but phase 1 drugs need not be discontinued.

Intrinsic side-effects of amantadine hydrochloride also include a peculiar but apparently harmless livedo reticularis, with red-purple venous marbleizing of the skin of the legs,[47, 59] and ankle edema in the absence of cardiac or renal disease or electrolyte imbalance.[47] These signs have not interfered with amantadine therapy.

Neurochemistry and Neurophysiology of Parkinson's Syndrome

The third and most promising phase of medical therapy is based on a series of neurochemical discoveries involving catecholamines, chiefly dopamine.[1] Dopamine, the direct precursor of norepinephrine, is synthe-sized in the body from the amino acid, tyrosine, by way of the in-termediary compound dopa (3,4-dihydroxyphenylalanine) with pyri-doxal as cofactor in the decarboxylation of dopa to dopamine. Dopamine can be hydroxylated to norepinephrine, diverted to melanin synthesis, or degraded to a biologically inactive compound, homovanillic acid (Fig. 1). Dopa metabolism occurs both in the brain and in extracerebral tissues, including the heart, liver, and kidneys.

The occurrence of dopamine in the brain was discovered in 1957, and about 80 per cent of brain dopamine and homovanillic acid were found to reside in the basal ganglia complex, chiefly in the striatum (caudate nucleus and putamen); here, dopamine is the predominant cate-cholamine, existing in concentrations of more than 100 times that of norepinephrine.[27] The pertinence of these data for diseases of the basal ganglia was strengthened by observations that reserpine, which is capa-ble of producing a clinical syndrome similar to parkinsonism, depletes the brain of dopamine. By 1960, necropsy analysis of human parkin-sonian brains confirmed a severe deficiency of dopamine in the substan-tia nigra and striatum, paralleling the sites of melanin pigment loss and cellular degeneration, and leading Hornykiewicz to refer to Parkinson's syndrome as "the striatal dopamine deficiency syndrome."[29]

The substantia nigra contains cell bodies of dopaminergic neurones which terminate in the striatum, where variable cell loss suggests the possibility of interruption of nigrostriatal projections with trans-synaptic

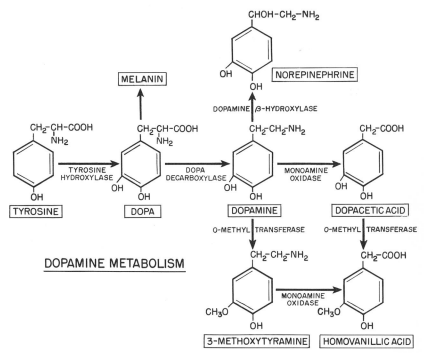

Figure 1. Dopamine metabolism. Dopamine can be hydroxylated to norepinephrine, diverted to melanin synthesis, or degraded to a biologically inactive compound, homovanillic acid.

degeneration. Dopamine has been identified as a neurotransmitter in this pathway, mediating an inhibitory function.[28] This system is thought normally to balance a facilitatory basal ganglia cholinergic pathway; in patients with Parkinson's syndrome, the striatum appears to be released from the effect of the inhibitory dopaminergic neuronal system, permitting the passage of extraneous motor impulses that produce some of the characteristic parkinsonian motor symptoms. As a result of this postulated cholinergic-dopaminergic imbalance, cholinergic hypersensitivity exists, with the administration of physostigmine aggravating the signs and symptoms of Parkinson's syndrome but not producing such adverse effects in normal subjects.[15] Scopolamine and benztropine mesylate (Cogentin)[15] and levodopa[63] block the physostigmine effect.

Insight into the mechanism of action of phase 1 antiparkinsonian drugs is provided by this demonstration of central reduction in synaptic acetylcholine activity, partially correcting cholinergic-dopaminergic imbalance. In addition to this basically negative effect, phase 1 drugs have also been shown to have a potentially positive action on dopaminergic pathways. Phase 1 drugs of groups A, B, and C inhibit dopamine uptake into neurones of rat striatum, thereby directly potentiating the action of dopamine released at striatal synapses by delaying the inactivation of this neurotransmitter by way of neuronal uptake.[14]

A related mechanism of action has been suggested for amantadine hydrochloride. While amantadine hydrochloride has no intrinsic anticholinergic activity in animal studies, small intravenous doses may release dopamine from neuronal storage sites, thus potentiating the action of dopamine.[25]

Drugs of phase 1 and especially phase 2 depend on a partially functional dopaminergic system for their effectiveness. This hypothesis helps to explain the clinical observation that patients with increasingly severe Parkinson's syndrome become progressively refractory to drug treatment; such patients with progressive nigrostriatal degeneration have insufficient intrinsic dopamine and reduced dopaminergic pathways for potentiation by antiparkinsonian drugs. The additional anticholinergic action of phase 1 drugs permits them to continue at partially effective levels, but the deficiency of chemical and neuronal substrate more seriously limits the long-term efficacy of amantadine hydrochloride, whose rapid onset of action depends on dopamine release. Phase 1 drugs are most effective in treating drug-induced Parkinson's syndrome, as such patients presumably have intact dopaminergic neuronal systems with adequate amounts of dopamine available for potentiation.[14]

Medical Treatment — Phase 3

In view of the imposing and well-documented theoretical background, initial trials of catecholamine therapy were both disorganized and disappointing. The inability of exogenous dopamine to enter the brain necessitated the use of its precursor, dopa. Relatively small doses of racemic D,L-dopa and levodopa were administered by way of various routes and dose schedules, usually totaling less than 1 gm. a day with slight and transient benefit in rigidity and akinesia.[1] The courageous administration of massive oral doses of D,L-dopa, ranging from 3 to 16 gm.

a day, by Cotzias and associates[12] produced "striking" improvement, somewhat greater for rigidity than for tremor, in more than half the patients treated for 1 to 8 months; reversible granulocytopenia was the major side-effect. With the subsequent use of levodopa,[11] marked benefits in bradykinesia, rigidity, and tremor were sustained in more than 70 per cent of patients for periods of observation up to 2 years without significant hematologic toxicity; side-effects consisted of mild nausea and vomiting which could be controlled by very slow increases in daily doses, and mild to moderate insomnia and involuntary movements which were dose-dependent and reversible. The sequence of events suggested that saturation of peripheral tissues by way of extracerebral dopa decarboxylation preceded the response of neurologic signs, and that improvement in bradykinesia was followed by response in rigidity and finally tremor.

Subsequent reports of large series of patients in the United States,[35, 36, 41, 69] Canada,[1] and Great Britain[4, 47] have documented improvement exceeding that obtained with any other antiparkinsonian medication, although individual investigators differ in describing extent of improvement ranging from mild to dramatic. Unlike amantadine hydrochloride, levodopa-induced benefits do not seem to diminish with time; rather, a constant dose may increase in efficacy over a period of months, and the maintenance dose often can be lower than the maximum tolerated dose. Progression of the disease may actually be slowed or halted in some patients.

PATIENT SELECTION. No absolute contraindications exist to the use of levodopa. However, levodopa should never be given to a patient within 4 weeks of the use of a monoamine oxidase inhibitor because of the risk of precipitating hypertensive crisis.[33] The presence of hypertensive, cardiovascular, renal, hepatic, hematologic, or psychiatric disorders does not prevent treatment, but such patients should be treated initially in a hospital to permit close observation. Others may safely be treated as outpatients, unless hospitalization is required for intensive physical therapy.

Patients with all degrees of severity of disease are benefited, but those with mild to moderately severe disease derive greater benefit than those with severely disabling Parkinson's syndrome.[35, 36] Patients with the mildest degree of disease who require treatment should not receive levodopa as the initial drug. Amantadine hydrochloride, with or without a phase 1 drug, is preferable in such patients whose disability is not sufficient to justify the initial use of levodopa with its attendant side-effects.[47]

ADMINISTRATION. Cotzias[9] has emphasized the necessity for a very gradual increase in levodopa dosage to therapeutic levels both to minimize side-effects and to overcome the characteristic time lag of several days between reaching a certain dose level and inducing benefit. To minimize gastrointestinal irritability, the oral medication must be taken immediately after a meal or snack, literally "for dessert," even though the presence of food has been shown to impede gastrointestinal absorption.[45] Therapy is begun with a single 250 mg. dose after breakfast, and an additional 250 mg. dose is added, after a meal or snack, in sequence every second or third day. The usual minimum dose range at which improvement first appears is 2 to 3 gm. a day, attained after 2 to 3 weeks of administration. The appearance of side-effects is the signal to proceed with smaller increments, of 100 mg., to halt increases temporarily, or to retreat to a lower dose level. The maximum dose at any hour should not exceed 1 gm. Should an interval of 4 or 5 hours between doses result in rapid loss of effect, small doses between meals may be added. It is rarely necessary or desirable to exceed a daily dose of 6 gm. on a schedule of 1 gm. after breakfast, in mid morning, after lunch, in mid afternoon, after supper, and in mid evening.

COMBINED THERAPY.   Especially in early stages of levodopa treatment, phase 1 drugs should not be discontinued; to do so would rob the patient of the often unrecognized benefits of these drugs before the full effect of levodopa has been obtained.[62]

Although multiple uncontrolled variables exist, it appears that the combination of either phase 1 or 2 drugs with levodopa exerts a synergistic effect.[47] This is especially desirable in permitting the use of a lower maintenance dose of levodopa, thereby decreasing the risk of dose-related side-effects.

LAHEY CLINIC FOUNDATION SERIES.   Between August 1, 1969, and September 1, 1971, 154 patients with Parkinson's syndrome began levodopa treatment at the Lahey Clinic Foundation.[62] Of the 154 patients, 79 were men and 75 were women. Ages ranged from 39 to 82 years, averaging 61 years. Parkinsonian symptoms had been present in 10 per cent for less than two years, in 70 per cent from 2 to 10 years, and in 20 per cent for more than 10 years. Clinical evaluation, performed before treatment and periodically during the course of therapy, followed a modification of the New York Hospital scoring system for severity of symptoms and impairment of activities.[41] *Tremor* was moderate to severe in degree in 20 per cent of the patients before treatment and mild in 35 per cent; *rigidity* was moderate to severe in 60 per cent and mild in 25 per cent; *bradykinesia* was moderate to severe in 25 per cent and mild in 60 per cent; and *impairment of daily activities* was severe in 50 per cent, moderate in 33 per cent, and mild in 15 per cent. The total score of all parameters before treatment indicated that 37 per cent of patients had severe disease, 35 per cent moderate disease, 26 per cent mild disease, and 2 per cent minimal disease. Details of administration of treatment conformed to the description given in preceding sections of this paper.

At the time of this report, 26 patients had received levodopa for less than 3 months, a period considered too brief to be fully effective; these patients have been excluded from the current analysis of results. Of the remaining 128 patients, 27 have been treated for less than 6 months, 54 up to 1 year, 29 up to 18 months, and 18 for as long as 2 years. Table 2 summarizes the results for the group of 128 patients. Less than 10 per cent improvement, in comparison to pretreatment scores, was considered a *poor* result; 10 to 30 per cent improvement was rated *fair;* 31 to 60 per cent improvement was rated *good;* and greater than 60 per cent was considered an *excellent* result.

To assess the benefits over longer periods of treatment, Table 3 presents the results for the 47 patients under treatment longer than 1 year.

Table 2. *Results of Levodopa Treatment for Three Months or Longer in 128 Patients*

CATEGORY	PER CENT OF PATIENTS SHOWING RESULT			
	Excellent	Good	Fair	Poor
Tremor	26	40	9	25
Rigidity	20	36	11	33
Bradykinesia	23	33	23	21
Daily activities	18	36	31	15
Total score	16	41	28	15

For all parameters except tremor, significant progress was achieved with longer duration of treatment, with the greatest improvement occurring in performance of daily activities. In each category, a trend was found to better results in patients with disease of moderate severity; the most severely disabled did significantly less well.[62] However, no correlation was found between duration of disease and response to levodopa.

SIDE-EFFECTS. In the Lahey Clinic Foundation series, 25 per cent of patients were totally free of side-effects. An additional 25 per cent experienced only one side-effect, and 50 per cent reported two or more. However, 10 per cent of patients were unable to continue treatment because of intolerable or uncontrollable side-effects. Table 4 lists significant side-effects with their time of onset for the total population of 154 patients.

Gastrointestinal. Anorexia, nausea, and vomiting are experienced by about 50 per cent of patients, usually within the first weeks of treatment.[39] Such symptoms are more likely to occur with the administration of large initial doses or after too rapid an increase in dosage, and they may be minimized by using small dose increments, taking medication with food and antacids, and temporarily reducing the dose in severe instances. Local gastric irritation is thought to be the primary factor in such symptoms, but dopaminergic stimulation of brain stem vomiting centers has also been suggested. Significantly less frequent are abdominal cramps and change in bowel function to either constipation or diarrhea. Activation of peptic ulcer is a rare but potentially treatment-limiting complication.[39]

Cardiovascular. On theoretical grounds, dopa might be expected to produce hypertension by way of alpha-adrenergic vasoconstriction. In

Table 3. *Results of Levodopa Treatment for One Year or Longer in 47 Patients*

CATEGORY	PER CENT OF PATIENTS SHOWING RESULT			
	Excellent	Good	Fair	Poor
Tremor	27	41	10	22
Rigidity	45	33	5	17
Bradykinesia	38	26	26	10
Daily activities	53	30	5	12
Total score	36	37	17	10

Table 4. *Side-Effects During Treatment with Levodopa in
154 Patients*

| SYMPTOM | NUMBER OF PATIENTS EXPERIENCING SYMPTOMS | | | | | | | |
| | Dose of Levodopa (gm.) | | | | | | Time of Treatment | |
	1	2	3	4	5	6	First Month	Later
Anorexia, nausea, or vomiting	15	26	12	18	9	3	68	15
Cramps or diarrhea	0	1	6	2	1	1	8	3
Dizziness or hypotension	6	8	4	5	3	0	20	6
Confusion or agitation	3	4	6	7	5	5	14	16
Depression	4	2	1	2	2	1	7	5
Dyskinetic movements	0	0	5	11	8	15	6	33

practice, this effect is encountered only with massive doses above the therapeutic range, and is clinically overshadowed by dopaminergic renal and mesenteric vasodilation, tending to produce an orthostatic hypotensive effect of varying degree.[23] Modulation of the rate of renin secretion by the sympathetic nervous system has also been proposed.[3] Levodopa has been found to augment renal sodium and potassium excretion, further contributing to orthostatic hypotension.[22] The effect of antihypertensive medications may be potentiated, and frequently the need for such agents disappears during levodopa treatment. Up to 33 per cent of patients may exhibit asymptomatic orthostatic hypotension, most often during the first month of treatment at doses less than 4 gm. In a minority, symptoms of orthostatic dizziness develop. To combat this problem, it may be necessary to increase dietary sodium, prescribe elastic stockings, or temporarily decrease the dose of levodopa.

Transient palpitations and flushing may be experienced, especially early in treatment and with rapid dose increase; these are benign. More ominous are disturbances in cardiac rate and rhythm, including ectopic activity and atrial fibrillation. Patients with preexisting disturbances of cardiac conduction and, to a lesser extent, those receiving sympathomimetic amines, such as epinephrine or isoproterenol, are at greatest risk and should be observed daily, preferably in a hospital, during early stages of levodopa treatment. Cardiac treatment, if necessary, may include the beta-adrenergic blocking agent propranolol hydrochloride or anti-arrhythmic agents such as procainamide and diphenylhydantoin.[23]

Psychiatric. Restlessness, hyperactivity, irritability, and insomnia may be experienced to varying degrees by up to 50 per cent of patients, and a smaller number may manifest depressive symptoms. Both types of affective response are somewhat more common in older age groups.[39] Frank psychotic episodes with delusions, hallucinations, distortion of reality, and gross behavioral disorders were seen in more than 17 per cent of patients in one series, many of whom had preexisting symptoms of mild chronic brain syndrome.[7] In each patient, the psychotic episode cleared on reduction or withdrawal of levodopa, independent of other antiparkinsonian medications. An unusually long average latency period of 4 months elapsed between onset of treatment and beginning of psychosis, usually after weeks of maintenance on a dose which had initially been well tolerated. A total of 75 per cent of patients with psychosis also had associated dyskinetic movements.[7]

The neurochemical mechanism by which psychiatric symptoms are produced cannot yet be stated, and in many instances the symptoms may actually represent exaggeration of preexisting mental disturbances, reacting to a change in the patient's chronic disease state. It has been speculated that modification of catecholamine metabolism may be a common denominator in Parkinson's syndrome, certain psychoses, and the action of psychoactive drugs.[39]

Neurologic. Dyskinetic movements are the only significant type of neurologic side-effect but may constitute the major limiting factor in treatment success. They appear to be dose related and tend to develop after several months of therapy, usually at dose levels yielding optimal improvement, in up to 50 per cent of patients. Barbeau[1] has catalogued more than 40 separate types of movement disorders, involving eyes, face, tongue, neck, respiratory muscles, truncal posture, and any limb. Of these, oral-facial dyskinesias are most common, with tongue protrusion, grimacing, and mouth movements. More severe and generalized choreoathetoid trunk and limb movements occur less frequently.

Attempts to control such movements with phenothiazines, neostigmine, and pyridoxine result in decrease of both dopa effect and dyskinesias, and the persistence of abnormal movements requires a compromise with therapeutic effectiveness at lower doses of levodopa.

Choreo-athetoid movements do not occur in normal control subjects receiving levodopa or in patients with dystonia musculorum deformans or spastic torticollis receiving levodopa treatment.[38] The movements occur more frequently on the abnormal side in patients with asymmetric disease, unless unilateral thalamic surgery had previously been performed.[44] Thalamotomy appears to offer some protection against the development of drug-induced dyskinesias in contralateral limbs.[30] It has been postulated that in parkinsonian patients with degeneration of nigrostriatal connections, exogenously administered levodopa may function as a false transmitter by way of other extrapyramidal pathways,[50] producing various dyskinetic movements, unless some of the alternate pathways have been blocked by destructive thalamic surgery.

Clinical Laboratory Abnormalities. No characteristic or significant changes in clinical laboratory tests of hematologic, renal, hepatic, or endocrine function are seen during levodopa treatment.[40] Granulocytopenia, a problem with racemic dopa, is not encountered with levodopa. Change in urine color, producing orange stains on undergarments of incontinent patients and causing urine to darken after exposure to air, is produced by catecholamine metabolites. Slight elevation in blood urea nitrogen levels is not reflected in abnormalities of serum creatinine or in clinical assessment of renal function. Spurious elevations of uric acid may be obtained with the standard colorimetric methods employed in automated testing; a dilute solution of levodopa in water also gives positive results for uric acid by these methods.[6] The more specific uricase method yields uric acid determinations within the normal range. Testing of urine with ferric chloride solution of Phenistix is positive in patients receiving 2 gm. or more of levodopa.[65]

DRUG INTERACTIONS. *Antidepressants.* Monoamine oxidase inhibitors potentiate the pressor effect of levodopa, presumably by decreasing the rate of metabolism of dopamine.[23] The combined use of levodopa and a monoamine oxidase inhibitor under controlled conditions precipitated a rapid and dramatic rise in blood pressure, terminated by the intravenous administration of phentolamine (Regitine).[33] Confusion and paranoia have been observed when levodopa was given 2 weeks after monoamine oxidase inhibitor treatment had been discontinued; it is recommended that at least 1 month elapse before levodopa is given.[33] If patients receiving levodopa require antidepressant medication, any of the tricyclic agents may safely be used. Dextroamphetamine in small doses also appears to be without hazard.[32]

Tranquilizers. Temporary decrease in effect of levodopa has followed the use of chlordiazepoxide (Librium),[55] diazepam (Valium), and a variety of phenothiazine compounds. The use of barbiturates and chloral hydrate has caused no problems.[32]

Vitamins. Because the decarboxylation of dopa to dopamine depends on pyridoxal as cofactor, it was thought that concomitant administration of pyridoxine (vitamin B_6) would enhance the therapeutic effect of levodopa. The opposite is true. The administration of pyridoxine in daily doses as low as 50 mg. produces partial reversal of dopa effect within 1 day and complete abolition of benefits after 3 to 4 days. As little as 5 mg. of pyridoxine a day produces significant decrease in the beneficial effects of levodopa.[17] The mechanism of this adverse effect is thought to be acceleration of the peripheral decarboxylation of dopa, at the expense of brain dopamine metabolism; the result is equivalent to reducing the dose of levodopa. Many multivitamin preparations contain 5 mg. or more of pyridoxine. Such compounds should not be taken by patients receiving levodopa. At least one multivitamin formula completely free of pyridoxine is now available (Larobec). The dietary consumption of certain foods high in pyridoxine content should be limited, including sweet potatoes, lima beans, avocados, wheat germ, oatmeal, walnuts, and most pork products.

Medical Treatment—Phase 4

Levodopa is definitely superior to any other antiparkinsonian drug currently available. However, significant problems limit its efficacy: (1) side effects frequently limit dosage or require termination of treatment; (2) clinical response at a fixed dose may fluctuate from day to day or even hour to hour; (3) only a minute fraction of administered levodopa actually reaches the brain (in experimental mice this fraction was 0.1 per cent;[66] (4) eliminating from consideration those patients unable to tolerate therapeutic doses because of side-effects and those with atypical or misdiagnosed disease, a small percentage of patients simply fail to improve.[43] This fact challenges the postulated mechanism of action of levodopa.

Approaches to these problems have centered about the development of adjunctive treatment measures. Gastrointestinal and cardiovascular side-effects represent peripheral actions of levodopa and dopamine, occurring at the expense of central metabolism. Gastrointestinal absorption of ingested levodopa is subject to fluctuations and is partly inhibited by the necessity of administration with food in an attempt to limit nausea and vomiting; absorption of levodopa is more rapid in a fasting than in a fed patient.[45] Central side-effects of behavioral alterations and dyskinetic movements, in contrast to peripheral symptoms, are dose related and frequently coexistent.

These observations point to the desirability of diminishing peripheral and enhancing central dopa metabolism while administering a smaller therapeutic dose. To accomplish this end, a compound which can inhibit the peripheral decarboxylation of levodopa, without affecting its central actions, is essential. Two such compounds are currently undergoing clinical trials, MK-485 (alpha-methyldopa hydrazine, Merck Sharp and Dohme)[8, 11] and Ro 4-4602 (seryl-trihydroxybenzyl hydrazine, Hoffmann-LaRoche).[2, 61] With such compounds, the average therapeutic dose of levodopa may be reduced fivefold. Intestinal absorption may be improved both because of the elimination of the need to administer such small levodopa doses with food to prevent nausea and also because of inhibition of intestinal dopa decarboxylase. With improved absorption, fluctuations in response may be better controlled. Other extracerebral side-effects may be diminished by reduction of catecholamine formation in extracerebral organs.

The problem of central side-effects remains. Pyridoxine reliably controls dyskinetic movements at the expense of a loss of beneficial effect of levodopa.[17, 34] The combination of levodopa plus a peripheral decarboxylase inhibitor and pyridoxine has been utilized in an attempt to deliver effective doses of vitamin B_6 directly to the brain and thereby further enhance central metabolism of smaller doses of levodopa.[10] The effect on movement disorders is under study.[68] Synthetic analogs of dopamine, similar to apomorphine, are also being developed.[13]

The critical question regarding the mechanism of action of levodopa is not yet answered. The theory of simple replacement of striatal dopamine deficiency is challenged by histochemical demonstration of neuronal degeneration in the pathways supposedly being replenished by exogenous dopa and by neurochemical evidence of changes in other catecholamines, notably serotonin and tryptamine, produced by exogenous dopa.[1]

Surgical Treatment

The rationale of stereotactic thalamic surgery in Parkinson's syndrome is the production of a lesion in a healthy area of the brain for the purpose of halting the propagation of incorrect motor information onward to the motor cortex and then to the spinal cord; such errant impulses would normally have been filtered out at a lower brain level.[5] A destructive lesion in the ventrolateral nucleus of the thalamus can alleviate the tremor and rigidity caused by disease farther down in the brain stem in substantia nigra and striatum.[53]

Critical reviews of the results of thalamic surgery agree on the following conclusions:[18, 37, 57, 60] (1) Case selection is of vital importance. The best candidate for surgery has unilateral or significantly asymmetric tremor and some rigidity but little or no bradykinesia or other parkinsonian features, is in good general health, and is physiologically, if not chronologically, fairly youthful. Not more than 1 in 10 patients with Parkinson's syndrome is suited for surgery. (2) Of such selected patients, 80 to 90 per cent will obtain good to excellent relief of tremor and rigidity; patients in poorer health or with other parkinsonian signs fare significantly less well. (3) Bradykinesia, impaired posture, abnormalities in speech and handwriting, and autonomic symptoms, including abnormal righting reflexes, are not benefited by surgery. (4) The inexorable progression of disease characteristically continues, with bradykinesia usually producing increasingly greater disability with the passage of years, negating the benefits in decreased tremor and rigidity. Successful thalamotomy does not necessarily prevent spread of tremor and rigidity to the initially uninvolved opposite side of the body, nor does it affect the rate of progression of the disease.

Recent analysis of surgical results[57, 58] has identified a small group of patients with unilateral tremor and rigidity whose thalamotomy was successful and whose tremor and rigidity did not spread to the opposite side of the body after more than 10 years of disease. These patients had no significant signs or symptoms of Parkinson's syndrome more than 5 years after surgery. They appear to have a relatively benign form of disease which would not have spread to the opposite side regardless of treatment. Patients in this group have a fairly early onset of disease, averaging 37 years of age, and frequently give a history of severe febrile illness preceding the onset of parkinsonian symptoms by up to 30 years. However, the average age at onset is almost 10 years older than that for postencephalitic parkinsonism, and the antecedent febrile illnesses are not forms of encephalitis, consisting instead of disorders such as severe pneumonia, scarlet fever, or malaria. Patients in this group have none of the typical stigmata of postencephalitic illness, such as oculogyric crises, dystonic phenomena, tics, or behavioral disorders. Unilateral thalamic surgery appears to be the treatment of choice in this select group, who can be spared the potential risks and expense of long-term treatment with levodopa.[56]

The advent of phase 3 medical treatment has markedly curtailed surgery for Parkinson's syndrome. The experience at the Lahey Clinic Foundation is illustrative; the number of stereotactic thalamic operations has declined from an average of almost 30 a year during 1964 through 1968[20] to less than 6 a year in the past 3 years.[19] Eighteen patients with previous thalamic surgery subsequently received levodopa at the Lahey Clinic Foundation with somewhat poorer results in the 5 patients with bilateral thalamotomies than in the 13 with unilateral surgery.[62] In a comparable study at Newcastle, however, it was concluded that previous ventrolateral thalamotomy, whether unilateral or bilateral, produced no apparent modification in the time course or extent of response to levodopa in comparison to a similar group of nonsurgical patients.[30]

CONCLUSIONS

In the evolution of medical treatment for Parkinson's syndrome, current methods are developing directly from basic scientific discoveries concerning catecholamines. Patients with only the mildest degree of parkinsonian involvement should be treated initially with amantadine hydrochloride (Symmetrel) with or without anticholinergic drugs or benztropine (Cogentin). Levodopa may be added later if necessary. Disease of greater degrees of severity merits initial treatment with levodopa. Pending the availability of peripheral dopa decarboxylase inhibitors or other adjunctive measures for the control of side-effects, patients whose levodopa therapy is limited by side-effects must depend on amantadine hydrochloride and anticholinergic drugs or benztropine. Thalamic surgery continues to have a limited role in treatment and is reserved for patients with nonprogressive unilateral tremor and rigidity. Physical therapy and supportive informal psychotherapy remain vital in the management of Parkinson's syndrome.

ACKNOWLEDGMENTS

The author is grateful to H. Stephen Kott, M.D., and Charles A. Fager, M.D., for their participation in the clinical evaluation and treatment of patients with Parkinson's syndrome in the Lahey Clinic Foundation series.

A portion of the levodopa administered in the Lahey Clinic Foundation series was supplied through the courtesy of Hoffmann-LaRoche, Inc., Nutley, New Jersey. The New England Deaconess Hospital Neurosurgical Research Fund defrayed some of the expenses for the remaining supplies of levodopa.

REFERENCES

1. Barbeau, A.: L-dopa therapy in Parkinson's disease: a critical review of nine years' experience. Canad. Med. Assoc. J. 101:59–68 (Dec. 27) 1969.
2. Barbeau, A., Gillo-Joffroy, L., and Mars, H.: Treatment of Parkinson's disease with levodopa and Ro 4-4602. Clin. Pharmacol. Ther. 12(pt. 2):353–359 (March-April) 1971.
3. Barbeau, A., Brossard, Y., Kuchel, O., et al.: Dopamine and blood pressure. Trans. Amer. Neurol. Assoc. 95:69–72, 1970.
4. Calne, D. B., Stern, G. M., Laurence, D. R., et al.: L-dopa in postencephalitic parkinsonism. Lancet 1:744–746 (April 12) 1969.
5. Carman, J. B.: Anatomic basis of surgical treatment of Parkinson's disease. N. Eng. J. Med. 279:919–930 (Oct. 24) 1968.
6. Cawein, M. J., and Hewins, J.: False rise in serum uric acid after L-dopa. N. Eng. J. Med. 281:1489–1490 (Dec. 25) 1969.
7. Celesia, G. G., and Barr, A. N.: Psychosis and other psychiatric manifestations of levodopa therapy. Arch. Neurol. 23:193–200 (Sept.) 1970.
8. Chase, T. N.: Cerebrospinal fluid monoamine metabolites and peripheral decarboxylase inhibitors in parkinsonism. Neurology 20:Suppl:36–40 (Dec.) 1970.
9. Cotzias, G. C.: Metabolic modification of some neurologic disorders. J.A.M.A. 210:1255–1262 (Nov. 17) 1969.
10. Cotzias, G. C., and Papavasiliou, P. S.: Blocking the negative effects of pyridoxine on patients receiving levodopa. J.A.M.A. 215:1504–1505 (March 1) 1971.

11. Cotzias, G. C., Papavasiliou, P. S., and Gellene, R.: Modification of parkinsonism – chronic treatment with L-dopa. New Eng. J. Med. *280*:337–345 (Feb. 13) 1969.
12. Cotzias, G. C., Van Woert, M. H., and Schiffer, L. M.: Aromatic amino acids and modification of parkinsonism. New Eng. J. Med. *276*:374–379 (Feb. 16) 1967.
13. Cotzias, G. C., Duby, S., Gincs, J. Z., et al.: Dopamine analogues for studies of parkinsonism. New Eng. J. Med. *283*:1289 (Dec. 3) 1970.
14. Coyle, J. T., and Snyder, S. H.: Antiparkinsonian drugs: inhibition of dopamine uptake in the corpus striatum as a possible mechanism of action. Science *166*:899–901 (Nov. 14) 1969.
15. Duvoisin, R. C.: Cholinergic-anticholinergic antagonism is parkinsonism. Arch. Neurol. *17*:124–136 (Aug.) 1967.
16. Duvoisin, R. C., and Yahr, M. D.: Encephalitis and parkinsonism. Arch. Neurol. *12*:227–239 (March) 1965.
17. Duvoisin, R. C., Yahr, M. D., and Coté, L. D.: Pyridoxine reversal of L-dopa effects in parkinsonism. Trans. Amer. Neurol. Assoc. *94*:81–84, 1969.
18. England, A. C., and Schwab, R. S.: Parkinson's syndrome. New Eng. J. Med. *265*:785–792 (Oct. 19) and 837–844 (Oct. 26) 1961.
19. Fager, C. A.: Personal communication.
20. Fager, C. A.: Evaluation of thalamic and subthalamic surgical lesions in the alleviation of Parkinson's disease. J. Neurosurg. *28*:145–149 (Feb.) 1968.
21. Fahn, S., Craddock, G., and Kumin, G.: Acute toxic psychosis from suicidal overdosage of amantadine. Arch. Neurol. *25*:45–48 (July) 1971.
22. Finlay, G. D., Whitsett, T. L., Cucinell, E. A., et al.: Augmentation of sodium and potassium excretion, glomerular filtration rate, and renal plasma flow by levodopa. New Eng. J. Med. *284*:865–870 (April 22) 1971.
23. Goldberg, L. I., and Whitsett, T. L.: Cardiovascular effects of levodopa. Clin. Pharmcol. Ther. *12*(pt. 2):376–382 (March-April) 1971.
24. Greenfield, J. G.: Neuropathology. Baltimore, Williams and Wilkins Co., 1963, pp. 582–585.
25. Grelak, R. P., Clark, R., Stump, J. M., et al.: Amantadine-dopamine interaction: possible mode of action in Parkinsonism. Science *169*:203–204 (July 10) 1970.
26. Hoehn, M. M., and Yahr, M. D.: Parkinsonism: onset, progression and mortality. Neurology *17*:427–442 (May) 1967.
27. Hornykiewicz, O.: Metabolism of brain dopamine in human parkinsonism: Neurochemical and clinical aspects. *In* Costa, E., Côté, L. J., and Yahr, M. D. (Eds.): Biochemistry and Pharmacology of the Basal Ganglia. New York, Raven Press, 1966, pp. 171–185.
28. Hornykiewicz, O.: Dopamine (3-hydroxytyramine) and brain function. Pharmacol. Rev. *18*:925–964 (June) 1966.
29. Hornykiewicz, O.: How does L-dopa work in parkinsonism? *In* Barbeau, A., and McDowell, F. H. (Eds.): L-dopa and Parkinsonism. Philadelphia, F. A. Davis Co., 1970, pp. 393–399.
30. Hughes, R. C., Polgar, J. G., Weightman, D., et al.: L-dopa in parkinsonism and the influence of previous thalamotomy. Brit. Med. J. *1*:7–13 (Jan. 2) 1971.
31. Hunter, K. R., Stern, G. M., Laurence, D. R., et al.: Amantadine in parkinsonism. Lancet *1*:1127–1129 (May 30) 1970.
32. Hunter, K. R., Stern, G. M., and Laurence, D. R.: Use of levodopa with other drugs. Lancet *2*:1283–1285 (Dec. 19) 1970.
33. Hunter, R. R., Boakes, A. J., Laurence, D. R., et al.: Monoamine oxidase inhibitors and L-dopa. Brit. Med. J. *3*:388 (Aug. 15) 1970.
34. Jameson, H. D.: Pyridoxine for levodopa-induced dystonia. J.A.M.A. *211*:1700 (March 9) 1970.
35. Keenan, R. E.: The Eaton collaborative study of levodopa therapy in parkinsonism: a summary. Neurology *20*:Suppl.:46–65 (Dec.) 1970.
36. Langrall, H. M., and Joseph, C.: Status of the clinical evaluation of levodopa in the treatment of Parkinson's disease and syndrome. Clin. Pharmacol. Ther. *12* (pt. 2):323–331 (March-April) 1971.
37. Markham, C. H.: Medical and surgical treatment of Parkinson's disease. MED. CLIN. N. AMER. *47*:1591–1601 (Nov.) 1963.
38. Markham, C. H.: The choreoathetoid movement disorder induced by levodopa. Clin. Pharmacol. Ther. *12* (pt. 2):340–343 (March-April) 1971.
39. Martin, W. E.: Adverse reactions during treatment of Parkinson's disease with levodopa. J.A.M.A. *216*:1979–1983 (June 21) 1971.
40. McDowell, F.: Clinical laboratory abnormalities. Clin. Pharmacol. Therapeut. *12* (pt. 2):335–339 (March-April) 1971.
41. McDowell, F., Lee, J. E., Swift, T., et al.: Treatment of Parkinson's syndrome with L-dihydroxyphenylalanine (levodopa). Ann. Intern. Med. *72*:29–35 (Jan.) 1970.
42. Merritt, H. H.: A Textbook of Neurology. Philadelphia, Lea & Febiger, 1967, pp. 473–482.
43. Mones, R. J.: Absence of response to levodopa in Parkinson's disease. J.A.M.A. *217*:1245 (Aug. 30) 1971.

44. Mones, R. J., Elizan, T. S., and Siegel, G.: L-dopa induced dyskinesias in 152 patients with Parkinson's disease. Trans. Amer. Neurol. Assoc. 95:286–287, 1970.
45. Morgan, J. P., Bianchine, J. R., Spiegel, H. E., et al.: Metabolism of levodopa in patients with Parkinson's disease. Arch. Neurol. 25:39–45 (July) 1971.
46. Nobrega, F. T., Glattre, E., Kurland, L. T., et al.: Comments on the epidemiology of parkinsonism. In Excerpta Medica International Congress Series No. 175, Progress in Neuro-Genetics, Vol. 1, Proceedings of the Second International Congress of Neuro-Genetics and Neuro-Ophthalmology. Montreal, September, 1967, pp. 474–485.
47. Parkes, J. D., Baxter, R. C., Curzon, G., et al.: Treatment of Parkinson's disease with amantadine and levodopa. A one-year study. Lancet 1:1083–1086 (May 29) 1971.
48. Parkes, J. D., Calver, D. M., Zilkha, K. J., et al.: Controlled trial of amantadine hydrochloride in Parkinson's disease. Lancet 1:259–262 (Feb. 7) 1970.
49. Parkes, J. D., Zilkha, K. J., Marsden, P., et al.: Amantadine dosage in treatment of Parkinson's disease. Lancet 1:1130–1133 (May 30) 1970.
50. Poirier, L. J., Parent, A., Ohye, C., et al.: The striopallidal system and its accessory morphological components: Some functional implications. In Barbeau, A., and McDowell, F. H. (Eds.): L-dopa and Parkinsonism. Philadelphia, F. A. Davis Co., 1970, pp. 125–132.
51. Rao, N. S., and Pearce, J.: Amantadine in parkinsonism. An extended prospective trial. Practitioner 206:241–245 (Feb.) 1971.
52. Ribera, V. A.: Movement disorders. MED. CLIN. N. AMER. 53:633–644 (May) 1969.
53. Schwab, R. S.: Limitations in treatment of Parkinson's disease. New Eng. J. Med. 279:943–944 (Oct. 24) 1968.
54. Schwab, R. S., England, A. C., Poskanzer, D. L., et al.: Amantadine in the treatment of Parkinson's disease. J.A.M.A. 208:1168–1170 (May 19) 1969.
55. Schwartz, G. A., and Fahn, S.: Newer medical treatments in parkinsonism. MED. CLIN. N. AMER. 54:773–785 (May) 1970.
56. Scott, R. M., and Brody, J. A.: Benign early onset of Parkinson's disease: a syndrome distinct from classic postencephalitic parkinsonism. Neurology 21:366–368 (April) 1971.
57. Scott, R. M., Brody, J. A., and Cooper, I. S.: The effect of thalamotomy on the progress of unilateral Parkinson's disease. J. Neurosurg. 32:286–288 (March) 1970.
58. Scott, R. M., Brody, J. A., Schwab, R. S., et al.: Progression of unilateral tremor and rigidity in Parkinson's disease. Neurology 20:710–714 (July) 1970.
59. Shealy, C. N., Weeth, J. B., and Mercier, D.: Livedo reticularis in patients with parkinsonism receiving amantadine. J.A.M.A. 212:1522–1523 (June 1) 1970.
60. Stellar, S., Mandell, S., Waltz, J. M., et al.: L-dopa in the treatment of parkinsonism; a preliminary appraisal. J. Neurosurg. 32:275–280 (March) 1970.
61. Tissot, R., Bartholini, G., and Pletscher, A.: Drug-induced changes of extracerebral dopa metabolism in man. Arch. Neurol. 20:187–190 (Feb.) 1969.
62. Wanger, S. L., Kott, H. S., and Fager, C. A.: Parkinson's disease: Treatment with L-dopa. Lahey Clin. Found. Bull. 20:1–9 (Jan.-March) 1971.
63. Weintraub, M. I., and Van Woert, M. H.: Reversal by levodopa of cholinergic hypersensitivity in Parkinson's disease. New Eng. J. Med. 284:412–415 (Feb. 25) 1971.
64. Wilkins, R. H., and Brody, I. A.: Parkinson's syndrome. Arch. Neurol. 20:440–441 (April) 1969.
65. Wolcott, G. J., and Hackett, T. N., Jr.: Levodopa and tests for ketonuria. New Eng. J. Med. 283:1522 (Dec. 31) 1970.
66. Wurtman, R. J., Rose, C. M., Matthysse, S., et al.: L-dihydroxyphenylalanine: Effect on S-adenosylmethionine in brain. Science 169:395–397 (July 24) 1970.
67. Yahr, M. D., and Duvoisin, R. C.: Medical therapy of parkinsonism. Mod. Treat. 5:283–300 (March) 1968.
68. Yahr, M. D., and Duvoisin, R. C.: Pyridoxine, levodopa, and L-α-methyldopa hydrazine regimen in parkinsonism. J.A.M.A. 216:2141 (June 28) 1971.
69. Yahr, M. D., Duvoisin, R. C., Schear, M. J., et al.: Treatment of parkinsonism with levodopa. Arch. Neurol. 21:343–354 (Oct.) 1969.

605 Commonwealth Avenue
Boston, Massachusetts 02215

The Treatment of Multiple Sclerosis

H. Stephen Kott, M.D.

To recount the history of the various treatments advocated for multiple sclerosis would be an exercise in futility. The nature of the disease, with its long course and good chance for remission early in the illness, makes it difficult to obtain an accurate objective assessment of any therapeutic agent.

It is also well recognized that a high percentage of patients will show improvement with any new medication or method. It may be difficult for the clinical researcher to accept the presence of placebo effect. The patient is, of course, even more convinced of the value of the treatment. I still see an occasional patient whose long remission is attributed to tolbutamide, a drug long ago cast aside as worthless for multiple sclerosis.

Unfortunately, until the exact etiology is established, it will be necessary to continue with empirical trials of various agents and methods. Thus, it is exceedingly important that worthwhile and reliable methods of assessing any treatment be utilized.

In 1961 a symposium[10] recognized the difficulties with clinical trials in multiple sclerosis and established the framework for a suitable protocol for clinical trials.[18] This protocol was utilized in a cooperative study of the evaluation of ACTH in multiple sclerosis. The results of this study will be discussed later. Hopefully, future treatment trials will use these guidelines.

Although we must be cautious in the evaluation of treatment for multiple sclerosis, we must not be therapeutic nihilists. The patient with multiple sclerosis requires significant emotional support in order to function at his best possible level. He often feels that "something" should be done for him, whether it be a physical therapy program at home or a placebo such as vitamin B_{12} or nicotinic acid. He needs to feel that he can call his physician to ask about a particular symptom that has him frightened. He has the right to feel that his physician is keeping up on the latest developments that might lead to effective treatment. The patient requires reassurance, and if he is supported sympathetically, his adjustment to the illness will be much more satisfactory. Many neurologists now believe that it is just as great a mistake to dismiss a patient, offering no hope, as it is to entice him with unrealistic anticipation of the results of treatment in vogue at the time.

Unfortunately, few treatment programs that can hope to influence the course of multiple sclerosis are available at this time. For any agent to have a significant influence, it must prevent exacerbation. Thus it would require long-term controlled studies to substantiate any results. In this article we will discuss some of the programs now in use and will touch on hopes for the future.

STEROIDS

The medications most commonly used in the past decade for the treatment of multiple sclerosis are the corticosteroids and ACTH. Much debate still exists concerning their usefulness. Several studies indicated that long-term prednisone or related drugs were not successful in affecting the course of the disease.[13, 14, 20] Alexander and associates,[1, 7] on the other hand, believe that high dose initial treatment with ACTH followed by long-term maintenance at lower doses produces significant improvement when compared to results in untreated controls. Others have believed that short-term ACTH was beneficial in terms of shortening an exacerbation and perhaps leaving less residua. Indeed, Miller et al.[15] reported that ACTH was beneficial for the acute attack.

In 1956 the cooperative study on the evaluation of ACTH in multiple sclerosis was launched. The effort was undertaken at 10 university centers and a double-blind ACTH-placebo procedure was utilized. The results of the study of 197 patients were first presented in 1969 and published in 1970.[17] One of the important results was that with a double-blind technique and randomization, it was considered possible to evaluate an agent in the treatment of multiple sclerosis exacerbation. In terms of ACTH it was found that the drug in short-term high dose use was slightly superior to placebo in its beneficial effects. ACTH hastened the improvement of signs and symptoms *but* it could not be stated that the ultimate improvement was greater than with the placebo. That is, if the study were continued longer, the placebo group may have been equal to the treatment group. Finally, no major complications occurred with the ACTH dosage used, namely, 80 units intramuscularly daily for 7 days, 40 units daily for 4 days, and 20 units daily for 3 days. A low-sodium diet, antacids, and potassium chloride were utilized in conjunction with the ACTH.

This, then, is a rather guarded, cautious recommendation for the use of ACTH, and one cannot help but wonder if the results are worth the cost, time, and inconvenience to the patient involved in hospitalization.

At the Lahey Clinic Foundation it has been our general policy to treat a functionally disabling or partially disabling attack with ACTH. Thus, for example, an attack consisting of paresthesia without ataxia or motor weakness would not necessarily require ACTH. Sensory attacks are known to have a fairly high rate of remission. Most of the patients with disabling attacks would fall into groups with motor weakness, ataxia, significant brain stem symptoms, and optic neuritis, especially in the rare bilateral instance. Some attacks of optic neuritis alone have been treated with retro-orbital injection of steroids or with orally administered pred-nisone. When possible in certain selected patients I have supervised a course of ACTH with the patient at home.

We have used dosages similar to those used by the cooperative study, although we have often carried treatment to 3 weeks. In 100 consecutive treatments, I found no instance of gastrointestinal hemorrhage, toxic psychosis, or adrenal exhaustion. Edema, insomnia, restlessness, and tachycardia were not uncommon but responded to dose reduction and symptomatic treatment.

We have also empirically treated a few patients with exacerbations that have been prolonged for several weeks or months beyond the normal expectation for remission. On occasion we have pleasantly been sur-prised that the use of ACTH was *associated* with a remission or signifi-cant improvement.

Many of our patients have heard about the use of intrathecal steroids in the treatment of multiple sclerosis and ask us about the efficacy of such a program. Boines[2, 3] is the champion of this method and has written extensively about it. He believes that a course of 3 weekly injections of methylprednisolone (60 mg., 80 mg., and 100 mg. for the third week) is indicated, and that this should be followed by booster injections every 2 months for a total of 6 months. After that, boosters are used as needed for exacerbation. Boines claims good to excellent improvement in 75 per cent of 450 patients. This includes patients who have never had a remis-sion. He believes the drug acts to suppress immune responses and to relieve spasticity.

It is generally accepted that steroids do loosen spasticity, but whether they work better intrathecally is dubious. The Lahey Clinic experience with intrathecal steroids has been limited to patients with progressively deteriorating disease and to instances of a steady plateau with consider-able disability. Worthwhile improvement has been almost nonexistent. In addition we have seen 3 patients in whom a fairly severe spastic para-paresis was altered by intrathecal methylprednisolone to a flaccid para-plegia. Spasticity was ameliorated to such an extent that it was no longer useful in holding the patient erect. Fortunately this complication was only temporary.

In summary, it is our feeling that steroids, and ACTH in particular, are useful in the symptomatic treatment of multiple sclerosis but do not pass the test in terms of preventing exacerbation or progression. We have witnessed new exacerbations while the patient has been receiving high doses of ACTH for a previous attack.

DIET

Although variations in dietary habits have been considered in the past as a possible factor in the latitudinal differences in multiple sclerosis prevalence, few investigators have advocated dietary treatment. Swank,[19] in trying to explain the paucity of multiple sclerosis in Korea, Japan, and some other northern latitude areas, thought that the low-fat diet in these countries might play a role. Some 20 years ago he began to advocate a low-fat diet for his patients. Other investigators generally dismissed his theories, but he recently reported the results of 20 years of treatment.

He found that those patients who remained on the diet had a lower exacerbation rate than reported series of nontreated patients. Exacerbation rates have varied with different authors from 0.2 per patient per year to 1.2. Some of this variation is the result of differing definitions of exacerbation and to different techniques in data gathering. Swank's patients had an exacerbation rate of about 1.0 per patient per year before treatment. This dropped to 0.3 in the first year of treatment, then to 0.05 over the next 5 years, and remained near or below that level during the last 14 years of the study.

In addition, patients on the low fat diet were reported to be functionally better for longer periods when compared to patients in other studies[11, 12] of the natural history of the disease. Finally, the death rate in the untreated patients was apparently 3 to 4 times higher than those following the Swank diet over a 20 year period. Unfortunately a randomized control was not used so that some room for questioning all of Swank's results may remain. At least one study, however, lends some circumstantial supporting evidence to Swank's theory that a low saturated fat and normal or high unsaturated fat diet helps multiple sclerosis. This is the experimental observation that rats, bred on a diet deficient in unsaturated fatty acids, exhibited an increased susceptibility to experimental allergic encephalomyelitis.[8] This condition is regarded by many to be similar to multiple sclerosis.

The Swank diet consists essentially of restricting saturated fats to less than 15 gm. a day. Unsaturated fats in the form of oils are allowed up to 50 gm.

The Swank diet does not meet the cardinal objective of preventing exacerbation or progression, but if the results are valid, it may retard the disease. Rather than incriminate fats or lack of saturated fats as a causal factor, it is more rational to think perhaps a low saturated, high unsaturated fat diet somehow protects against demyelination triggered by other agents.

IMMUNOSUPPRESSANTS

In recent years much interest has centered on immunologic mechanisms in multiple sclerosis. It is possible that multiple sclerosis is an autoimmune disease or that it is a viral illness with secondary autoimmune reactions.

Steroids, of course, might be expected to suppress immune responses, but we have already indicated that most long-term steroid studies have failed to show slowing of progression or arrest of the disease. Here, Alexander and associates[1, 7] are in disagreement.

Azathioprine (Imuran) and methotrexate were logical choices, then, to use in an attempt to halt the disease. Bornstein[5] initially believed that azathioprine in doses of 1.5 mg. per kg. of body weight was successful in arresting some progressive cases. Poskanzer[16] at the Massachusetts General Hospital and Ziegler[21] at the University of Kansas have been involved in the clinical study of azathioprine, 6-mercaptopurine, and methotrexate, and they have failed to observe beneficial effects in studies lasting as long as 2 years.

The Lahey Clinic experience includes 15 patients using azathioprine in doses of 1.5 mg. per kg. of body weight for 2 years. No problem occurred with marrow suppression, and no infectious complications were noted. Two patients stopped the drug because of nausea and vomiting. Four continued their previous pattern of steady, slow deterioration. Four other patients remained unchanged although each experienced one or more exacerbations, which subsequently cleared during the course of treatment. Finally 5 patients were unchanged or improved. We thought these results were not sufficient to justify continued trials in the face of reported increased incidence of reticuloendothelial system malignancies in patients receiving long-term immunosuppressive treatment. The final word on azathioprine or methotrexate is not in, but to date the results are not encouraging.

THE FUTURE

A great deal of evidence has been accumulating that multiple sclerosis involves the activation of immune mechanisms, both cellular and circulating. Experimental allergic encephalomyelitis and multiple sclerosis seem to have many similarities. Bornstein[4] found a similar demyelinating factor in the blood of patients with multiple sclerosis and animals with experimental allergic encephalomyelitis. Campbell[6] found that the serum of patients with multiple sclerosis contained an antibody that was directed against the myelin sheath and cytoplasm of oligodendroglia. This action is blocked by absorption with myelin protein obtained by acid extraction of human brain.

If, indeed, experimental allergic encephalomyelitis and multiple sclerosis have a similar pathophysiology, then some of the methods used to protect animals from experimental allergic encephalomyelitis may apply to humans. For instance, if the experimental animal is desensitized by using encephalitogenic myelin protein *without* adjuvant, experimental allergic encephalomyelitis can be prevented. This effect can also be achieved by using human myelin protein to hyposensitize the experimental animal.

The next step would be to attempt hyposensitization of patients having multiple sclerosis with the human encephalitogenic myelin protein. Trials are underway now, but they will not be effective, however, if the antigen-antibody phenomenon in multiple sclerosis is secondary to damage from another agent such as a slow virus. Indeed, many believe that the ultimate etiology is viral. In such a case the viral protein would have to be isolated in order to prepare an effective vaccine.

SUMMARY

At the present time no drug therapy of great value in the treatment of multiple sclerosis exists. A low saturated and high unsaturated fat diet may retard the progress somewhat, and ACTH in high dose, short-term usage may be effective for the acute exacerbation. To date, long-term immunosuppression with steroids or agents such as azathioprine, methotrexate, and cyclophosphamide has not been very effective. Physical therapy, control of infection, and emotional balance are all important adjunctive treatments not discussed here but familiar to all physicians who deal with this disease.

Hopes for the future depend on establishing the cause of multiple sclerosis. Currently, autoimmune disease and slow viral infection are the foremost theories.

REFERENCES

1. Alexander, L., and Cass, L. J.: The present status of ACTH therapy in multiple sclerosis. Ann. Intern. Med. 58:454–471 (March) 1963.
2. Boines, G. J.: Remissions in multiple sclerosis following intrathecal methylprednisolone acetate. Delaware Med. J. 33:230–235 (Aug.) 1961.
3. Boines, G. J.: The management of the multiple sclerosis patient. Behav. Neuropsychiatry 1 (No. 3):29–32 (June) 1969.
4. Bornstein, M. B.: Quoted by Merritt, H. H.: Multiple sclerosis. Med. World News, July 24, 1970, pp. 29–39.
5. Bornstein, M.: Personal communication, 1968.
6. Campbell, B.: Quoted by Merritt, H. H.: Multiple sclerosis. Med. World News, July 24, 1970, pp. 29–39.
7. Cass, L. J., Alexander, L., and Enders, M.: Complications of corticotropin therapy in multiple sclerosis. J.A.M.A. 197:173–178 (July 18) 1966.
8. Clausen, J., and Moller, J.: Allergic encephalomyelitis induced by brain antigen after deficiency in polyunsaturated fatty acids during myelination. Is multiple sclerosis a nutritive disorder? Acta Neurol. Scand. 43:375–388, 1967.
9. Davis, L., Lynch, R., Little, L. M., et al.: Viral infections in multiple sclerosis patients on low-dose immunosuppression: a prospective study. Neurology 21:765–768 (July) 1971.
10. Forster, F. M. (ed.): Report of the Panel on Multiple Sclerosis in Evaluation of Drug Therapy. Madison, Wisconsin, University of Wisconsin Press, 1961, 228 pp.
11. McAlpine, D.: The benign form of multiple sclerosis: results of a long-term study. Brit. Med. J. 2:1029–1032 (Oct. 24) 1964.
12. MacLean, A. R., and Berkson, J.: Mortality and disability in multiple sclerosis; statistical estimate of prognosis. J.A.M.A. 146:1367–1369 (Aug. 11) 1951.
13. Merritt, H. H., Glaser, G. H., and Herrmann, C., Jr.: Study of short- and long-term effects of adrenal steroids on clinical patterns of multiple sclerosis. Ann. N.Y. Acad. Sci. 58:625–632 (July 28) 1954.
14. Miller, H., Newell, D. J., and Ridley, A.: Multiple sclerosis. Trials of maintenance treatment with prednisolone and soluble aspirin. Lancet 1:127–129 (Jan. 21) 1961.
15. Miller, H., Newell, D. J., and Ridley, A.: Multiple sclerosis. Treatment of acute exacerbations with corticotrophin (A.C.T.H.). Lancet 2:1120–1122 (Nov. 18) 1961.
16. Poskanzer, D.: Personal communication, 1971.
17. Rose, A. S., Kuzma, J. W., Kurtzke, J. F., et al.: Cooperative study in the evaluation of therapy in multiple sclerosis. ACTH vs. placebo—final report. Neurology 20:1–59 (May) 1970.
18. Schumacker, G. A., Beebe, G., Kibler, R. F., et al.: Problems of experimental trials of therapy in multiple sclerosis: report by the panel on the evaluation of experimental trials of therapy in multiple sclerosis. Ann. N.Y. Acad. Sci. 122:552–568 (March 31) 1965.
19. Swank, R. L.: Multiple sclerosis: twenty years on low fat diet. Arch. Neurol. 23:460–474 (Nov.) 1970.
20. Tourtellotte, W. W., and Haerer, A. F.: Use of an oral corticosteroid in the treatment of multiple sclerosis; a double-blind study. Arch Neurol. 12:536–545 (May) 1965.
21. Ziegler, D.: Personal communication, 1971.

605 Commonwealth Avenue
Boston, Massachusetts 02215

Hyperthyroidism

Henry E. Zellmann, M.D.

It is not surprising that the various forms of hyperthyroidism fascinate many physicians, for herein lies something for almost everyone. For the scientist, there is the challenge that more than a half century of medical progress has added little to our knowledge of the etiology of the hyperthyroid states. For the clinician, there is almost always a colorful, even dazzling array of signs and symptoms or its counterpart, an obscure subtle illness which tests his diagnostic skill. For the clinical pathologist, there is a surfeit of laboratory tests, and for the therapist, a dilemma of three powerful modalities, with the problem of when and how and on whom to use them. Since it is with therapy that we are chiefly concerned in this volume, it is fortunate that these diseases are not so rare as to have given us little opportunity for their management. Instead, experience has been extensive with all modes of therapy. The fact that probably no more controversial area exists in medicine emphasizes that the ideal method has yet to be discovered. A rigid, unitarian program, however skillfully executed, will surely be a disservice to at least some patients. What we propose is a balanced approach fitting the treatment to the patient rather than the reverse.

GRAVES' DISEASE

Although treatment is most effective when directed toward etiology, no such plan is available in Graves' disease. This condition is best viewed as a familial immunologic disorder.[6] Lymphocytes and plasma cells, in response to an antigen as yet unidentified but presumably of thyroid origin, produce a variety of antibodies directed against one or several target tissues. The thyroid gland responds by secreting an excess of its hormones, thyroxine and triiodothyronine (T-4 and T-3). Thyroid-stimulating hormone (TSH) is not detectable in the serum because the thyroid-pituitary feedback mechanism is intact. TSH will reappear if therapeutic myxedema ensues. Orbital tissues react with the usual picture of thyroid ophthalmopathy, and the skin of the legs, feet, and rarely of the hands shows the changes of infiltration known as "pretibial myxedema."

The thyroid-stimulating antibody has been identified and termed long-acting thyroid stimulator (LATS). It is a 7-S globulin of the IgG class that, in the mouse bioassay model, induces secretion of radioiodinated thyroxine later than does TSH.[8] The immunologic identity of the dermal or ocular factors, if indeed they are antibodies, remains elusive.

Medical Treatment

Our most potent weapons are directed against the hypermetabolic component of this illness. We have much less to offer patients with dermopathy and ophthalmopathy. The rationale of medical therapy alone is based on the premise that the thyroid stimulator, which originates outside the thyroid and outside the pituitary gland, will eventually cease to be produced and TSH will resume its physiologic role. Whatever substance acts on the eyes and skin tends to run a more or less self-limiting course of 1 to 5 or more years and then remits. LATS apparently behaves in a similar manner. The goal, then, is to curtail T-3 and T-4 synthesis with antithyroid drugs and wait until the various stimulators no longer act.

Ideally, we would like to be able to select candidates who would enter a remission in 1 or 2 years and subject only them to the discipline required for prolonged medical therapy. Thus, we would reduce by perhaps one half to three quarters the number of patients at risk, however small, from surgical and radioiodine treatment. Alexander and associates[1] have outlined a technique that shows great promise. A 20 minute intravenous uptake of [132]I, which assesses only the trapping mechanism, since it is a short-lived isotope, may be used while the patient is taking both thyroid and antithyroid drugs. Suppression of [132]I uptake after an interval of 6 months of medical therapy is a favorable prognostic sign. Lack of suppression indicates that a remission is unlikely.

Prospects for long-term therapy are children and young adults with small goiters who can be persuaded to follow the program. Frequently, they lack motivation. Anyone familiar with the vicissitudes of inducing young persons to do anything can envision pitfalls in this plan. It is not difficult to judge favorable progress. Clinical improvement, maintenance of normal weight, ability to function in life, school, and work, supplemented when necessary by laboratory confirmation with serum protein-bound iodine (PBI) or T-4, indicate the metabolic trend. Shrinkage of the goiter is an encouraging prognostic sign.

A single drug is sufficient in most instances. Added thyroid substance makes metabolic balance easier in unstable hyperthyroidism. Education of the patient and family is perhaps emphasized less than in chronic diseases such as rheumatoid arthritis and diabetes but is just as important. We ask that any indication of infection, localized or generalized, be reported. This is the first line of defense against the complications of agranulocytosis.

The choice of drugs is simple enough. Propylthiouracil and methimazole appear to have equal incidence of agranulocytosis, 1 in 300 to 500 patients. The latter is more likely to produce minor reactions involving the skin and joints. All that need be said regarding dosage is to be certain to give enough. Often doubling or tripling the customary amount is sufficient for control of what seems to be intractable hyperthyroidism. We must be certain that the patient takes the appropriate drug faithfully, and our lines of communication must be open. We should be realistic and flexible enough to admit medical failure and to move on to an alternate method. Young, poorly motivated persons with inadequately controlled hyperthyroidism easily lose scholastic momentum and may fall behind a year or two. A career may be jeopardized. From the physical standpoint, inordinate growth in height can be distressing, particularly among girls. Paradoxically, some of these youths become obese during this period of hypermetabolism.

Surgery

It goes without saying that thyroidectomy in the hands of skilled surgeons has an impressive record.[4] It is decisive, morbidity is minimal, the complications of hypoparathyroidism and vocal cord paralysis are uncommon, recurrence is rarely seen, and mortality is virtually zero. It is the treatment of choice if the patient lives in an area remote from medical attention. Thyroidectomy should be performed on children and young adults with goiters of moderate to large size or those with unstable hyperthyroidism. Adolescence itself is challenge enough without the burden of a quickly curable metabolic disease that, if unchecked, can seriously interfere with psychologic and physical function. Surprisingly perhaps, a person with a large goiter and significant heart disease is often best managed by thyroidectomy. It is a precise, rapidly executed treatment. These recommendations are contingent on the availability of an expert thyroid surgeon and a well prepared euthyroid patient. Thyroid storm, associated with thyroidectomy, should remain an historical entity. In the absence of the optimal conditions mentioned, alternative approaches of radioiodine and drugs are safer.

Radioiodine

Radioiodine therapy was greeted with enthusiasm in 1941. It circumvented the shortcomings of long-term medical treatment and avoided the admittedly few complications of thyroid surgery. It was simple, painless, bloodless, and not at all expensive. Initial fears of leukemogenesis, carcinogenesis, and genetic mutations were not borne out. Sustained enthusiasm, however, is never easy, and here there was no exception. Its power was unquestioned; precision is what it lacked. Failure to respond could be traced almost always to an inadequate dose or to compromise of thyroid uptake by exogenous iodine. The more elaborate formulas proved no better than rather crude empiric choices when it came to selecting the proper dosage.

A mood of disillusionment with radioactive iodine therapy began in the early 1960's.[5] Myxedema was too often the outcome when conventional amounts of radioactive iodine were used. Halving the customary dose and supplementing the program with stable iodine or an antithyroid drug for a few years does, it is true, reduce the incidence of myxedema, but in many persons it just as surely postpones a final resolution of the problem.

Myxedema is not such a dreadful disease either to treat or to have.

Much less is made, it seems, of hundreds of thousands of patients whose adrenal glands have been rendered atrophic by corticosteroid therapy than of the few thousand made myxedematous by radioactive iodine. A plan that includes a little radioiodine and a little antithyroid drug or iodine and a long, long time appears to differ little from prolonged medical treatment, except that it is more complicated and adds the uncertainty of radiation. No one can say that a small dose of radioactive iodine plus adjuvant therapy, which will achieve a euthyroid state in 5 or 10 years, will not induce myxedema in 15, 20, or more years. We, at the Lahey Clinic Foundation, tend to be almost as decisive in using radioiodine as surgery, and we depend on the supervision and education of the patient to avoid the complications of myxedema.

Pregnancy

The proper management of a hyperthyroid patient when she is pregnant is no less controversial than when she is not, except no one recommends radioiodine. Proponents of medical therapy stress combined treatment using the smallest possible dose of antithyroid drugs supplemented by thyroid substance.[7] Their aim is to prevent even a brief period of hypothyroidism in the fetus whose nervous system requires thyroid hormones for maximal protein synthesis, growth, and maturation. The central problem is the ease with which antithyroid drugs traverse the placenta to the fetal circulation and the relative impermeability of the placenta to maternal thyroxine and triiodothyronine, whether endogenous or exogenous. In other words, the fetus depends on its own T-3 or T-4 for neural development. Comparable results in terms of fetal mortality, that is, living infants, can be achieved by either medical or surgical means. The crucial question, which the medical therapist finds difficult to answer, was asked by Werner:[13] how will we ever know if the infant, who now has an IQ of 105, was destined for 160 before he experienced "mild" hypothyroidism in utero? We believe that this problem is, at present, unsolved, and we recommend thyroidectomy for most patients in the first or second trimester[3] of pregnancy. There is a singular advantage to this plan—the fetus in the current pregnancy, and those in all subsequent pregnancies, is protected from the potential central nervous system effects of hypothyroidism. Less troublesome complications during pregnancy are neonatal goiter with respiratory obstruction and goiter, and exophthalmos resulting from transplacental passage of maternal LATS.

TOXIC NODULAR GOITER

Far less is known about the cause of this disease than diffuse toxic goiter. In all likelihood, it is a stage in the evolution of nodular goiter. Miller and Block[9] outlined several levels of development from a localized area of concentration of radioactivity on scintiscan suppressible by exogenous thyroid hormone through an autonomous stage of nonsuppressibility yet with normal serum tests of thyroid function and no symptoms, to overt hyperthyroidism, namely, an increase in T-3 and T-4 in the serum as well as an appropriate clinical picture. LATS, dermopathy, and oph-thalmopathy are uniformly absent. Remission does not occur except in a rare instance when the nodule becomes infarcted. Although pure Plummer's disease with a single hyperfunctional nodule and toxic multinodular goiter may seem superficially different, they are probably the same entity. In the former, paranodular tissue is completely suppressed; in the latter, an irregular pattern of radioactivity with one or occasionally more than one dominant nodule is present. The pathologist can help us little. His diagnosis is usually adenomatous goiter, at times showing hyperplasia but more often not.

T-3 THYROTOXICOSIS

Clinicians noted soon after protein-bound iodine (PBI) determinations were introduced 20 years ago that now and then a patient with goiter and convincing clinical evidence of thyrotoxicosis had completely normal serum levels of thyroid hormone. Intuitively, they treated these persons as if they had hyperthyroidism and were gratified when they showed appropriate response. The concept of hypermetabolism caused by excess secretion of triiodothyronine not measured in routine serum test (PBI and the later T4I, T4D, and RT3) slowly emerged. The characteristic features of this disease are the clinical picture of hyperthyroidism in the presence of goiter, usually nodular, with uptake of radioactive iodine not suppressible below 50 per cent of its baseline value by 1 week of triiodothyronine therapy, 100 micrograms a day. Sterling and associates[11] described a technique for measuring serum levels of T-3, which are elevated in this syndrome, termed T-3 thyrotoxicosis. Radioimmunoassay of T-3 will soon be widely available.

Therapy

Antithyroid drugs alone will relieve the symptoms of hyperthyroidism even though response is slower than in diffuse toxic goiter presumably because a good deal of hormone is stored in the nodular gland. Since relapse is the rule after discontinuing therapy, definitive control should be sought unless life expectancy is short. Radioiodine is feasible and effective, although we do not believe it to be ideal. Because the 24-hour uptake of radioactive iodine is either normal or not strikingly elevated, the dose is large, from 10 to 20 millicuries, for single hyperfunctioning nodules (compared with 4 to 10 millicuries for diffuse toxic goiter) to as much as 40 to 50 millicuries for multinodular goiter. Single nodules shrink slowly in size. Many can no longer be felt in 1 to 2 years. The size of multinodular goiter remains virtually unchanged. Myxedema is an unusual outcome because the resting paranodular tissue is spared radiation and easily responds when necessary to endogenous TSH. Since these patients are usually older than 50 years, pregnancy does not influence our decision. For the same reason, carcinogenesis is unlikely.

Surgery

We urge all patients with multinodular toxic goiter and most of those with single hyperfunctioning nodules to accept thyroidectomy. It guarantees complete, rapid control of hypermetabolism. Patients tolerate the operation remarkably well. Perhaps the illness itself is more or less a stress test, so that when euthyroid, the patients find surgery a lesser stress than their initial symptoms. Since the extent of dissection in the neck is less for a multinodular goiter than for diffuse goiter and still less for single nodules, the already small risk to local structures, laryngeal nerves and parathyroids, is further reduced. Persistent and recurrent hyperthyroidism should not occur.

Ancillary Drugs and Procedures

Antithyroid drugs act on the thyroid follicular cell within 30 minutes after ingestion. Yet, clinical improvement is delayed for a week or more until pathologic amounts of free and bound thyroid hormones approach physiologic levels. As a rule, no hardship is incurred, and the patient is content to wait. When more rapid action is essential, the beta-adrenergic blocking agent, propranolol hydrochloride,[12] is important in controlling distressing peripheral manifestations, such as tachycardia, sweating, and tension signs and symptoms. Its chief place, however, is in managing thyroid storm or crisis. Although experience with the technique is limited, plasmapheresis[2] or exchange transfusion offers promise of the most rapid reduction of plasma levels of thyroid hormones in life-threatening storm.

On a less heroic note, the course of therapy in hyperthyroidism is smoother in patients who have adequate amounts of rest, relative freedom from stress, and who avoid or sharply restrict their use of coffee, tea, tobacco, and alcoholic beverages.

An all but forgotten, simple, safe, inexpensive drug for control of mild hyperthyroidism with a small diffuse goiter is iodide. Both synthesis and secretion of T-3 and T-4 are inhibited. Remission may be long-lasting or permanent. Iodides, of course, are contraindicated as the sole agent in more severe degrees of hyperthyroidism.

IATROGENIC AND FACTITIOUS HYPERTHYROIDISM

It is not widely known that classic Graves' disease may follow the unnecessary although well intended use of thyroid hormones in euthyroid persons.[10] Although uncommon, it is probably more frequent than the rare case reports would suggest. The mechanism is unknown. These individuals are believed to be genetically vulnerable, and the clinical illness comes to the surface when the thyropituitary axis is disturbed.

Diagnosis and treatment of hyperthyroidism can be difficult enough without the added handicap of surreptitious thyroid administration. This is usually a manifestation of severe psychosis, neurosis, or situational reaction. Often the psychodynamic structure is an elaborate one. A good deal must be gained by the illness, that is, coping with life in a euthyroid state must be so threatening that escape by way of the inconvenience of hypermetabolism is an acceptable alternative. The diagnosis is not always obvious, for these patients are often crafty and resourceful. Features of the syndrome include clinical evidence of hyperthyroidism without goiter, ophthalmopathy, or dermopathy, with the hallmark being elevated serum tests and zero uptake of radioactive iodine. If triiodothyronine is the drug used, both the serum levels of thyroid hormone and the uptake of radioactive iodine will be low in the presence of hypermetabolism.

ASSOCIATED PSYCHOSIS AND NEUROSIS

Hyperthyroidism may be associated with troublesome symptoms of psychosis or neurosis. It is metabolic stress which causes the breakdown. Past and subsequent history will often reveal decompensation following stress of other sorts, loss of esteem, job, or loved one. It is important to recognize that if disabling nervous symptoms persist, when from a clinical and laboratory standpoint a euthyroid state is reached, additional antithyroid measures are futile and must be supplemented by psychologic ones, either drugs or formal psychiatric assistance or both. At times, nervous symptoms overshadow those of hypermetabolism and interfere with successful resolution of the underlying thyroid problem.

SUMMARY

Until more logical avenues open before us, our options in dealing with hyperthyroidism remain limited by our ignorance of its etiology. For toxic multinodular goiter, thyroidectomy offers an immediate curative solution. The large dose of radioactive iodine required, the delayed response, and the residual goiter make radioiodine less than an ideal choice. A single hyperfunctioning nodule may be excised easily and quickly; radioiodine here is usually just as effective, but its action is slower. Except as a temporizing measure where life expectancy is short, prolonged medical therapy should not be offered to these patients.

Subtotal thyroidectomy has and deserves its enduring reputation as excellent treatment for diffuse toxic goiter from childhood through youth to middle age. When performed during the first two trimesters of pregnancy, subtotal thyroidectomy should protect against fetal hypothyroidism.

When thyroid enlargement is minimal and the patient is cooperative, preferably in fact a bit compulsive, a trial of medical therapy is justified. Radioiodine is easily the simplest permanent way to deal with diffuse toxic goiter after the age of 40. We avoid using it during pregnancy and in fact do not recommend it enthusiastically for women in their childbearing years.

Fear of leukemia and thyroid cancer has not, so far, materialized. Radioiodine is, however, an imprecise tool, tending to induce myxedema if it is relied upon as the sole agent. A multifaceted plan, including a small dose of radioiodine, antithyroid drugs, or iodine, and the passage of a long, long time, may delay the end point interminably and still carry the risk of ultimate myxedema. For this reason, we plan to give enough radioiodine to control the hyperthyroid process with one dose, supplemented when necessary by a few weeks or months of antithyroid therapy.

As to the future, little improvement can be expected in the management of toxic nodular goiter lest it be in the area of prevention. Hopefully, Graves' disease may someday yield to an immunologic attack. A limited trial of immunosuppressive drugs has thus far been disappointing. The ultimate weapon against hyperthyroidism remains to be discovered.

REFERENCES

1. Alexander, W. D., Harden, R. M., Shimmins, J., et al.: Treatment of thyrotoxicosis based on thyroidal suppressibility. Lancet 2:681–684 (Sept. 30) 1967.
2. Ashkar, F. C., Katims, R. B., Smoak, W. M., 3d, et al.: Thyroid storm treatment with blood exchange and plasmapheresis. J.A.M.A. 214:1275–1279 (Nov. 16) 1970.
3. Bell, G. O., and Hall, J.: Hyperthyroidism and pregnancy. MED. CLIN. N. AMER. 44:363–367 (March) 1960.
4. Colcock, B. P., and King, M. L.: The mortality and morbidity of thyroid surgery. Surg. Gynec. Obstet. 114:131–136 (Feb.) 1962.
5. Dunn, J. T., and Chapman, E. M.: Rising incidence of hypothyroidism after radioactive-iodine therapy in thyrotoxicosis. New Eng. J. Med. 271:1037–1042 (Nov. 12) 1964.
6. Hall, R.: Hyperthyroidism – pathogenesis and diagnosis. Brit. Med. J. 1:743–745 (March 21) 1970.
7. Herbst, A. L., and Selenkow, H. A.: Hyperthyroidism during pregnancy. New Eng. J. Med. 273:627–633 (Sept. 16) 1965.
8. McKenzie, J. M.: The long-acting thyroid stimulator: its role in Graves' disease. Recent Progr. Horm. Res. 23:1–46, 1967.
9. Miller, J. M., and Block, M. A.: Functional autonomy in multinodular goiter. J.A.M.A. 214:535–539 (Oct. 19) 1970.
10. Paz, A. T., Zellmann, H. E., and Bell, G. O.: Graves' disease following thyroid therapy. Lahey Clin. Found. Bull. 18:11–16 (Jan.–March) 1969.
11. Sterling, K., Refetoff, S., and Selenkow, H. A.: T-3 thyrotoxicosis. Thyrotoxicosis due to elevated serum triiodothyronine levels. J.A.M.A. 213:571–575 (July 7) 1970.
12. Vinik, A. I., Pimstone, B. L., and Hoffenberg, R.: Sympathetic nervous system blocking in hyperthyroidism. J. Clin. Endocrinol. 28:725–727 (May) 1968.
13. Werner, S. C.: Moderator: panel discussions on hyperthyroidism. I. Hyperthyroidism in the pregnant woman and the neonate. II, Etiology and treatment of hyperthyroidism in the adult. J. Clin. Endocrinol. 27:1637–1654 and 1763–1777 (Nov.) 1967.

605 Commonwealth Avenue
Boston, Massachusetts 02215

The Present Status of Chemotherapy in Dermatology

Samuel L. Moschella, M.D.

Topical application, intralesional administration, arterial infusion, regional perfusion, and systemic chemotherapeutic agents have been used in benign and malignant cutaneous conditions. They are effective through their cytotoxic, anti-inflammatory, or immunosuppressive effects (Table 1). Among the drugs used are:

Purine and pyrimidine analogues
    5-Fluorouracil (5-FU) – fluorinated pyrimidine; floxuridine (5-FUDR)
    5-iodo-2'-deoxyuridine (iodoxuridine)
    Cytarabine
    Azathioprine (Imuran)
    6-Mercaptopurine (6-MP)
Folic acid antagonist – methotrexate (Mtx)
Alkylating agents
    Nitrogen mustard – cyclophosphamide (Cytoxan), chlorambucil (Leukeran), phenylalanine mustard (Alkeran)
Triethylene thiophosphoramide (Thio-tepa)
    Dimethanesulfonoxybutane – busulfan (Myleran)
Antibiotics
    Bleomycin
    Streptonigrin
    Actinomycin-D (Cosmegen)
Miscellaneous
    Hydroxyurea (Hydrea)
    Azaribine (Triazure)
    Procarbazine
    Vinca alkaloid – leukocristine (Vincristine, VCR)
    Combined chemotherapy – "MOPP" (Mustargen, Oncovin, Procarbazine, Prednisone)

TOPICAL THERAPY

When systemic 5-fluorouracil (5-FU) was being evaluated, a disappearance of senile keratoses was noted. Topically applied 5-FU selectively affects actinic keratoses with relative sparing of normal skin and makes the subclinical keratoses apparent. 5-FU, 1 per cent, in propylene-

Table 1. *Chemotherapeutic Agents in Dermatology*

MODE OF ADMINISTRATION	DRUG	DISEASE	RELATIVE THERAPEUTIC EFFEC- TIVENESS
Topical	5-Fluorouracil (5-FU)	Actinic and senile keratoses	4+
		Keratoses of xeroderma pigmentosa and x-ray dermatitis	4+
		Superficial epitheliomas (Bowen's disease, super- ficial basal cell epithelioma, erythroplasia of Queyrat)	2+
		Inoperable solitary metastatic adenocarcinoma of skin	1+
	Nitrogen mustard (HN₂)	Lymphomatous process of skin	3+
		Psoriasis	2+
	5-Iodo-2'-deoxyuridine (Iodoxuridine)	Herpes simplex (corneal)	3+
		Skin	1+
	Cytarabine	Herpes simplex (corneal)	3+
		Skin	1+
Intralesional	Nitrogen mustard (HN₂)	Lymphoma cutis	2+
Regional perfusion	Alkylating agents	Epithelioma – Melanoma	2+
		Squamous cell carcinoma	2+
	Nitrogen mustard	Lymphoma cutis (solitary)	3+
	Cyclophosphamide (Cytoxan), phenylala- nine mustard (Alkeran)	Kaposi's sarcoma	2+
		Sarcoma (soft tissue)	1+
Arterial infusion	Methotrexate (Mtx)	Cutaneous lymphoma (localized)	3+
	5-Fluorouracil (5-FU) Floxuridine (5-FUDR)	Unresponsive or uncontrolled epitheliomas (squamous cell carcinoma, satellitosis of melanoma)	2+
		Kaposi's sarcoma	2+
		Midline lethal granuloma	1+
		Wegener's granulomatosis (facial)	1+
		Carcinoid involvement of liver	1+
Systemic administration	Methotrexate	Mycosis fungoides	3+
		Psoriasis	3+
		Pemphigus vulgaris	3+
		Bullous pemphigoid	3+
		Vasculitis	3+
		Allergic vasculitis	2+
		Wegener's granulomatosus	2+
		Systemic lupus erythematosus	2+
		Reiter's syndrome	2+
		Letterer-Siwe's disease	2+
		Behçet's disease	1+
	Azathioprine (Imuran)	Mycosis fungoides	2+
		Pemphigus vulgaris	3+
		Bullous pemphigoid	2+
		Mycosis fungoides	2+

Table 1. *Chemotherapeutic Agents in Dermatology* (Continued)

MODE OF ADMINISTRATION	DRUG	DISEASE	RELATIVE THERAPEUTIC EFFEC- TIVENESS
		Vasculitides – Allergic	2+
		Wegener's granulomatosis	2+
		Systemic lupus erythematosus	2+
		Crohn's disease	1+
	Hydroxyurea (Hydrea)	Psoriasis	3+
		Melanoma	±
	Azaribine (Triazure)	Mycosis fungoides	3+
		Psoriasis	3+
	Cytarabine	Severe herpes simplex, varicella, disseminate herpes zoster	2+
Alkylating agents			
	Cyclophosphamide (Cytoxan)	Pemphigus vulgaris	3+
		Wegener's granulomatosis	2+
		Systemic lupus erythematosus	2+
		Behçet's disease	1+
	Chlorambucil (Leukeran)	Letterer-Siwe's disease	2+
		Primary macroglobulinemia	2+
	Phenylalanine mustard (Alkeran)	Multiple myeloma	2+
		Melanoma	1+
Antibiotics			
	Bleomycin	Mycosis fungoides	2+
		Squamous cell carcinoma	2+
		Lymphoma and lymphosarcoma	2+
		Reticulum cell sarcoma	2+
	Streptonigrin	Mycosis fungoides	2+
		Lymphoma cutis	2+
Miscellaneous			
	Procarbazine hydrochloride (Matulane)	Mycosis fungoides	2+
	Vincristine (Oncovin)	Mycosis fungoides	2+
	MOPP	Mycosis fungoides	2+

glycol has been used most frequently; concentrations up to 5 per cent have been incorporated and used in hydrophilic ointment.[13] The medication is applied twice a day over the involved face except the periorbital and oral areas. When a brisk inflammatory reaction occurs, usually 7 to 21 days after the institution of therapy and with the treatment of thicker keratoses 28 to 60 days, the drug is discontinued, and an anti-inflammatory program in the form of cool compresses, followed by corticosteroid creams three or four times a day is begun. Sunlight may have a phototoxic effect on the treated skin, with a resultant diffuse erythematous reaction. The therapy can aggravate an existing rosacea. Patients with the greatest amount of therapeutically induced inflammation experience the best results with the fewest recurrences.

The keratoses of xeroderma pigmentosa and radiation dermatitis can similarly and effectively be treated. This type of therapy may be useful in superficial epithelial malignancies such as Bowen's disease, basal cell epithelioma, and erythroplasia of Queyrat. Klein et al.[25] treated two metastatic adenocarcinomas and a keratoacanthoma with 20 per cent 5-FU in a hydrophilic ointment with selective tumor necrosis. One of our patients, a middle-aged woman, had the unpleasant experience of a severe persistent aggravation of an accompanying rosacea during 5-FU therapy for a moderate number of senile keratoses.

Topical nitrogen mustard[28, 39] has been most effective in lymphoma cutis and reportedly effective in psoriasis. In lymphoma cutis, the topical nitrogen mustard is unexplainably effective especially when used on the early lesion. It has been most effective in erythematous areas with or without induration and inflammatory infiltrated plaques, and causes generally insignificant reduction of tumid, nodular, or ulceronodular lesions.

The medicament is applied as a dilute nonvesicating aqueous solution of 10 mg. nitrogen mustard (HN_2) in 20 to 50 ml. of tap water when it is to be used to cover large areas, and 2.5 mg. in 10 ml. for a few lesions. These are applied daily for 4 to 7 days, or one to two times a week, using plastic or rubber gloves to protect the fingers. The treatment may cause a little erythema and discomfort; however, in more than 50 per cent of the patients an allergic dermatitis develops which can result in precipitous improvement. When this reaction occurs, the treatment is continued with a more dilute solution, and a topical corticosteroid may be added for symptomatic relief.

The treatment is continued until a response is appreciated, and these remissions usually last 2 weeks to 4 months. Treatment is given again when recurrence is evident, and only after the accompanying reaction has subsided. Other than pigmentation, no other cutaneous changes, such as are seen as complications of radiotherapy, are appreciated. The carcinogenic effect of this form of therapy has not been established.

Mandy et al.[28] reported the essentially complete clearing of psoriatic lesions within 3 weeks with the daily application of 10 mg. of nitrogen mustard (mechlorethamine) in 50 ml. of tap water, but the complicating contact dermatitis led to poor patient acceptance.

Topical 5-iodo-2'-deoxyuridine (iodoxuridine)[2] for herpes simplex of the skin is of questionable value; further trials of the use of 1 per cent iodoxuridine in dimethylsulphoxide (DMSO) in early mild cases may be indicated; it is most effective in superficial corneal infections. Systemic iodoxuridine should be administered early in herpes simplex encephalitis.

Cytarabine[23, 24] (arabinofuranosylcytosine, cytosine arabinoside) is a pyrimidine nucleoside analogue that interferes with the synthesis of DNA through the inhibition of the reduction of cytodine diphosphate and its incorporation into DNA molecules. Cytarabine is water soluble. It is being used in adults to induce remissions in acute granulocytic leukemia and other acute leukemias in adults and children; occasional responses have been described in patients with lymphoma and Hodgkin's disease. It has been found to be effective against a number of DNA viruses such as vaccinia and herpes simplex in cell culture.

Topical cytarabine, 5 per cent, in saline has been found as effective as iodoxuridine in the treatment of herpetic keratitis.[23, 24] Early application (within 24 hours on onset) of cytarabine, 1 per cent, in cream for local and cutaneous herpes simplex can result in a rapid remission of less than 1 week.

Patients with an altered immunologic state secondary to lymphoma, leukemia, and multiple myeloma are susceptible to disseminated infections with the DNA viruses of herpes simplex and zoster varicella. Intravenous cytarabine, 2 mg. per kilogram per day for 5 days, has been successfully used, especially if initiated early in these infections. Protracted rather than bolus infusion seems to be more effective and requires smaller doses. It has also been effective systemically in severe local herpetic lesions of the mouth, pharynx, and lung; the dose schedules were 0.2 to 3 mg. per kilogram per day for 5 days, with the disappearance of the virus in 1 to 7 days.[23, 24] If chickenpox or herpes zoster becomes life threatening, systemic cytarabine in adequate dosage should be considered.

The toxic effects of systemic administration of cytarabine are leukopenia, thrombocytopenia, bone marrow suppression, megaloblastosis, anemia, vomiting, diarrhea, oral inflammation or ulceration, thrombophlebitis, hepatic dysfunction, and fever.

INTRALESIONAL THERAPY

Intralesional chemotherapy has limited usefulness for cutaneous malignancies and may cause some temporary regression of these tumors, for example lymphoma cutis treated with nitrogen mustard. The nitrogen mustard is prepared for intralesional therapy by dissolving it in sterile distilled water to the concentration of 0.01 mg. per ml. The tumor receives multiple injections, 0.04 to 0.1 ml. at each site (0.0005 to 0.01 mg. HN_2). The treatment is repeated at weekly intervals until the desired effect occurs or there is failure to respond. One of our patients has experienced temporary regression of several nodules of Kaposi's sarcoma involving several toes.

REGIONAL PERFUSION

Regional perfusion[38] is a closed, extracorporeal (utilizing motor pumps and oxygenator), superlethal chemotherapeutic perfusion of an isolated anatomic area containing an epithelioma, for example melanoma or squamous cell carcinoma, lymphoma, or sarcoma, for up to 1 hour. Since the extremities are more successfully isolated, they are more suitable for perfusion, although lesions of the chest wall and head have also been effectively treated. The most frequently used chemotherapeutic agents are phenylalanine mustard (Alkeran), methyl-bis-(B-chloroethyl) amine (Mustargen), cyclophosphamide (Cytoxan), and actinomycin-D (Cosmegen) or a combination of any or all of them.

Perfusion is a valuable adjunct to surgical treatment of melanomas which arise on the upper extremity in the epitrochlear region and below it and on the lower extremities. It is useful in local recurrences of cutaneous malignancies and is effective for Kaposi's sarcoma of extremities. The combination of regional perfusion, radiation, and simple local excision is superior to any one of the modalities for local sarcoma, and reduces greatly the necessity for amputation. The complications of this type of therapy are local—inflammatory edema, persistent oozing from the operative site, blistering of the skin, and nerve pressure from the tourniquet; and systemic—hemolysis, red blood cells in urine, and a rise in free hemoglobin in the plasma.

ARTERIAL INFUSION

Continuous arterial infusion[15] is a continuous 24-hour infusion of a drug through a catheter intubating an artery supplying blood to the tumor. Positioning of the catheter into the vessel is aided by the injection of fluorescent dye; fluorescence of the involved skin by Wood's light indicates that the tumor-bearing area is within the blood supply.

An electrically driven pump or a clock-driven portable apparatus[41] is the method of infusion. The antimetabolites used are methotrexate, fluorouracil (5-FU), and floxuridine (5-FUDR). A chemotherapeutic agent such as methotrexate can be given in superlethal doses because the appropriate antidote, leucovorin, administered systemically neutralizes the antitumor agent as it returns by way of the venous circulation. The duration of continuous therapy with the portable ambulatory pump has varied from 3 weeks to 3 months.

This therapeutic modality has been used for localized cutaneous lymphoma, progressive unresponsive epitheliomas, and Kaposi's sarcoma, particularly of the head, neck, and extremities. The complications are inaccurate catheter placement, premature catheter displacement or leakage, hemorrhage usually associated with infection in the catheter tract, and rarely thrombosis of vessel associated usually with the development of mycotic aneurysm.

SYSTEMIC CHEMOTHERAPY[1, 18, 33]

A number of dermatologic disorders and systemic diseases with significant cutaneous involvement have been classified as autoimmune diseases and require treatment with corticosteroids for a long period with the inevitable development of a hypercorticoid state and other significant complications. Cytotoxic drugs, because of their immunosuppressant or anti-inflammatory effects or both, have been used in these disorders to control the underlying process and to obviate the undesirable and sometimes fatal complications of the diseases or corticosteroid therapy.

Guidelines,[34] which have been recommended for the selection of patients for the use of cytotoxic agents are: (1) presence of a life-threatening or potentially disabling disease; (2) lesions should be reversible; (3) failure to respond or intolerance to conventional therapy must be demonstrated; (4) no clinically active infection should be present; (5) hematologic contraindications must be absent; (6) close and careful follow-up for acute and long-term toxicity is mandatory; (7) clinical and laboratory means must be used to evaluate objectively the course of the disease; (8) reasons for therapy and its complications must be explained to each patient and written permission obtained for same is advisable, and (9) a peer group should review the results of therapy.

When it has been decided to use a potentially toxic drug for the treatment of benign conditions which have, because of their nature, severe socioeconomic effects, the drug must be effective and capable of inducing worthwhile remissions, have a low incidence of side-effects, and have a low, if any, chance of fatality. With the increased use of immunosuppressive agents for benign conditions, the probability of increased risk of cancer or its metastasis in the patients so treated should be appreciated. The most frequent and current systemic cytotoxic drugs being used dermatologically are methotrexate, azathioprine, and hydroxyurea.

Methotrexate

Methotrexate[7] has been the drug most frequently used, but because of the increasing reports of toxicity or fatality or both, other chemotherapeutic agents are being used and evaluated. Methotrexate is an analogue of folic acid which blocks the enzyme, folic acid reductase, thereby preventing the conversion of dehydrofolic acid to tetrahydrofolic acid, an enzyme, which participates in the various transmethylation reactions; as a result, there is a defective synthesis of purines and certain amino acids with resultant inhibition of DNA synthesis and cell division. It may be administered *orally* at 2.5 mg. every 8 hours for 4 doses, or a daily dose of 2.5 to 5.0 mg. for 6 to 12 days, or at a once weekly dose of 25 to 30 mg., and *parenterally* at a once weekly dose of 15 to 50 mg.[31] The most safe and effective therapeutic schedule is not known.

Methotrexate has been effective in psoriasis, especially psoriatic arthropathy, keratosis blenorrhagicum,[21] pemphigus,[21, 27] bullous pemphigoid, pityriasis rubra pilaris, Wegener's granulomatosis,[10] dermatomyositis,[36] Hand-Schüller-Christian disease, and mycosis fungoides.[19] Methotrexate has been used with variable and limited success in cases of multiple keratoacanthomas and basal cell carcinomas. It is probably the most effective systemic drug available, but unfortunately it has the most adverse reactions, especially irreversible liver damage.

Methotrexate has been effective as an adjunct and rarely as a solitary therapeutic drug for the treatment of pemphigus and bullous pemphigoid. Because of the slow response of both diseases to these immunosuppressants, the corticosteroids are given initially in large doses then reduced, and occasionally discontinued when the antimetabolites become effective. In psoriasis,[4] it is effective in 60 to 80 per cent of patients, with 20 to 30 per cent of patients experiencing some evidence of toxicity. The duration of treatment may be as responsible as the concentration of the drug in the production of toxicity. Since a higher proportion of a large oral dose is excreted, this mode of administration may be less toxic. Aspirin potentiates toxicity by reducing renal excretion and protein binding of methotrexate. Among the toxic effects of methotrexate are mouth ulcers, soreness and erosion of skin, toxic epidermal necrolysis, delay in skin healing, breaking of hair, nausea, abdominal cramps, elevated serum glutamic oxaloacetic transaminase (SGOT), headache, ataxia, malaise, fatigue, manic-depressive behavior, renal damage, chromosomal gaps, and teratogenicity. The principal side-effects are susceptibility to infections, megaloblastic anemia, gastrointestinal ulceration, pneumonitis, and cirrhosis. The administration of citrovorum factor after each dose may permit administration of larger doses of methotrexate with fewer side-effects.

Azathioprine (Imuran)

Azathioprine (Imuran)[1, 11] is a purine analogue which is derived from 6-mercaptopurine by the addition of an imidazole ring and is largely converted to 6-mercaptopurine in the body. It acts mainly by blocking purine synthesis, resulting in inhibition of DNA and RNA synthesis.

Of the antimetabolites (methotrexate, 6-mercaptopurine and related compounds, and alkylating agents), azathioprine has the greatest therapeutic index, expressed as the ratio of immunosuppressive activity to cytotoxicity,[3] and has a relatively acceptable level of toxicity. Because of increasing resistance to the use of methotrexate, this drug is being used for pemphigus[42] and bullous pemphigoid[16] with the same therapeutic approach and comparable success. It has also been used in allergic vasculitis, Wegener's granulomatosis,[20] systemic lupus erythematosus, and Crohn's disease of the rectum.[5]

The initial daily dose of azathioprine is 2 to 3 mg. per kilogram of body weight with a daily maintenance dose of 1 to 2 mg. per kilogram. The principal side-effects of therapy are infections, leukopenia, and thrombocytopenia. There are increased blood levels of the drug in the presence of azotemia or with the use of allopurinol (Zyloprim).

Hydroxyurea

Hydroxyurea (Hydrea)[26, 37] is a simple compound which has a cytotoxic effect; it has been hypothesized that hydroxyurea causes an immediate inhibition of DNA synthesis without interfering with the synthesis of ribonucleic acid or of protein. It has been used to treat inoperable malignant melanoma, resistant chronic myelocytic leukemia, and solid tumors; the usual daily dose is 20 to 30 mg. per kilogram of body weight. The drug has been and is being investigated as an oral chemotherapeutic agent for psoriasis;[17] it appears to be effective and less toxic than methotrexate. The dose is 1 gm. a day for 3 to 6 weeks, and the remissions induced in about 60 per cent of cases vary from 2 weeks to 4 months.[17] The drug is administered intermittently to treat recurrent flares; attempts to find and utilize a maintenance suppressive dose are not recommended. The adverse side-effects are bone marrow suppression (leukopenia is first, and later thrombocytopenia and anemia), gastrointestinal disturbances, alopecia, maculopapular eruption, and fever with or without a "flu" syndrome and vasculitis.

Azaribine (Triazure)

Azaribine (Triazure)[8] is an orally absorbable triacetyl derivative of 6-azauridine which inhibits orotidylic acid decarboxylase, a key enzyme in the de novo biosynthesis of pyrimidines. Like the other systemic chemotherapeutic agents, it is contraindicated in pregnancy and in potential childbearing women. It has been used in mycosis fungoides[9] and presently is being used and evaluated in the treatment of psoriasis.[40]

The dose is 250 to 270 mg. per kg. of body weight daily in three or more divided administrations every 6 or 8 hours for 2 to 3 weeks and is regulated according to response and accompanying toxicity. If the patient responds within the prescribed first 3 weeks, the drug is discontinued; if there is an associated decrease in the level of hemoglobin or hematocrit, the dosage should be cut in half and continued for 4 weeks.

Azaribine is available in 500 mg. tablets; the therapeutic number of tablets, which depends on the weight of the patient, is between 24 and 51 tablets for patients between 100 and 240 lbs. The cost and number of tablets to be taken affect adversely the patient's attitude and acceptance.

Toxic reactions include an anemia which antedates the occasional leukopenia, nausea, vomiting, diarrhea, lethargy or drowsiness, fever, "flu" syndrome, and exacerbation of an accompanying rheumatoid arthritis. No disturbance of the liver or kidney function has been reported. Azaribine has been reported to be a weak immunosuppressant. Mutagenicity and possible carcinogenicity have not so far been demonstrated experimentally.

Alkylating Agents

Alkylating agents[1, 18, 30, 33] (cyclophosphamide, Cytoxan; chlorambucil, Leukeran; and phenylalanine nitrogen mustard, Melphalan and Alkeran) have high chemical reactivity with negatively charged zones within a molecule (nucleophilic centers). Because of the widespread nucleophilic centers within cells, the cytotoxicity of these agents results probably from the inhibition of diverse enzyme systems, cross-linking effects on DNA, and possibly reactions with other molecules such as RNA and proteins. They are only partially radiomimetic, producing chiefly the lymphoid effects of x-radiation.

Cyclophosphamide has been used in pemphigus vulgaris,[14] Behçet's disease, Wegener's granulomatosis,[29] systemic lupus erythematosus, and mycosis fungoides; chlorambucil in Letterer-Siwe's disease and primary macroglobulinemia; and phenylalanine nitrogen mustard in melanoma and multiple myeloma. In mycosis fungoides, the alkylating agents are temporarily effective but cannot be given repeatedly because of their hematopoietic toxicity.

Like the other previously mentioned effective systemic chemotherapeutic agents, cyclophosphamide can reduce the suppressive and maintenance dose of prednisone, thereby reducing the latter's adverse side-effects. The dosage of cyclophosphamide is 30 to 50 mg. orally over 5 days, then 2 to 3 mg. per kilogram of body weight a day to maintain the white blood count below 4000 per cubic millimeter; that of chlorambucil is 6 to 10 mg. initially with 2 to 4 mg. as maintenance; and that of Melphalan is 6 mg. daily for 2 to 3 weeks, then 2 mg. per day for maintenance. The adverse effects are infections, bone marrow depression (leukopenia with a relative sparing of platelets), mucosal damage, alopecia, sterile hemorrhagic cystitis, and rarely hepatitis.

Antibiotics

Streptonigrin[35] is an antibiotic which is isolated from broth filtrates of Streptomyces flocculus; it inhibits DNA synthesis, and can be administered orally, intravenously, or intra-arterially. A favorable response to the drug has been described in advanced Hodgkin's disease, mycosis fungoides, chronic myelogenous leukemia, carcinoma of the colon, and sarcomas. The oral dose varies from 0.2 to 0.4 mg. a day and is modified according to its effect on the bone marrow. The dose for continuous intravenous and intra-arterial infusion has been 7 mcg. per kilogram of body weight a day for 6 days.

The toxic gastrointestinal manifestations of the drug are nausea, anorexia, dyspepsia, vomiting, oral ulcers, and diarrhea; the bone marrow toxic signs are leukopenia and thrombocytopenia which are delayed in onset, occur 5 to 6 weeks after treatment, and are prolonged; and the cutaneous evidence of toxicity is alopecia and an erythematous eruption.

Bleomycin[32] is a new experimental antineoplastic antibiotic isolated from Streptomyces verticillus in Japan. It inhibits the incorporation of thymidine into DNA and the activity of DNA polymerase in cells sensitive to this antibiotic. In animals and man, the drug is concentrated by squamous epithelium, especially in the tissues producing keratin. It is effective in the therapy of squamous cell carcinoma of the skin and the anogenital system, and carcinona of the head, neck, and esophagus, and to a lesser degree for melanoma, mycosis fungoides, lymphoma, and bronchogenic and cervical carcinoma. The dose is 1.25 to 26 mg. per square meter of the body surface area, given twice a week for 6 weeks. Complete regression has been observed in squamous cell carcinoma of skin, mycosis fungoides, and cancer of the penis. It is very effective in arterial perfusion therapy of oropharyngeal tumor.

The drug is especially important because of the absence of a toxic effect on the hematopoietic system and of any immunosuppressive action. Major toxicity is seen in the skin and lungs. The mucocutaneous changes which occur in 10 to 30 per cent of patients are ulcerative stomatitis, brawny edema and swelling of the interphalangeal joints, discoloration and tightening of the palmar and plantar skin with or without ulceration, cutaneous polymorphous erythema and keratosis which may also undergo necrosis and involve not only the hands but also the elbows and back, dermatographia, desquamation, and alopecia. Interstitial pneumonia occurs infrequently in elderly patients or those on high doses and may progress to pulmonary fibrosis and death. Other toxic manifestations are low-grade fever, anorexia, and weight loss.

Miscellaneous (Other Useful Solitary or Combined Therapeutic Agents)

Procarbazine hydrochloride (Matulane)[6] is an antineoplastic drug which is cytotoxic probably owing to its inhibition of protein and RNA and DNA synthesis. It is effective against Hodgkin's disease and useful in advanced mycosis fungoides. The drug is given in single or divided doses of 100 to 200 mg. daily for the first week and then maintained at 300 mg. daily until the white blood cell count is below 4000 and stopped upon the appearance of hematologic toxicity. Upon the maximum response or hematologic recovery or both, the maintenance dose is 50 to 100 mg. daily. Hemoglobin, hematocrit, and platelet determinations should be obtained every 3 or 4 days; urinalysis, SGOT, alkaline phosphatase, and blood urea nitrogen levels should be determined every 2 weeks.

The drug should be discontinued when central nervous system signs or symptoms (paresthesias, neuropathies, or confusion), leukopenia (white blood cell count less than 4,000), thrombocytopenia (platelets less than 100,000), or hemorrhagic or bleeding tendencies appear. Nausea and vomiting are the most common side-effects; diarrhea, flushing, alopecia, hyperpigmentation, and jaundice are also seen. Ethyl alcohol should not be used, since there may be a disulfiram (Antabuse)-like reaction. Since procarbazine possesses some amine oxidase inhibitory activity, sympathomimetic and tricyclic antidepressant drugs and foods with high tyramine content should be avoided.

Vincristine (Oncovin)[22] is used adjunctively in multiple drug therapy for advanced (systemic) mycosis fungoides or its transition to or association with another lymphoma. The amount of the intravenous dose is determined by body weight and is usually 2 mg. weekly. The adverse reactions are alopecia (application of a scalp tourniquet affords protection), leukopenia, neuromuscular problems (sensory loss, paresthesia, slapping gait, loss of tendon reflexes, muscle wasting), fever, oral ulceration, headache, vomiting, diarrhea, and constipation. It does not appear to have a significant effect upon platelets or red blood cells.

Combination chemotherapy has been used for mycosis fungoides when there is visceral involvement or the disease has another lymphomatous component or when it is resistant to all other therapeutic measures. One of the common multiple chemotherapeutic programs (MOPP) is that outlined by Devita et al.,[12] which consists of Mustargen, 6 mg. per square meter of body surface, and Oncovin, 2 mg., given on days 1 and 8, procarbazine, 100 mg. per square meter of body surface, and prednisone, 40 mg. per square meter of body surface, for a 10 day course. This program is initiated every 28 days for a total of 6 courses.

SUMMARY

In the constant struggle against cancer, the use of systemic chemotherapy has been useful as an adjunctive measure, but unfortunately it is usually of limited usefulness and success and causes potential and frequent toxic reactions. The topical application of 5-fluorouracil for actinic, senile, and radiodermatitis keratoses and nitrogen mustard for mycosis fungoides are significant therapeutic advances. The therapeutic value of cytarabine, especially in virus infections, is being further investigated. Regional perfusion and arterial infusion are relatively effective but unfortunately temporary palliative measures for localized malignant disease. Systemic chemotherapy with methotrexate, hydroxyurea, and azaribine has been effective in severe debilitating and incapacitating psoriasis, and methotrexate or azathioprine has been helpful in Wegener's granulomatosis. Among the so-called immunosuppressant drugs, methotrexate and azathioprine have been very effective in pemphigus vulgaris and bullous pemphigoid. Combination chemotherapy appears to reduce temporarily the morbidity and to extend life in the advanced cases of lymphoma cutis.

REFERENCES

1. Ashton, H., Beveridge, G. W., and Stevenson, C. J.: Therapeutics XI. Immunosuppressive drugs. Brit. J. Dermatol. 83:326–329 (Aug.) 1970.
2. Ashton, H., Frenk, E., and Stevenson, C. J.: Therapeutics XIV. Herpes simplex virus infections and idoxuridine. Brit. J. Dermatol. 84:496–499 (May) 1971.
3. Bach, J. F., Dardenne, M., and Fournier, C.: In vitro evaluation of immunosuppressive drugs. Nature 222:998–999 (June 7) 1969.
4. Baker, H.: Some hazards of methotrexate treatment of psoriasis. Trans. St. John's Hosp. Dermatol. Soc. 56:111–116, 1970.
5. Brooke, B. N., Hoffman, D. C., and Swarbrick, E. T.: Azathioprine for Crohn's disease. Lancet 2:612–614 (Sept. 20) 1969.
6. Brunner, K. W., and Young, C. W.: A methylhydrazine derivative in Hodgkin's disease and other malignant neoplasms. Therapeutic and toxic effects studied in 51 patients. Ann. Intern. Med. 63:69–86 (July) 1965.
7. Burrows, D., Shanks, R. G., and Stevenson, C. J.: Methotrexate in dermatology. Brit. J. Dermatol. 80:348–352 (May) 1968.
8. Calabresi, P.: Current status of clinical investigations with 6-azauridine, 5-iodo-2'-deoxyuridine, and related derivatives. Cancer Res. 23:1260-1267 (Sept.) 1963.
9. Calabresi, P., and Turner, R. W.: Beneficial effects of triacetyl azauridine in psoriasis and mycosis fungoides. Ann. Intern. Med. 64:352–371 (Feb.) 1966.
10. Capizzi, R. L., and Bertino, J. R.: Methotrexate therapy of Wegener's granulomatosis. Ann. Intern. Med. 74:74–79 (Jan.) 1971.
11. Corley, C. C., Jr., Lessner, H. E., and Larson, W. E.: Azathioprine therapy of "autoimmune" diseases. Amer. J. Med. 41:404–412 (Sept.) 1966.
12. DeVita, V. T., Serpick, A., and Carbone, P. P.: Combination chemotherapy of advanced Hodgkin's disease (HD): The NCI program, a progress report. Abstract 73. Proc. Amer. Assoc. Cancer Res. 10:19 (March) 1969.
13. Dillaha, G. J., Jansen, G. T., and Honeycutt, W. M.: Topical therapy with fluorouracil. Prog. Dermatol. 1:1-2 (Nov.) 1966.
14. Ebringer, A., and Mackay, I. R.: Pemphigus vulgaris successfully treated with cyclophosphamide. Ann. Intern. Med. 71:125–127 (July) 1969.
15. Fromer, J. L., and Sullivan, R. D.: Continuous arterial infusion chemotherapy for lymphoma and other cutaneous malignant tumors. Arch. Dermatol. 95:111–120 (Jan.) 1967.
16. Greaves, M. W., Burton, J. L., Marks, J., et al.: Azathioprine in treatment of bullous pemphigoid. Brit. Med. J. 1:144–145 (Jan. 16) 1971.
17. Greenwald, M. A., and Moschella, S. L.: The treatment of psoriasis with hydroxyurea: A preliminary report of 40 cases. Arch. Dermatol. (in press).
18. Grieco, M. H.: Immunosuppressive drug therapy. Drug Therapy, pp. 9–16 (April) 1971.
19. Haynes, H. A., and Van Scott, E. J.: Therapy of mycosis fungoides. Prog. Dermatol. 3:1–5 (March) 1968.
20. Israel, H. L., and Patchefsky, A. S.: Wegener's granulomatosis of lung: diagnosis and treatment. Ann. Intern. Med. 74:881–891 (June) 1971.
21. Jetton, R. L., and Duncan, W. C.: Treatment of Reiter's syndrome with methotrexate. Ann. Intern. Med. 70:349–351 (Feb.) 1969.
22. Johnson, I. S., Armstrong, J. C., Gorman, M., and Burnett, J. P., Jr.: The vinca alkaloids: A new class of oncolytic agents. Cancer Res. 23:1390–1427 (Sept.) 1963.

23. Juel-Jensen, B. E.: Varicella and cytosine arabinoside. Lancet *1*:572 (March 14) 1970.
24. Juel-Jensen, B. E.: Severe generalized primary herpes treated with cytarabine. Brit. Med. J. 2:154–155 (April 18) 1970.
25. Klein, E., Milgrom, H., Helm, F., et al.: Tumors of skin: Effects of local use of cytostatic agents. Skin *1*:81–87 (April) 1962.
26. Leavell, U. W., Jr., and Yarbro, J. W.: Hydroxyurea: A new treatment for psoriasis. Arch. Dermatol. *102*:144–150 (Aug.) 1970.
27. Lever, W. F., and Goldberg, H. S.: Treatment of pemphigus vulgaris with methotrexate. Arch. Dermatol. *100*:70–78 (July) 1969.
28. Mandy, S., Taylor, J. R., and Halprin, K.: Topically applied mechlorethamine in the treatment of psoriasis. Arch. Dermatol. *103*:272–276 (March) 1971.
29. McIlvanie, S. K.: Wegener's granulomatosis. Successful treatment with chlorambucil. J.A.M.A. *197*:90–92 (July 11) 1966.
30. Oberfield, R. A.: Alkylating agents. *In* Sullivan, R. D. (Ed.): Clinical Cancer Chemotherapy Including Ambulatory Infusion. Springfield, Illinois, Charles C Thomas, 1970, pp. 55–67.
31. Roenigk, H. H., Jr., Fowler-Bergfeld, W., and Curtis, G. H.: Methotrexate for psoriasis in weekly oral doses. Arch. Dermatol. *99*:86–93 (Jan.) 1969.
32. Rosenbaum, C., and Carter, S. K.: Bleomycin (NSC 125066, "Bleo," BLM). Clinical brochure. National Cancer Institute, March, 1970.
33. Schwartz, R. S.: Immunosuppressive drugs. Progr. Allergy *9*:246–303, 1965.
34. Schwartz, R. S., and Gowans, J. D.: Guidelines for the use of cytotoxic drugs in rheumatic diseases. Arthritis Rheum. *14*:134 (Jan.-Feb.) 1971.
35. Smith, G. M., Gordon, J. A., Sewell, I. A., et al.: A trial of streptonigrin in the treatment of advanced malignant disease. Brit. J. Cancer *21*:295–301 (June) 1967.
36. Sokologg, M. C., Goldberg, L. S., and Pearson, C. M.: Treatment of corticosteroid-resistant polymyositis with methotrexate. Lancet *1*:14–16 (Jan. 2) 1971.
37. Squibb: Hydroxyurea (hydrea). Clin. Pharmacol. Ther. *10*:142–146 (Jan.-Feb.) 1969.
38. Stehlin, J. S., Jr.: Perfusion of extremities for cancer. Proc. Natl. Cancer Conf. 6:617–620, 1970.
39. Van Scott, E. J., and Winters, P. L.: Responses of mycosis fungoides to intensive external treatment with nitrogen mustard. Arch. Dermatol. *102*:507–514 (Nov.) 1970.
40. Vogler, W. R., and Olansky, S.: A double-blind study of azaribine in the treatment of psoriasis. Ann. Intern. Med. 73:951–956 (Dec.) 1970.
41. Watkins, E., Jr.: Chronometric infusor – an apparatus for protracted ambulatory infusion therapy. New Eng. J. Med. 269:850–851 (Oct. 17) 1963.
42. Wolff, K., and Schreiner, E.: Immunosuppressive Therapie Pemphigus vulgaris. Vorlaufige Erfahrungen mit Azathioprin (Imurel). Arch. Klin. Exp. Dermatol. *235*:63–77, 1969.

605 Commonwealth Avenue
Boston, Massachusetts 02215

Chemosurgery (Mohs' Technique) in the Treatment of Epitheliomas

E. Laurie Tolman, M.D.

The standard modalities of curettage and electrodesiccation, scalpel excision, or radiation therapy are all used for the treatment of basal cell epitheliomas. Since the cure rates with these modalities approach 95 per cent, we tend to regard these tumors as relatively nonaggressive.

However, this high cure rate falls to about 50 per cent when the small percentage of recurrent lesions are retreated by the same modalities. This is true even if the method used is different from that used for the original tumor. When dealing with such tumors, therefore, a more radical or completely different mode of therapy must be employed. An example of this is Mohs' chemosurgical technique.

In 1936, Mohs first used the term chemosurgery to describe a new method whereby cancer of external surfaces could be excised completely and with assurance by the use of microscopic control.[5] This control is achieved by the use of in situ tumor fixation with zinc chloride paste and, later, excision of the fixed tissue in a precise manner with detailed mapping of the tissue sections.[3-6, 9] The excised tissue is then prepared by a frozen section technique for almost immediate examination to determine the presence or absence of tumor. If tumor is found, the process is repeated serially until a cancer-free plane is achieved. The following case report illustrates these points.

REPORT OF A CASE

A 68 year old man had had a malignant lesion on his chest excised 8 years previously. Four to 5 years later the lesion recurred and was excised again with a wider margin. Two years ago, it recurred again and was treated with liquid nitrogen.[8] The same lesion recurred once again this past year.

Physical examination revealed a clinically apparent basal cell carcinoma on the chest measuring 18 by 4 by 3 by 2 cm. in an elongate manner from left to right (Fig. 1). The entire area was treated chemosurgically; initial excision required 21 individual specimens. As can be noted on a replica of the map made at excision, cancer was found in parts of almost every section (Fig. 2). The paste was reapplied to involved areas (Fig. 3), and a second chemosurgical excision was performed with 20 separate sections; all sections were found to be free of cancer. Ten days

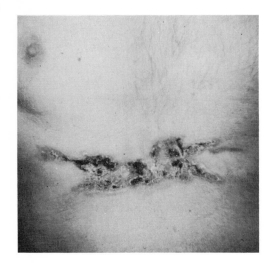

Figure 1. Before chemosurgery, clinical appearance of the lesions, measuring 18 by 4 by 3 by 2 cm.

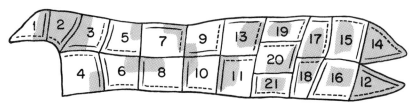

Figure 2. Map of first chemosurgical excision; solid lines indicate red dye and dashed lines blue dye. Shaded areas represent cancer found on microscopic examination.

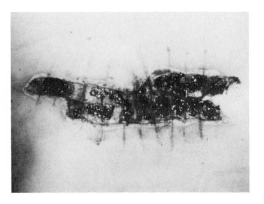

Figure 3. Clinical picture after reapplication of zinc chloride paste to areas that contain cancer after first excision.

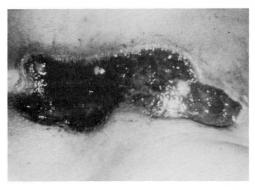

Figure 4. Clinical picture 10 days after completion of chemosurgery. Final fixed layer had spontaneously separated, leaving a base of granulation tissue.

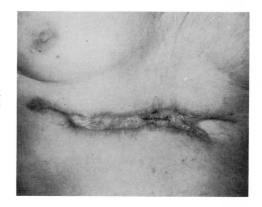

Figure 5. Two months later, area had healed completely with a soft pliable scar.

later, the final fixed layer had separated spontaneously leaving a clean granulating base (Fig. 4). Two months later (Fig. 5) the area had healed completely with a soft pliable scar.

METHOD

The chemosurgical technique consists of three basic steps: (1) in situ fixation, (2) excision of fixed tissue with detailed mapping, and (3) microscopic examination of fixed tissue prepared by frozen sections.

The involved areas are prepared by the application of dichloracetic acid which penetrates the keratin layer and turns the skin white. This destroys the barrier function of the skin and allows penetration of the fixative chemical.

The zinc chloride fixative, which kills the tissue but preserves the microscopic structure, is incorporated in a paste of Stibonite, 80 mesh sieve, 40.0 gm.; Sanguinaria canadensis, 10.0 gm.; and zinc chloride, saturated solution, 34.5 cc. This paste was specifically designed to carry the fixative to the tissue and then to release it.[3]

The paste is applied to the involved area, and the thickness of this application may range from a portion of 1 mm. to 3 to 4 mm. The thickness is determined by the depth of penetration, the size of the lesion, the duration of the exposure to the paste, and the type of tissue involved. In practice, one develops an intuition for what thickness to use.

An occlusive dressing is then applied on the treated area. Occlusion is necessary to prevent liquefaction or desiccation of the paste, which would affect its fixative properties. The dressing is kept in place until adequate fixation has occurred, usually about 4 to 24 hours.

After fixation has taken place, a layer of tissue, 1 to 2 mm. thick, is excised. Since this is through fixed tissue, no pain or bleeding is involved. If the excised tissue exceeds the fixed area, small amounts of bleeding are controlled by applying zinc chloride paste-impregnated gauze squares to the bleeding part for a few moments to achieve a bloodless field.[3] If the involved area is greater than 1 cm. square, the excision is performed by removing specimens about 1 cm. square and 2 mm. deep. These specimens are sketched on a map as each is removed, to show their relationship to one another and to the excisional area as a whole. The specimens are numbered consecutively as are the corresponding areas on the map.

As each specimen is excised, adjacent edges are marked with red (mercurochrome, 10 per cent) and blue (washing bluing) dyes for orientation purposes. These markings are also recorded on the map.

The excised specimens are then treated by frozen section. They are placed upside down, and the sections are cut horizontally from the undersurface of each specimen. The sections are stained and mounted for microscopic reviewing. The dyed edges are preserved through the staining and this enables the chemosurgeon to locate precisely any tumor in the specimen. By marking the locations of any remaining tumor on the map, a diagram is obtained that shows where any further chemosurgery, if any, need be done. This is accomplished by constant repetition of the steps outlined until a cancer-free plane is reached.

The thin layer of fixed tissue that has been left in place after a cancer-free plane has been reached is sloughed off spontaneously in 5 to 10 days. Healthy granulation tissue is revealed beneath; granulation will occur in 4 to 12 weeks. If the defect is too great or is in such an area that primary healing cannot take place, the patient can be referred to a plastic surgeon for repair. The post chemosurgically treated area is a healthy granulative area that has been proved cancer free. Reconstruction of this area can take place without concern of the possibility of a hidden or undetected focus of tumor.

INDICATIONS

Since chemosurgery has been shown to produce cure rates higher than those usually obtained by radiation or other excisional or destructive modalities,[2, 3, 10] it seems to be the procedure of choice and should be considered first for the treatment of recurrent cutaneous epitheliomas, especially recurrent basal cell epitheliomas, regardless of the previous treatment.[1, 2, 4, 7, 9]

The technique is also indicated for skin cancer under the following conditions:[7]

Primary basal cell epitheliomas
Unusual locations, such as eyelids, canthus, pinna, nasolabial fold, or ala nasi
Aggressive clinical histopathologic types, such as morphea-like, infiltrating, or
  fibrotic
Poorly demarcated clinical borders
Unusually large diameters
Primary squamous cell carcinoma
Same as with primary basal cell epithelioma
Bowen's disease and tumor
Erythroplasia of Queryrat

Mohs has extended the use of chemosurgery to other cancerous and noncancerous conditions. In treating melanomas, he tends to cut at least a 1 cm. wider area after a cancer-free plane has been achieved. He reports a series of 66 patients with melanoma, of which 61 had been followed at least 5 years with a cure rate of 47.5 per cent.[4] Some chemosurgeons have also extended the indications to include chemosurgical amputation for gangrene and other vascular-related problems of the extremities. Mohs, in particular, has had good success with this method. In a series of 500 cases of gangrene, he indicated a healing rate of 72 per cent.[3, 7]

In addition to its direct uses as a therapeutic modality, the technique has been employed to verify complete histologic removal of tumor by other methods, especially curettage and electrodesiccation.[7, 11] When chemosurgery is used in this manner, a good and reliable histologic scan of the margins and base of the treated area is obtained. If the tumor persists, the chemosurgical technique is then completely performed.

ADVANTAGES

The method offers its greatest advantages in an unprecedented reliability. This is evidenced by the unusually high 5 year cure rates, which surpass those attained by standard surgical and radiation modalities in series comparably weighed with recurrent and advanced lesions. Mohs reported a 5 year cure rate of 99.1 per cent in a series of 4159 determinant basal cell carcinomas, and a 5 year cure of 92.3 per cent in a series of 1330 determinant cases of squamous cell carcinoma.[4] Both of these surveys contained a high proportion of recurrent and advanced cases. Similarly, Tromovitch et al.[10] reported a 5 year cure rate of 93.1 per cent in a series of 102 recurrent cutaneous carcinomas. Robins and Menn[7] reported on a series of 713 cases over a 5 year period and have noted only 14 recurrences for a 98 per cent cure rate.

Because of the microscopic control offered by chemosurgery, conservation of normal tissue is an important feature. Only 2 to 3 mm. of normal tissue beyond the border of the cancer need be removed at any point. Most lesions will granulate spontaneously but, should repair be needed, preservation of well vascularized normal tissue maximizes cosmetic and functional results.

The operative mortality is extremely low, less than one third of 1 per cent in the large series of skin cancer.[3–5] The fact that no general anesthesia is used and that the wound tends to heal well without breakdown or infection contributes to this low mortality. This is true even though the precise nature of the technique allows its use in patients previously believed to have cancer too extensive for hope of cure with other methods.

Chemosurgeons have found excellent healing after chemosurgical treatment. The resultant scars tend to be soft, smooth, and pliable. Should plastic repair be needed, the well vascularized tissues heal well. Because all extensions of cancer have been searched out and destroyed by the treatment, there is no danger of later ulcerative or malignant change developing in the scar or the plastic repaired area.

DISADVANTAGES

While the concept of chemosurgery is simple to understand, its practice requires time, knowledge, and experience. The chemosurgeon must know exactly how much fixative to use for a given purpose, he must develop skill in removing the specimen, and he must learn to interpret carefully the microscopic sections. The procedure can sometimes be quite time consuming.

In the treatment of advanced cancer considerable pain may be present during penetration of the fixative, especially in sensitive areas.

The preparation of the frozen sections in the technique requires a specially trained technician and facilities for preparing the frozen sections that should be kept in the area where the surgery is performed.

Occasionally, loss of conservatism and destruction of too much tissue may occur, especially around the nose and ears.[1]

Limited availability[4–6] is another disadvantage; approximately 50 chemosurgeons have been trained in this field and they are unevenly distributed geographically.

CONCLUSIONS

Mohs' chemosurgical technique has a definite place among modalities for the therapy of cutaneous cancers. It should be considered first in the treatment of recurrent epitheliomas, regardless of the previous type of therapy used, in view of its proved ability to produce significantly higher cure rates than with other techniques. Other situations occur where primary epitheliomas may be treated by chemosurgery.

Chemosurgery is not to be undertaken lightly. Prior training in the technique is necessary, and the procedure can be both time-consuming and arduous. A need exists for a trained assistant to process the frozen sections and produce good microscopic sections.

Awareness by nonchemosurgeons of the technique and its place among other modalities for treatment of recurrent and certain primary epitheliomas will extend to many patients a chance for cure of such lesions that previously would have required extensive surgery or just palliative procedures.

REFERENCES

1. McDonald, R., Nichols, L. M., and Pitts, R.: Proceedings of Tenth Advanced Seminar in Dermatology. Cutis 8:151–169 (Aug.) 1971.
2. Menn, H., Robins, P., Kopf, A. W., and Bart, R. S.: The recurrent basal cell epitheliomas. Arch. Dermatol. 103:628–631 (June) 1971.
3. Mohs, F. E.: Chemosurgery in Cancer, Gangrene and Infections. Springfield, Illinois, Charles C Thomas, Publisher, 1956, p. 112.
4. Mohs, F. E.: Chemosurgery for the microscopically controlled excision of cutaneous cancer. In Epstein, E. (ed.): Skin Surgery. Springfield, Illinois, Charles C Thomas, Publisher, 1970, pp. 295–310.
5. Mohs, F. E.: Chemosurgery for the Microscopically Controlled Excision of Skin Cancer. Sixth National Cancer Conference Proceedings. Philadelphia, J. B. Lippincott Co., 1970, pp. 517–525.
6. Phelan, J. T., and Milgrom, H.: The use of Mohs' chemosurgery technique in the treatment of skin cancers. Surg. Gynec. Obstet. 125:549–560 (Sept.) 1967.
7. Robins, P., and Menn, H.: Chemosurgery of the treatment of skin cancer. Hosp. Prac. 5:40–50 (Dec.) 1970.
8. Tromovitch, T. A.: Mohs' technique. In Maddin, S., and Brown, T. H. (eds.): Current Dermatologic Management. St. Louis, The C. V. Mosby Company, 1970, pp. 20–23.
9. Tromovitch, T. A., Beirne, G. A., and Beirne, C. G.: Cancer chemosurgery. Cutis 1:523–529 (Nov.) 1965.
10. Tromovitch, T. A., Beirne, G. A., and Beirne, C. G.: Mohs' technique (cancer chemosurgery). Treatment of recurrent cutaneous carcinomas. Cancer 19:867–868 (June) 1966.
11. Zacarian, S. A.: Cryosurgery of Skin Cancer and Cryogenic Techniques in Dermatology. Springfield, Illinois, Charles C Thomas, Publisher, 1969, 224 pp.

605 Commonwealth Avenue
Boston, Massachusetts 02215

Immunologic Deficiency States

John M. O'Loughlin, M.D.

Abnormalities of the immunologic system vary in their manifestations and present in a wide range of disease patterns. To understand more clearly the underlying mechanisms, it should be recalled that two basic types of immunologic processes occur, those which are cell mediated and those which involve the secretion of humoral antibody. Deficiency states may involve either system or occasionally combinations of both; they may be congenital and inheritable, following genetic rules, or secondary or acquired often resulting from another disease process.

IMMUNE RESPONSE

Humoral Antibody Response

The humoral factors are serum proteins which run electrophoretically as gamma globulins. These antibodies can react directly with antigens and are serum proteins known as immunoglobulins—IgG, IgA, IgD, IgE, and IgM. IgA has been separated further to a secretory IgA and serum IgA, each with specific characteristics. IgG, IgA, and IgD have a molecular weight of approximately 150,000; IgE, 200,000; and IgM, about 900,000. Properties of the specific antibodies are listed in Table 1.

Ordinarily the newborn infant is supplied with maternal IgG so that cord serum closely approximates maternal IgG. Practically no maternal IgA and very little IgM crosses the placenta into the fetus. Passage of gamma globulin begins about the fourth month of gestation and appears to involve an active transport system. The newborn child synthesizes IgM antibodies at birth. Levels rise rapidly and reach about 75 per cent of adult level by the end of the first year of life. IgA synthesis begins a few weeks later and reaches 75 per cent of adult level about the end of the second year. IgG received from the mother is gradually catabolized so that by the end of the third month of life levels are very low. Just before this, at the beginning of the third month, IgG synthesis occurs and about this time is a period of physiologic hypogammaglobulinemia. Levels rise rapidly to achieve close to adult values by the end of the first year. The structure of IgG is shown in Figure 1.

Table 1. *Properties of Specific Antibodies*

	IgG (γG)	IgA (γA)	IgM (γM)	IgD (γD)	IgE (γE)
Molecular weight	160,000	170,000 (serum) 390,000 (secretory)	900,000	160,000	200,000
Sedimentation coefficient	7S	7S, 11S	19S	7S	8S
Electrophoretic mobility	γ	Slow β	Between β and γ	Between β and γ	Slow β
Nomenclature heavy chains (subclasses)	γ (1,2,3,4)	γ (1,2)	μ (1,2)	δ	ε
Number of heavy chains	2	2	10	2	2
Number of light chains	2κ or 2λ	2κ 2λ	10κ 10λ	2κ 2λ	2κ 2λ
Bind complement	+	−	+	−	−
React with rheumatoid factor	+	−	−	−	−
Carbohydrate, percent	2.5	5–10	5–10	...	10
Synthetic rate (gm./day/70 kg.)	2.3	2.7	0.4	0.03	
Half-life (days)	25	6	5	3	2–3 (serum) 9–10 (skin)

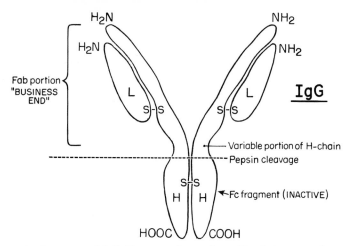

Figure 1. Structure of IgG illustrates four polypeptide chains, two of approximate molecular weight of 25,000 (light chains) and two of 50,000 molecular weight (heavy chains).

The immunoglobulins are made by cells of the plasma cell series, and it is believed that one cell makes only one type of globulin. Ordinarily no plasma cells can be found in the normal newborn child, however as the infant matures immunologically, maturation of the lymphoid tissue occurs with organization of follicles and the appearance of plasma cells during the third month of life. A comparison of the proportion of different immunoglobulins in the serum with approximate normal values is given in Table 2.

Cell-Mediated Immunity

When antigen is fixed in tissues, such as a solid tissue homograft, or is a modified part of the body's own tissues, such as areas of skin treated with a chemical sensitizing agent, the response is different from that of the humoral antibody production. In the former, small lymphocytes passing through tissues are sensitized in the periphery and pass down to the local lymph node where they enter the free area of the cortex between lymph follicles. In the process of proliferation, this area is enlarged to become known as the "paracortical area." The sensitized cells differen-

Table 2. *Comparison of Immunoglobulins in Serum*

	NORMAL RANGE (MG./100 ML.)	PERCENTAGE IMMUNOGLOBULINS IN SERUM
IgG	1240 (±220)	70–80
IgA	390 (±90)	5–25
IgM	120 (±35)	5–10
IgD	3 (±3)	0.2–1.0
IgE	0.05	0.002

tiate into large cells, reaching their peak concentration 3 to 4 days after sensitization, and then divide into a new population of lymphocytes, part of which are immunologically active and leave the local lymphatic tissue to proceed to other lymph nodes to continue propagation. The cell-mediated immune response is dependent upon the integrity of the thymus during embryonic and early neonatal life. If the thymus is removed experimentally in early neonatal life in mice or rats, cell-mediated immune responses will be unable to develop.

Reactions in tissues mediated by humoral antibodies are:

1. Passive sensitization (Prausnitz-Küstner reaction);
2. Anaphylactic antibodies
   a. Mild reactions, that is, conjunctivitis, rhinorrhea secondary to pollens, animal dander;
   b. Systemic anaphylaxis, that is, drug injection (penicillin), foreign sera, stinging insect;
   c. Blocking antibodies
      Desensitization of anaphylactic individuals by regular and repeated injections of antigen, which results in formation of blocking antibodies (IgG);
3. Arthus reaction—takes 2 to 8 hours to begin, lasts 12 to 24 hours; occurs in walls of small blood vessels as a result of antibody from the circulation, meeting antigen diffusing inward from the extravascular space; and
4. Serum sickness—reactions occurring are the result of IgG or IgM; however, if antibodies are mainly anaphylactic, IgE. The symptoms will be mainly anaphylactic because of reactions taking place on the cell surface.

CELL-MEDIATED IMMUNE REACTIONS (DELAYED HYPERSENSITIVITY). Once the individual is sensitized, it takes 24 to 48 hours for the reaction to develop on subsequent contact with the antigen. Reactions caused by cell-mediated immune response are:

1. Delayed hypersensitivity to heterologous serum proteins (foreign serum, that is, horse serum);
2. Delayed hypersensitivity to microbial antigen
   a. Tuberculin;
   b. Vaccinia—"reactions of immunity;"
   c. Diphtheria toxoid—"pseudo" Schick reaction;
   d. Fungal antigen—Coccidioidal mycosis, histoplasmosis;
   e. Protozoal antigens—Leishmaniasis (Montenegro test);
3. Insect bites;
4. Chemical contact sensitivity;
5. Homograft reaction; and
6. Skin reactions to homologous tissue in allergic autoimmune states.

Remembering that immunologic mechanisms are of the two previously mentioned types (cell-mediated and humoral antibody), deficiency states may involve either type alone or a combination of both. Also, cells involved in secreting one type of immunoglobulin can be involved without affecting the secretion of others. Finally, while the amount of immunoglobulins may not be affected, a qualitative defect may be present, reducing the body's effectiveness in controlling infection. As stated previously, defective immunologic mechanisms may be congenital and inherited or secondary.

In order to clarify some of the confusion regarding primary immune deficiencies, World Health Organization investigators proposed the following classification:[2]

1. Infantile x-linked agammaglobulinemia,
2. Selective immunoglobulin deficiency (IgA),
3. Transient hypogammaglobulinemia of infancy,
4. X-linked immunodeficiency with hyper-IgM,
5. Thymic hypoplasia (pharyngeal pouch syndrome, DiGeorge),
6. Episodic lymphopenia with lymphocytotoxin,
7. Immunodeficiency with normal or hyperimmunoglobulinemia,
8. Immunodeficiency with ataxia telangiectasia,
9. Immunodeficiency with thrombocytopenia and eczema (Wiskott-Aldrich),
10. Immunodeficiency with thymoma,
11. Immunodeficiency with short-limbed dwarfism,
12. Immunodeficiency with generalized hematopoietic hypoplasia,
13. Severe combined immunodeficiency (autosomal recessive, x-linked, sporadic),
14. Variable immunodeficiency (largely unclassified). This will become more widely accepted and understood as time passes. For the present, a brief discussion of congenital defects will be presented followed by a discussion of primary or secondary acquired deficiencies.

CONGENITAL DEFICIENCIES

Swiss-type agammaglobulinemia or combined immune deficiency syndrome is characterized by defects in both cell-mediated immunity and immunoglobulin synthesis. It can be either autosomal recessive or sex-linked to the X chromosome, in which case it is found only in men. Most of these patients are sick in the early months of life and die within the first 2 years. Generally there is absence of all the immunoglobulins, and the lymphocyte count is less than 1500 per cu. mm. Lymphoid tissue is virtually absent in the body. The thymus is underdeveloped, often weighing less than 1.0 gm., and is extremely difficult to find. These patients readily accept skin grafts and cannot be sensitized to produce contact sensitivity with 2,4 dinitrofluorobenzene (2,4 DNFB). They suffer repeated bacterial, viral, and fungal infections. Clinically these patients are far worse off than those with defective immunoglobulin synthesis, only because the latter group can deal with viral infections.

More than 100 cases have been described, with many names, including hereditary thymic dysplasia.[4] Intractable diarrhea with frequent Salmonella and enteropathic E. coli strains are found, together with thrush and morbilliform rash. Pneumonia caused by Pseudomonas or Penumocystis carinii is a frequent cause of death. Death has also resulted from generalized varicella, rubeola pneumonitis, and occasionally progressive, fatal vaccinia if vaccination is given.

Gamma globulin therapy is not helpful in these inevitably fatal situations, and attempts to restore immunologic competence with thymus graft and bone marrow transplants have uniformly failed. The pathogenesis of this disorder is believed to involve a deficient immunoblast stem cell line or absence of this cell type.

DEFECT IN IMMUNOGLOBULIN SYNTHESIS ONLY

This disorder, first described by Bruton in 1952, is found in boys and is inherited as an x-linked recessive characteristic. Afflicted individuals usually remain well during the first 9 months of life, being protected by maternal gamma globulin. Their susceptibility to infection becomes manifest during the second year of life, when circulating IgG is usually less than 100 mg. per 100 ml. While these boys do not have excessive susceptibility to common childhood viruses and exanthems, they do have frequent pyogenic infection with staphylococci, streptococci, pneumococci, and hemophilus influenzae, and fail to develop immune responses to diphtheria, pertussis, and tetanus toxoid. Anti-A and anti-B isohemagglutinin levels are low or absent. The ability to reject homografts and develop delayed hypersensitivity is retained. The sine qua non of this disease is failure to demonstrate plasma cells in lymph nodes stimulated with antigen. These patients are highly susceptible to disabling collagen disorders.

Patients with this entity usually reject skin grafts, and delayed reactions to mumps, candida, streptokinase-streptodornase, and 2,4 dinitrofluorobenzene develop. In vitro lymphocyte transformation and proliferation induced by phytohemagglutinin, allogeneic cells, and antigen to which the patient has previously been stimulated are normal.

DEFECT IN CELL-MEDIATED IMMUNITY ONLY

In this problem, thymic dysplasia, lymphoid tissue depletion, and lymphopenia are present; immunoglobulin levels, however, are normal. Patients are unable to reject skin homografts or to develop contact sensitivity to 2,4 DNFB. While they produce humoral antibodies there is probably a qualitative defect in these, since they are unable to cope with virtually any viral infection.

A variant of this problem, the DiGeorge's syndrome, is characterized by a defect in the third branchial arch with absence of the parathyroid glands as well as thymic dysplasia.

DYSGAMMAGLOBULINEMIAS

Partial defects in immunoglobulin synthesis have been described when one or more elements are lowered or absent. Most commonly found is a deficiency of IgA and IgG, with increased amounts of IgM. The condition is inherited as an x-linked phenomenon, and the patients are unduly susceptible to infection.

Another variant is deficiency of IgA and IgM with normal IgG. This is extremely rare and has many features in common with Wiskott-Aldrich syndrome to be discussed later.

Last, the isolated absence of IgA and normal IgG and IgM has been described. This occurs in a small portion of otherwise normal persons and is of no clinical significance. It has, however, been described in patients with nontropical sprue and steatorrhea.

Recently it has been shown that a group of patients with selective IgA deficiency and normal cellular immunity have a greater incidence of autoimmune diseases, especially rheumatoid arthritis, systemic lupus erythematosus, thyroiditis, and pernicious anemia.[1] Many of these patients had recurrent sinus and upper respiratory tract infections. Hence, a thorough investigation is in order in patients with selective IgA deficiency.

About 80 per cent of patients with hereditary ataxia-telangiectasia lack both serum and secretory IgA. Signs may begin in infancy, with choreoathetoid movements. This is followed by telangiectasias between 6 and 14 years of age which involve the conjunctivae and exposed body areas, such as the face, arms, and eyelids. Frequent and progressive infections of the sinuses, middle ear, and lungs appear, and death from respiratory infection or lymphoreticular malignancy is common. The relation between absent IgA levels and respiratory tract infections is unclear. Patients with this disorder frequently have a defect in cellular immunity.

Wiskott-Aldrich syndrome is an x-linked disease in which boys rarely survive to the second decade. It is characterized by eczema, thrombocytopenia, and frequent infections. Cellular immunity is defective and appears to be progressive. Serum IgG and IgA levels are normal, but IgM levels are low. Death usually ensues either from overwhelming infection or lymphoreticular malignancy. Presently, no rational explanation exists to unite the varying elements of this problem.

ACQUIRED DEFECTS OF THE IMMUNOLOGIC SYSTEM

Primary acquired hypogammaglobulinemia can be found in adults. Usually the level of circulating IgG is less than 500 mg. per 100 ml. It affects both men and women and is probably not inherited. Associated with this disorder are other immunologic disorders, such as systemic lupus erythematosus, hemolytic anemia, and thrombocytopenia. Steatorrhea is frequently found, as well as lymph nodes which usually reveal decreased plasma cells. Noncaseating granulomas of the lungs, spleen, liver, or skin are also found. This is the most common immune deficiency disease and is classified by the World Health Organization[2] as idiopathic hypogammaglobulinemia of variable duration. The incidence of malignancy is high in these patients, and one can speculate whether the malignancy causes the hypogammaglobulinemia or the latter the malignancy.

In the secondary acquired defects, low levels of immunoglobulins can occur in a number of other disease states, including those in which loss of serum protein is excessive, such as in exfoliative dermatitis and renal and gastrointestinal disorders. It frequently occurs in diseases of the reticuloendothelial systems, such as Hodgkin's disease, chronic lymphatic leukemia, and lymphosarcoma. The causes of secondary hypogammaglobulinemia[3] are:

1. *Physiologic* — both of these can be distinguished from hereditary hypogammaglobulinemia since levels of IgA and IgM are normal (premature babies, delayed maturity);

2. *Catabolic* — increased turnover of protein; affects IgG but not IgM or IgA (nephrotic syndrome, protein-losing enteropathy, malnutrition, dystrophia myotonia, thoracic duct fistula);

3. *Marrow disorders* — IgM antibodies present against IgG antigens (hypoplasia, bony metastases, myelosclerosis, paroxysmal nocturnal hemoglobinuria);

4. *Toxic factors* — renal failure, high levels of steroids, cytotoxic therapy, gluten-sensitive enteropathy (IgM deficiency), thyrotoxicosis, diabetes mellitus without proteinuria, after severe infections, and congenital heart disease.

Levels of immunoglobulins in the diseases listed here will vary according to stage and severity: primary reticuloendothelial tumors, reticulum cell sarcoma, mycosis fungoides, Hodgkin's disease, lymphosarcoma, giant follicular lymphoma, chronic lymphatic leukemia, thymoma, malignant paraproteinemia, and macroglobulinemia. Usually, the more severe the disease, the lower the values. One might prognosticate on the course if serial determinations of the immunoglobulin levels were available.

CELLULAR IMMUNITY AND NEOPLASIA

While immunoglobulin level determinations may be helpful in the previously mentioned disease states from a prognostic point of view, cellular immunity has been noted to be of significance in determining the degree of severity and magnitude of spread of neoplasia. One might take a familiar problem, for example, Hodgkin's disease. This is characterized by progressive loss of cellular immune response while humoral antibody production is normal or near normal. The immune defect is demonstrable early in the disease, even in patients with asymptomatic stage 1 disease. As the disease progresses, the defect becomes more severe, and patients with disseminated disease have loss of cellular immune activity which runs the spectrum of relative anergy and poor sensitization response to chemicals such as 2,4 DNFB to failure to become positive even during active tuberculosis and most severely to the inability to reject a skin transplant from an unrelated donor. In many patients in remission, delayed hypersensitivity responses are returned. This return may be rapid after a course of chemotherapy. It has been shown that among patients whose deficiency had progressed to loss of capacity for 2,4 DNFB sensitization, it usually took several months of remission before the response returned. Therefore, loss of cellular immunity in Hodgkin's disease is reversible, but at some point in the end stages of the disease, becomes irreversible.

The consequences of immunologic defects in Hodgkin's disease or in other neoplasia are obvious. These patients are susceptible to infections requiring cellular immune response for control, that is, tuberculosis, fungal infections, some gram-negative infections, and certain viral infections, such as herpes zoster.

The intimate relationship between cellular immunity and the course of the disease has led to the postulate that measurement of cellular immune reactivity could provide significant prognostic information. In a series of patients studied by Sokal,[6] patients with a tuberculin negative response were given bacille Calmette Guérin (BCG) vaccination when the disease was under control. Of 9 patients who failed to convert their response to second strength purified protein derivative (PPD), 7 died within a year of the BCG vaccination. However, only 1 of 32 patients who converted the tuberculin response died during this interval, and the median survival of the latter group was more than 3 years from the tests.

DIAGNOSIS OF DEFICIENCY STATES

As noted previously, many of the disease states mentioned will be suspected at an early age. In addition to detecting deficiencies, one might suspect, in the newborn, congenital infection from an elevated IgM level (cord serum) usually greater than 20 mg. per 100 ml. This indicates that the child has responded to antigenic stimulus by accelerated IgM synthesis, the levels being those of the child since no placental transfer of maternal IgM takes place. Elevated levels are usually seen in congenital syphilis, rubella, toxoplasmosis, and cytomegalic inclusion disease.

Clues to the presence of deficiency states are frequent infections, diarrhea, failure to thrive, and so forth. Initial studies (Table 3) should

Table 3. *Studies to Diagnose Immunologic Deficiency Syndromes*

Humoral deficiency
  Schick test
  Total gammaglobulin level
  Isoagglutinin titers of anti-A or anti-B
  Quantitative immunoglobulin determination
  Recurrent severe bacterial infections

Cell-mediated deficiency
  Lymphopenia
  Severe viral infections
  Skin tests: Negative (PPD, histoplasmin,
        Coccidioides immitis blastomycosis,
        streptokinase-streptodornase)
    2,4 dinitrofluorobenzene skin test – no
        response after sensitization dose

include a Schick test which measures IgG neutralizing antibody to diphtheria toxin and should be negative after one or two diphtheria immunizations. Determination of total gamma globulin level by paper electrophoresis can be performed, and gamma globulin levels should be more than 400 mg. per 100 ml. or within two standard deviations of age-matched controls. Saline isoagglutinin titers of anti-A or anti-B or both are a measure of IgM antibodies. Titers should be more than 1 to 4 to A or B erythrocytes or both (depending on ABO blood groups) by 6 months and higher by 1 year. Except for the patient with AB blood type, low or absent isoagglutinin titers indicate poor IgM function.

If any of the preceding screening tests are abnormal, quantitative immunoglobulin determination is indicated. Measurement of IgA, IgG, and IgM can be performed with commercially available agar radial diffusion kits. Values are determined in per 100 milliliters and compared with age-matched controls. While IgE can now be measured also, its level is not significant in the deficiency states. If the immunoglobulins are abnormal, further evaluation of the immunologic abnormality is indicated before gamma globulin or other therapy is started.

Evaluation of cell-mediated deficiency should include skin tests for tuberculosis, histoplasmin, coccidioidin, blastomycin, mumps, and candida. Typically, these will show no delayed skin reaction. Phytohemmagglutination activity will show no stimulation of culture lymphocytes, and the absolute lymphocyte count is usually <1500 per cc. Poor sensitization response to 2,4 DNFB is also seen.

TREATMENT

In the combined form of immunologic deficiency, cell-mediated as well as immunoglobulin deficiency, gamma globulin therapy is of no help, and the process progresses to its inevitably fatal outcome. Restoration of immunologic competence has been attempted by thymus grafts, bone marrow transplants, and so forth, but has uniformly failed.

However, in contrast, those patients with congenital or acquired hypogammaglobulinemia have been helped with doses of gamma globulin. The effective prophylactic dose is empirical. Bacterial infection can often be prevented by raising the level 200 mg. per 100 ml. A loading dose in a newly diagnosed patient of 1.8 ml. per kg. of body weight in three divided doses (0.6 ml. or 100 mg. per kilogram of body weight) is given. The half-life of gamma globulin is about 1 month, and the initial boost raises serum concentration by about 300 mg. per 100 ml.; therefore, a monthly injection of 0.6 ml. (100 mg.) per kilogram of body weight is needed to maintain the approximate 200 mg. per 100 ml. serum level.[5] Antibiotic therapy is given only for specific infections.

Caution must be taken not to give gamma globulin intravenously since severe pyrogenic and cardiovascular reactions can take place. Injections have been given patients for many years without isosensitization. The severe reaction with intravenously administered gamma globulin has been attributed to aggregation of small amounts of globulin during preparation of the product. Commercially prepared gamma globulin usually contains trace amounts of IgA and IgM and is made from a pool of donor plasmas so that antibodies to many infectious agents will be present in adequate titer. The injections are given at multiple sites so that not more than 5.0 cc. is given at any one site.

SUMMARY

A brief review of the congenital and acquired forms of immunologic deficiency disorders shows that if a high index of suspicion is present, means are now available for the diagnosis and treatment of these disorders. While combined deficit disease is uniformly fatal, those with immunoglobulin deficiency can only be protected with periodic use of gamma globulin and appropriately selected antibiotics as the situation demands.

REFERENCES

1. Amman, A. J., and Hong, R.: Selective IgA deficiency: presentation of 30 cases and a review of the literature. Medicine 50:223–236 (May) 1971.
2. Fudenberg, H. H., Good, R. A., Hitzig, W., et al.: Classification of the primary immune deficiencies: WHO recommendation. New Eng. J. Med., 283:656–657 (Sept. 17) 1970.
3. Hobbs, J. R.: Disturbances of the immunoglobulins. Sci. Basis Med. Ann. Rev., 106–127, 1966.
4. Hoyer, J. R., Cooper, M. D., Gabrielsen, A. E., et al.: Lymphopenic forms of congenital immunologic deficiency diseases. Medicine 47:201–226 (May) 1968.
5. Medical Research Council Working-Party: Hypogammaglobulinemia in the United Kingdom. Lancet 1:163–168 (Jan. 25) 1969.
6. Sokol, J. E., and Aungst, C. W.: Response to BCG vaccination and survival in advanced Hodgkin's disease. Cancer 24:128–134 (July) 1969.

SELECTED REFERENCES

1. Holborow, E. J.: An ABC of Modern Immunology. Boston, Little, Brown and Company, 1968, 89 pp.
2. Samter, M. (ed.): Immunological Diseases. Boston, Little, Brown and Company, 1971, 966 pp.
3. Stiehm, E. R.: The gamma globulins. Brennemann's Practice of Pediatrics. Harper and Row Publishers, Inc., 1970, Vol. 2, Chap. 1B, pp. 1–9.
4. Turk, J. L.: Immunology in Clinical Medicine. New York, Appleton-Century-Crofts, 1969, 226 pp.

605 Commonwealth Avenue
Boston, Massachusetts 02215

Management of Patients with Chronic Obstructive Jaundice

Victor M. Rosenoer, M.D., and Gualberto Gokim, Jr., M.D.

The clinical syndrome of obstructive jaundice develops when bile, having passed through the hepatic cells, fails to be excreted by way of the biliary system into the duodenum. The sequelae may be considered in terms of the "forward failure" phenomena, the diminished excretion of bile salts into the intestinal lumen leading to failure of dietary fat absorption with the ensuing steatorrhea and malabsorption of fat-soluble vitamins and calcium, and in terms of the "backward failure" phenomena leading progressively to the fully developed picture of biliary cirrhosis with late portal hypertension and eventually hepatocellular failure.

ETIOLOGIC FACTORS

The causes of chronic obstructive jaundice persisting for more than 6 months are somewhat limited. Most commonly, *sclerosing cholangitis* occurs owing to prolonged extrahepatic obstruction from stones, to traumatic postoperative biliary stricture, or occasionally to a slowly growing primary hepatic duct carcinoma with infection of the dilated biliary tree. The intrahepatic bile ducts undergo progressive sclerosis. A predominantly polymorphonuclear inflammatory reaction surrounds the duct and infiltrates the wall. The annular sclerosis continues to advance slowly, presumably in relation to the direct effect of the gram-negative infection of the cholangiole together with the retention of toxic bile acids which excite a periductal reaction. *Primary sclerosing cholangitis* is far less common and in the majority of cases complicates long-standing ulcerative colitis. The histologic features are nonspecific, with chronic inflammation of the intrahepatic and extrahepatic ducts. Lymphoid aggregates, polymorphonuclear infiltration, and occasionally, eosinophils, are prominent. Pericholangiolar and peribiliary fibrosis develops. *Chronic nonsuppurative destructive cholangitis* (primary biliary cirrhosis) usually occurs in women 30 to 60 years of age and presents with pruritus followed by cholestatic jaundice of varying intensity, progressing insidiously over the succeeding 3 to 7 years. The septal and interlobular bile ducts are surrounded by a mononuclear reaction, the ductal epithelium being distorted and necrotic. Later, portal zone fibrosis becomes prominent and the bile ductules finally disappear. The last stage of all these cholangitides is biliary cirrhosis with the nodular regeneration essential for its diagnosis.

Biliary atresia will also lead to chronic obstructive jaundice, and when the ductules and interlobular ducts are involved, a picture resembling primary biliary cirrhosis can be produced. *The cholestatic reaction to drugs,* most commonly the phenothiazines, is usually acute and transient. Rarely, the cholestatic picture continues for many months. Read et al.[38] have reported persistence of the jaundice for as long as 3 years. In these cases initial hepatocellular damage disappeared, but the portal zones expanded with aggressive fibrosis and bile duct proliferation. Although recovery is usual, portal hypertension[31] and permanent biliary cirrhosis[54] have been reported.

NUTRITIONAL PROBLEMS

The general treatment in patients with chronic obstructive jaundice is particularly concerned with the control of the undesirable effects which follow the deficiency of bile salts in the intestine. The chief function of bile salts in fat absorption is now considered to be the molecular dispersion of the products of pancreatic lipolysis into a micellar phase in which the polymolecular aggregates of bile salts (micelles) incorporate less soluble or insoluble fatty acids and monoglycerides into their structure to form mixed micelles – slightly larger than the simple bile salt micelles but small enough to give clear solutions. The mixed bile salt-monoglyceride-fatty acid micelle appears to be an important transport phase for the passage of water-insoluble products of pancreatic lipolysis into the mucosal cell.

Conjugated bile salts enhance the activity of pancreatic lipase in triglyceride hydrolysis,[12] but they do not affect the activities of certain nonlipolytic digestive enzymes such as trypsin, chymotrypsin, amylase, and ribonuclease.[27] The transport of glucose or the incorporation of glucose into triglyceride or acetate into lipids is not affected by bile salts.[36] The intestinal uptake and esterification of palmitate[11] and of oleate[44] is increased by conjugated bile salts. A specific cholic acid-enzyme complex appears to exist for cholesterol esterification and absorption in which the esterase requires cholic acid or its conjugates, not only for significant activity but also to protect itself against the action of proteolytic enzymes.[53]

The lipid-soluble vitamins A, D, and K are almost completely dependent on the action of bile to facilitate their absorption. The uptake and central cleavage of carotene into two molecules of retinol (vitamin A aldehyde) requires bile salts,[15, 34] as does the absorption of vitamin D[16] and vitamin K.[37]

Calcium absorption is impaired in the absence of bile salts. Insoluble calcium soaps of unabsorbed fatty acid form in the intestinal lumen, thus making dietary calcium unavailable for absorption.[21] Bile salts enhance the solubility of calcium salts in lipid solvents in approximately the same proportion as they increase calcium absorption from the intestine, possibly by forming a calcium complex which diffuses more rapidly through the cell wall.[56]

The clinical consequences of the failure of bile salts to reach the intestinal lumen are clear. Steatorrhea develops and if jaundice is considered an indicator of the degree of cholestasis and of the failure of bile salt excretion, an inverse correlation exists between serum bilirubin values and the percentage of dietary fat absorbed. The stools are frequent, loose, bulky, and offensive. The patient loses weight, with an average fecal fat loss of 10 gm. a day on a dietary intake of 70 gm. of fat a day.[10, 51] Vitamin A deficiency rarely reaches clinical significance, although failure of dark adaptation occasionally develops in patients who have suffered from cholestasis for many years and who have never been given parenteral vitamin A supplements. Deficiency of vitamin K — required for the hepatic synthesis of prothrombin, factor VII and factor X — is commonly of clinical importance but is easily corrected. The problem of vitamin D and calcium deficiency in chronic cholestasis is, however, complex. Atkinson et al.[2] reported bone disease in patients with prolonged biliary obstruction and biliary cirrhosis. Osteomalacia with wide osteoid seams and osteoporosis with thinning of the bone trabeculae were both present. Of 25 patients studied, 7 had osteomalacia, 3 appeared to be suffering from osteoporosis, and 2 patients had both conditions. Bone pain was present in 5 patients. These patients, and 1 who had no bone pain, had a severe kyphosis. Spontaneous fractures occurred in 2 patients with osteomalacia and in 2 with osteomalacia and osteoporosis. Thoracic kyphosis with vertebral compression was seen in 2 patients with osteoporosis.

Ideally, the defect in fat digestion and vitamin and mineral absorption should be corrected by feeding adequate amounts of bile salts by mouth. Unfortunately, commercial preparations of human bile salts are not available. Animal preparations contain large amounts of unconjugated bile salts which are irritant to the bowel. Not only are they nauseating to ingest but they provoke diarrhea. Enteric-coated capsules tend to pass directly into the feces and are of little value.

In view of these problems, the nutritional approach is supplemental. A low neutral fat diet of about 30 gm. reduces the troublesome steatorrhea. Additional fats should be given as medium-chain triglycerides (octanoic to decanoic acids) prepared from coconut oil which are easily hydrolyzed in the absence of pancreatic lipase and are absorbed principally by way of the portal vein in the absence of bile salts. Linscheer et al.[26] have shown that they are absorbed in patients with cirrhosis and steatorrhea at the same rate as in normal subjects. Medium-chain triglycerides are of value in the treatment of patients with biliary steatorrhea.[6, 18]

Vitamin A deficiency is preventable by the administration of intramuscular injections of vitamin A, 100,000 I.U. monthly, while vitamin K deficiency is corrected readily by vitamin K1, 10 mg. intramuscularly daily for 7 days and thereafter 10 mg. intramuscularly monthly. The dose of vitamin D required is uncertain: 100,000 I.U. intramuscularly every 4 weeks has been shown to be effective but is greater than that required to correct nutritional vitamin D deficiencies, and it is possible that smaller doses might suffice.

Calcium supplementation is difficult, as the absorption of orally administered calcium salts is unpredictable while parenterally administered calcium supplements have marked side-effects when given in therapeutic doses. Medium-chain triglycerides may stimulate the calcium absorption while, at least in rats with a ligated common bile duct, olive oil may depress calcium absorption.[21] This suggests that low dietary neutral fats and supplemental medium-chain triglycerides with calcium between meals may be the optimal approach. The form in which the calcium supplement is given— as an effervescent calcium gluconate tablet or as an elixir of calcium glubionate (Neo-Calglucon)—deserves further study.

The recent progress in intracaval hyperalimentation provides yet another approach in the cachectic patient with chronic cholestasis and certainly should be considered if surgery is required. The technique consists of the intracaval infusion of a high caloric, hyperosmolar solution containing approximately 25 per cent glucose and 6.8 gm. of nitrogen as amino acids and peptides together with most of the essential vitamins and minerals (Table 1). After a cautious start with 1 to 2 liters per 24 hours to allow adaptation to the higher levels of carbohydrate, the infusion can be increased to 3 liters or even 4 liters a day (1000 calories per liter). Careful attention must be paid to the blood glucose concentration, especially in the diabetic patient. Hyperosmotic nonketotic coma has been reported, characterized by a depressed neurologic state, dehydration and blood glucose levels ranging from 500 to 1500 mg. per 100 ml. In most patients, however, blood glucose levels rarely are greater than 350 mg. per 100 ml. Above this level, the infusion should be slowed, and insulin should be used. With the usual attention to the central venous pressure, fluid overload is rarely a problem if renal function is adequate.

The most serious complications, septicemia and Candida fungemia, are best avoided by scrupulous care of the catheter. Should sepsis develop, the catheter should be removed and specific antibiotic therapy begun. Clearly, in the face of clinically obvious hepatic decompensation with fluid retention and incipient coma, intracaval alimentation will be approached with extreme caution especially with regard to the amino acid and sodium content of the infusion fluid.

RETENTION PROBLEMS

Pruritus is one of the most distressing symptoms of chronic cholestasis and has been related to the increased bile salt concentration in the blood and skin. Schoenfield et al.[47] demonstrated higher concentrations of bile salts in the skin of patients who itched than in those who did not. A reduction in the high skin bile salt concentrations in these patients, by relief of the obstruction, relieved the pruritus.

Table 1. *Preparation of Hyperalimentation Solution*

Single Unit Method
    500 ml. 50 per cent glucose added to
    500 ml. 10 per cent enzymatic casein hydrolysate (Hyprotigen, McGaw)

Volume	1,000 ml.
Calories	1,000 k cal.
Glucose	250 gm.
Casein hydrolysate	58 gm.
Nitrogen	
As free amino acids	4.1 gm.
As peptides	2.7 gm.
Sodium	25 mEq.
Potassium	18 mEq.
Calcium	5 mEq.
Magnesium	2 mEq.
Chloride	18 mEq.
Phosphate	25 mEq.

Electrolyte Additives to each Unit (According to Patient's Needs)
    Sodium (⅔ chloride to

⅓ bicarbonate)	25 mEq.
Potassium chloride	20 mEq.
Magnesium	2 mEq.
Calcium gluconate	4 mEq.

Vitamin Additives — Usually to First Unit each Day

Vitamin A	10,000 USP units	
Vitamin D (ergocalciferol)	1,000 USP units	
Ascorbic acid	500 mg.	
Thiamine hydrochloride	50 mg.	As 10 ml. multivitamin infu-
Riboflavin	10 mg.	sion, USV Pharmaceutical
Pyridoxine	15 mg.	Corporation
Niacinamide	100 mg.	
Dexpanthenol	25 mg.	
Vitamin E	5 I.U.	
Folic acid	1 mg.	
Vitamin B_{12}	10 μg.	
Phytonadione	1 mg.	

If the biliary obstruction is partial, pruritus can be relieved by the use of the anion exchange resin cholestyramine which exchanges chloride for bile acids. Serum bile salt concentrations fall and pruritus ceases when the serum bile salt concentrations approach normal levels. When cholestyramine is withheld, high serum concentrations are reached before pruritus begins. The lag period (one or more days) probably represents the time required for concentrations of bile salts sufficient to cause pruritus to accumulate in or leave the skin.[7]

The treatment is effective in the majority of patients with partial biliary obstruction. Datta and Sherlock[10] reported that 23 of 27 patients with chronic cholestasis were totally or partially relieved of pruritus. The optimal dose is uncertain: 12 gm. a day has been recommended although 6 gm. a day has been proved effective. Unfortunately, cholestyramine will increase the fecal fat loss,[10] while Gallo et al.[13] have demonstrated that cholestyramine impairs the absorption of digitoxin, aspirin, secobarbital, and phenylbutazone in animals. Northcutt et al.[33] found that the absorption of orally administered thyroxine and triiodothyronine is prevented by the ion exchange resin. Thus, care must be taken in the timing of drug administration in patients taking cholestyramine. At least 30 minutes should elapse after the drug is taken before the dose of cholestyramine is ingested.

If the biliary obstruction is complete, cholestyramine therapy will be ineffective since no bile salts reach the intestine. In this case pruritus is controlled by orally administered methyltestosterone, 25 mg. daily, in men, or by orally administered norethandrolone, 30 mg. daily, in women. Although these anabolic steroids may increase the jaundice—this is a dose-dependent phenomenon and probably will occur if the dose is sufficiently high in all normal persons so exposed—partial or complete relief of pruritus is usually obtained. In addition, the anabolic effect may be of value in slowing the development of osteoporosis in these patients.

It has been mentioned earlier that retention of bile salts may have an injurious effect on the liver. Javitt[19] showed that lithocholic acid which is formed in the intestine by bacterial 7 α dehydroxylation of chenodesoxycholic acid can cause cholestasis. In experimental animals, portal tract inflammation with hepatic ductular proliferation is produced and gallstones may develop.[35, 59] Carey et al.[8] have shown that raised serum lithocholic acid levels in patients with liver disease may be reduced by feeding neomycin which reduces the intestinal bacterial synthesis of lithocholic acid. Sharp et al.[50] reported improved liver function in children with a paucity of intrahepatic ducts but without cirrhosis or inflammatory changes in the liver receiving treatment with cholestyramine. In 3 of these patients, all previous abnormal liver function tests, apart from the alkaline phosphatase, returned to normal levels. The growth rates returned to normal levels when the serum bile salt concentrations were maintained at normal levels. However, Schaffner et al.[45] and Datta and Sherlock[10] noted no significant changes in liver function in adults with prolonged obstructive jaundice treated by long-term cholestyramine feeding.

Recently Smallwood et al.[52] have estimated the liver-copper concentrations in 95 patients with liver disease by neutron activation analysis of liver samples. The normal range was found to be 15 to 55 mcg. copper per gm. of dry liver. Levels of greater than 250 mcg. per gm. of dry liver were found only in Wilson's disease and long-standing intrahepatic (as in primary biliary cirrhosis) and extrahepatic biliary obstruction. No diagnostic confusion existed between these two groups of patients as those with biliary obstruction and high liver-copper levels had definite clinical and biochemical features of cholestasis. In the patient with biliary obstruction, the liver-copper level was related to the duration of symptoms. In other liver diseases, liver-copper levels were normal or only moderately increased. Since copper is mainly excreted in the bile,[4, 28, 32, 43] the high copper concentrations in chronic cholestasis would appear to be accounted for simply by failure of biliary excretion. If the high copper content of the liver in Wilson's disease is instrumental in producing cirrhosis and liver cell failure, then copper could play a role in the pathogenesis of liver cell failure in biliary cirrhosis.

Hunt et al.[17] treated two patients with primary biliary cirrhosis with penicillamine (the copper chelating agent) without noticeable benefit. However, they were patients with advanced disease with presumably irreversible liver damage, and a more extensive trial of penicillamine is warranted in chronic cholestasis. Any therapeutic trial of penicillamine should be controlled carefully, particularly in view of the variable course of chronic cholestasis (from whatever cause) and the different stages at which it is diagnosed. Unless the therapeutic effect was dramatic, the comparative rarity of this disease might require a trial extending over many years to allow any definite conclusions to be drawn. Penicillamine therapy is not entirely without hazard.[3, 46, 55] However, experience with penicillamine in Wilson's disease has been good, and penicillamine may well offer an approach to the prevention of liver failure in long-standing biliary obstruction.

DRUG ADMINISTRATION

The liver is important in the metabolism of foreign compounds and the duration and intensity of the action of many drugs are increased in some patients with liver disease.

Drug metabolism can be considered as a two-phase process. In the first phase the compound is oxidized, reduced, or hydrolyzed by the drug metabolizing enzymes of the hepatic smooth endoplasmic reticulum. A biologically active compound may be inactivated or an inactive compound may be transformed into an active metabolite in this phase. In the second phase, compounds are inactivated by conjugation reactions – glucuronide formation, methylation, acylation, mercapturic acid formation, or sulfate formation. In general, the products of the first phase tend to be polar (water-soluble) and those of the second phase even more polar. Highly polar compounds tend not to be metabolized, in part at least as a result of their inaccessibility to the liposoluble sites of the lipid layers of the smooth endoplasmic reticulum to which the drug metabolizing enzymes are attached.

The more polar compounds inactivated by conjugation are excreted either by the kidney or by way of the bile. Compounds with molecular weights greater than 200 tend to be excreted into the bile in amounts which increase with increasing molecular weight. An appropriately located polar group and the ability of the drug to form a conjugate, such as glucuronide, enhance the probability of its biliary excretion.[57]

The efficacy of drug metabolism in the liver is impaired in starvation,[20] or if animals receive a calorically sufficient but protein-free diet.[49] Clearly, this is of importance in the therapy of undernourished patients. However, the degree of individual variation in normally nourished patients may outweigh these effects. For example, the plasma half-life of diphenylhydantoin in epileptic subjects may vary between 8 and 50 hours. Remmer[40] reported that the plasma level in 50 patients receiving the recommended standard dose of 300 mg. daily varied from 4 to 60 mcg. per ml. It must be noted that below a plasma concentration of 10 mcg. per ml., diphenylhydantoin exerts no significant antiepileptic action, whereas toxic side-effects appear if levels above 20 mcg. per ml. are achieved. The rate-limiting step in diphenylhydantoin metabolism is the extremely slow hepatic hydrolysis of the drug.

A great variety of lipid-soluble drugs increase their own metabolism and the metabolism of compounds not related chemically or pharmacologically by inducing new synthesis of the drug hydroxylating system in the endoplasmic reticulum of the liver.[9] This nonspecific phenomenon can be regarded as an adaptive process to protect the organism against the overload of foreign compounds. About 200 compounds have been shown to induce these enzymes.

Enzyme induction by phenobarbital and other drugs has been used clinically to increase the activity of glucuronyl transferase in patients with severe congenital unconjugated hyperbilirubinemia and neonatal jaundice. In liver failure the activity of the hydroxylase system is probably decreased, but Levi et al.[25] have shown that even in the failing liver many drugs may stimulate the synthesis of microsomal drug metabolizing enzymes. However, since induction takes several days to develop, some drugs may still have an exaggerated effect, at least initially.

The study by Rubin et al.[42] on the effect of acute ethanol intoxication on drug metabolism is of great interest. Whereas chronic ingestion of ethanol induces hepatic microsomal drug metabolizing enzymes in both rats and man, with a concomitant increase in drug clearance from the blood, acute ethanol intoxication leads to increased sensitivity to the effects of barbiturates and tranquilizers. This is the result of the inhibition of the hepatic microsomal drug-metabolizing enzymes and explains in part the heightened sensitivity of inebriated persons to the effects of certain drugs.

Liver failure may be associated with impaired functions of other organs such as the kidneys or the brain, as in hepatic encephalopathy. In this situation altered responsiveness to drugs may have complex causes. For example, short-acting barbiturates and opiates can precipitate hepatic coma in patients with liver disease. Laidlaw et al.[24] reported that an injection of morphine, 8 mg., produces pathologic electroencephalographic changes in patients with a history of encephalopathy whereas patients with cirrhosis alone respond like normal subjects. The susceptibility to morphine is further increased by the addition of protein to the diet and decreased by the administration of neomycin. More recently Read et al.[39] reported that patients with cirrhosis were extremely sensitive to chlorpromazine; an oral dose of as little as 1 mg. per kilogram of body weight slowed the electroencephalogram for many hours. Patients with the most definite electroencephalographic changes were in general very sleepy and took several hours to recover. Although it was not possible to demonstrate impaired clearance of chlorpromazine from the blood in these patients, and the basal arterial ammonia concentration was not altered by the drug, the response to an oral ammonia load was modified. The 45 minute and 90 minute postload values were higher in chlorpromazine-treated patients. In this context Ritchie and Shead[41] have shown diminished removal of ammonia by the liver in dogs after an injection of morphine.

In general it may be stated that sedative drugs should be avoided if possible in patients with liver disease. Chloral hydrate is first converted to the active metabolite trichloroethanol in the liver, which is subsequently inactivated. Its effect in patients with liver disease is therefore difficult to predict. Patients with impaired liver functions are particularly susceptible to paraldehyde which, although in part excreted in the breath, is also metabolized in the liver. If sedation is required, phenobarbital has the advantage that it is excreted mainly by the kidneys. Chlordiazepoxide (Librium) or diazepam (Valium) can also be used in the treatment of convulsions but should be used cautiously.

The treatment of fluid retention associated with cirrhosis is difficult because excessive diuretic therapy can precipitate hepatic coma by increasing the ammonia concentration in the renal veins by causing hypokalemic alkalosis and by helping in the development of a dilutional hyponatremia. Restriction of the sodium intake to 10 to 20 mEq. daily will limit the need for a diuretic, but should it prove necessary, a thiazide together with spironolactone is a suitable combination. If this fails, furosemide with spironolactone or ethacrynic acid with spironolactone can be tried. Initially the dose should be small, and the serum electrolytes should be checked daily. Weight loss from diuresis should not exceed 0.5 kg. daily if problems are to be avoided. Potassium chloride should be given to prevent the development of hypokalemic hypochloremic alkalosis.

Cholestasis, produced in mice by bile duct ligation or by phenylisothiocyanate or alpha-naphthylisothiocyanate treatment, increases the lethality in mice of a number of drugs[5, 14] including ouabain, promazine, perphenazine, and meprobamate. The toxicity of chlorpromazine and phenobarbital was unaltered, while the toxicity of pentobarbital was reduced. Lahiri et al.[23] demonstrated that the LD 50 of a single intravenous dose of actinomycin D is significantly lower in rats subjected to bile duct ligation or to 70 per cent hepatectomy than in normal or sham-operated control animals; the enhanced toxicity following partial hepatectomy was paralleled by the impaired biliary excretion of tritiated actinomycin D.

These results underline the marked enhancement in the clinical toxicity of actinomycin D reported in children who have undergone hepatic lobectomy for the management of metastatic Wilms' tumor. A similar problem of enhanced toxicity is encountered when vincristine is administered to patients with obstructive jaundice. In animals, the vinca alkaloids appear to be excreted primarily by the liver into the biliary system. However, it must be stressed at this point that the results obtained in animal studies, while enjoining caution, cannot be transferred quantitatively to the clinic. Not only are there quantitative differences in drug metabolizing enzymes in different species but qualitative species variations make any prediction of the fate of a compound in man hazardous.[58] The speed and type of oxidation may vary considerably, and the metabolites formed may not be the same, because species hydroxylate preferentially at different sites of the drug molecule.

Liver function does not appear to be a critical factor in the handling of most antibacterial antibiotics, although the plasma half-life of chloramphenicol and rifamycin is prolonged in patients with cirrhosis.[1, 22] Antibiotics may be of value in managing the sclerosing cholangitis associated with prolonged choledocholithiasis, stricture, or primary sclerosing cholangitis. Tetracycline, ampicillin or rifamycin SV may be given at the beginning of a febrile attack — usually associated with a gram-negative septicemia. Prolonged prophylaxis has not been recommended as bacterial resistance develops, and long-term antibiotic therapy in patients with the hepatobiliary complications of ulcerative colitis has been shown to be ineffective.[30]

However, the bacterial population of infected bile can be enormous and can produce effects in the small intestine paralleling those following the infection of the small bowel in the "blind loop" syndrome — bacterial deconjugation of bile salts and impaired vitamin B_{12} absorption.[48] These results emphasize the importance of the control of bacterial cholangitis by surgical drainage and by antibiotics. If the patients have a positive vitamin B_{12} absorption test (Schilling test), supplemental parenteral vitamin B_{12} might be of value.

The place of immunosuppressant therapy in the treatment of chronic obstructive jaundice with immunologic disturbances has not been established. Corticosteroid therapy is of no value in the treatment of chronic chlorpromazine-induced jaundice. In primary sclerosing cholangitis it is of dubious value. In primary biliary cirrhosis, where the immunologic disturbance is demonstrably greater, corticosteroids and azathioprine have been used. However, without a controlled trial in a large number of patients over a prolonged period, definite conclusions cannot be drawn. Since most corticosteroids are metabolized in the liver, and since patients with cirrhosis and impaired liver function clear injected radioactive cortisol from the blood more slowly than normal, signs of hypercorticism, especially exacerbation of osteoporosis, may be anticipated even on relatively small doses. Azathioprine is a known hepatotoxin although Mistilis and Blackburn[29] reported that its toxic effects are largely avoided if the dose does not exceed 1.5 mg. per kg. of body weight daily.

REFERENCES

1. Acocella, G., Barion, G. C., and Muschio, R.: [Absorption and elimination of rifamycin SV in intramuscular administration.] G. Mal Infett., *14*:552–555 (Sept.) 1962.
2. Atkinson, M., Nordin, B. E. C., and Sherlock, S.: Malabsorption and bone disease in prolonged obstructive jaundice. Quart. J. Med., 25:299–312 (July) 1956.
3. Bearn, A. G.: Wilson's disease. *In* Stanbury, J. B., Wyngaarden, J. B., and Fredrickson, D. S. (eds.): The Metabolic Basis of Inherited Disease. New York, McGraw-Hill Book Co., 1966, 2nd ed., pp. 761–779.
4. Bearn, A. G., and Kunkel, H. G.: Metabolic studies in Wilson's disease using Cu_{64}. J. Lab. Clin. Med., 45:623–631 (April) 1955.
5. Becker, B. A., Hindman, K. L., and Gibson, J. E.: Enhanced mortality of selected central nervous system depressants in hypoexcretory mice. J. Pharm. Sci., 57:1010–1012 (June) 1968.

6. Burke, V , and Danks, D. M.: Medium-chain triglyceride diet: its use in treatment of liver disease. Brit. Med. J., 2:1050–1051 (Oct. 29) 1966.
7. Carey, J. B., Jr., and Williams, G.: Relief of the pruritus of jaundice with a bile-acid sequestering resin. J.A.M.A., 176:432–435 (May 6) 1961.
8. Carey, J. B., Jr., Wilson, I. D., Zaki, F. G., et al.: The metabolism of bile acids with special reference to liver injury. Medicine, 45:461–470 (Nov.) 1966.
9. Conney, A. H.: Pharmacological implications of microsomal enzyme induction. Pharmacol. Rev., 19:317–366 (Sept.) 1967.
10. Datta, D. V., and Sherlock, S.: Cholestyramine for long term relief of the pruritus complicating intraheptic cholestasis. Gastroenterology, 50:323–332 (March) 1966.
11. Dawson, A. M., and Isselbacher, K. J.: Studies on lipid metabolism in the small intestine with observations on the role of bile salts. J. Clin. Invest., 39:730–740 (May) 1960.
12. Desnuelle, P.: Pancreatic lipase. Advances Enzymol., 23:129–161, 1961.
13. Gallo, D. G., Bailey, K. R., and Sheffner, A. L.: The interaction between cholestyramine and drug. Proc. Soc. Exper. Biol. Med., 120:60–65 (Oct.) 1965.
14. Gibson, J. E., and Becker, B. A.: Demonstration of enhanced lethality of drugs in hypoexcretory animals. J. Pharm. Sci., 56:1503–1505 (Nov.) 1967.
15. Goodman, D. S., and Huang, H. S.: Biosynthesis of vitamin A with rat intestinal enzymes. Science, 149:879–880 (Aug. 20) 1965.
16. Greaves, J. D., and Schmidt, C. L. A.: The role played by bile in the absorption of vitamin D in the rat. J. Biol. Chem., 102:101–112 (Sept.) 1933.
17. Hunt, A. H., Parr, R. M., Taylor, D. M., et al.: Relation between cirrhosis and trace metal content of liver with special reference to primary biliary cirrhosis and copper. Brit. Med. J., 2:1498–1501 (Dec. 14) 1963.
18. Iber, F. L., Hardoon, E., and Sangree, M. H.: Use of eight and ten carbon fatty acids as neutral fat in the management of steatorrhea. Abstract. Clin. Res., 11:185 (April) 1963.
19. Javitt, N. B.: An experimental model for the study of cholestasis. Abstract. Gastroenterology, 50:394–395 (March) 1966.
20. Kato, R., and Gillette, J. R.: Effect of starvation on NADPH-dependent enzymes in liver microsomes of male and female rats. J. Pharmacol. Exper. Ther., 150:279–284 (Nov.) 1965.
21. Kehayoglou, A. K., Williams, H. S., Whimster, W. F., and Holdsworth, C. D.: Calcium absorption in the normal, bile-duct ligated, and cirrhotic rat, with observations on the effect of long- and medium-chain triglycerides. Gut, 9:597–603 (Oct.) 1968.
22. Kunin, C. M., Glazko, A. J., and Finland, M.: Persistence of antibiotics in blood of patients with acute renal failure. II. Chloramphenicol and its metabolic products in the blood of patients with severe renal disease or hepatic cirrhosis. J. Clin. Invest., 38:1498–1508 (Sept.) 1959.
23. Lahiri, S. R., Bolton, N., Brown, B. L., and Rosenoer, V. M.: The role of the liver in actinomycin-D metabolism. Abstract. Gastroenterology, 58:1021 (June) 1970.
24. Laidlaw, J., Read, A. E., and Sherlock, S.: Morphine tolerance in hepatic cirrhosis. Gastroenterology, 40:389–396 (March) 1961.
25. Levi, A. J., Sherlock, S., and Walker, D.: Phenylbutazone and isoniazid metabolism in patients with liver disease in relation to previous drug therapy. Lancet, 1:1275–1279 (June 15) 1968.
26. Linscheer, W. G., Patterson, J. F., Moore, E. W., et al.: Medium and long chain fat absorption in patients with cirrhosis. J. Clin. Invest., 45:1317–1325 (Aug.) 1966.
27. Lippel, K., and Olson, J. A.: The activity of non-lipolytic digestive enzymes of the pancreas in the presence of conjugated bile salts. Biochem. Biophys. Acta, 127:243–245 (Sept. 26) 1966.
28. Mahoney, J. P. and others: Studies on copper metabolism; excretion of copper by animals. J. Lab. Clin. Med., 46:702–708 (Nov.) 1955.
29. Mistilis, S. P., and Blackburn, C. R.: The treatment of active chronic hepatitis with 6-mercaptopurine and azathioprine. Austr. Ann. Med., 16:305–311 (Nov.) 1967.
30. Mistilis, S. P., Skyring, A. P., and Goulston, S. J.: Effect of long-term tetracycline therapy, steroid therapy and colectomy in pericholangitis associated with ulcerative colitis. Austr. Ann. Med., 14:286–294 (Nov.) 1965.
31. Myers, J. D., Olson, R. E., Lewis, J. H., and Moran, T. J.: Xanthomatous biliary cirrhosis following chlorpromazine, with observations indicating overproduction of cholesterol, hyperprothrombinemia, and the development of portal hypertension. Trans. Assoc. Amer. Physicians, 70:243–261, 1957.
32. Neumann, P. Z., Carr, R. I., and Sass-Kortsak, A.: The handling of a single intravenous dose of copper by the rat. Abstract. Can. Med. Assoc. J., 86:229 (Feb. 3) 1962.
33. Northcutt, R. C., Stiel, J. N., Hollifield, J. W., et al.: The influence of cholestyramine on thyroxine absorption. J.A.M.A., 208:1857–1861 (June 9) 1969.
34. Olson, J. A.: The effect of bile and bile salts on the uptake and cleavage of β-carotene into retinol ester (vitamin A ester) by intestinal slices. J. Lipid Res., 5:402–408 (July) 1964.
35. Palmer, R. H., and Ruban, Z.: Production of bile duct hyperplasia and gallstones by lithocholic acid. J. Clin. Invest., 45:1255–1267 (Aug.) 1966.

36. Pope, J. L., Parkinson, T. M., and Olson, J. A.: Action of bile salts on the metabolism and transport of water-soluble nutrients by perfused rat jejunum in vitro. Biochem. Biophys. Acta, 130:218–232, 1966.
37. Quick, A. J., Hussey, C. V., and Collentine, G. E., Jr.: Vitamin K requirements of adult dogs and influence of bile on its absorption from the intestine. Amer. J. Physiol., 176:239–242 (Feb.) 1954.
38. Read, A. E., Harrison, C. V., and Sherlock, S.: Chronic chlorpromazine jaundice: with particular reference to its relationship to primary biliary cirrhosis. Amer. J. Med., 31:249–258 (Aug.) 1961.
39. Read, A. E., Laidlaw, J., and McCarthy, C. F.: Effects of chlorpromazine in patients with hepatic disease. Brit. Med. J., 3:497–499 (Aug. 30) 1969.
40. Remmer, H.: The role of the liver in drug metabolism. Amer. J. Med., 49:617–629 (Nov.) 1970.
41. Ritchie, H. D., and Shead, G. V.: The effect of morphine on hepatic extraction of ammonium from canine portal blood. Abstract. Gut, 4:89–90 (March) 1963.
42. Rubin, E., Gang, H., Misra, P. S., and Liever, C. S.: Inhibition of drug metabolism by acute ethanol intoxication: hepatic microsomal mechanism. Amer. J. Med., 49:801–806 (Dec.) 1970.
43. Sass-Kortsak, A.: Copper Metabolism. Adv. Clin. Chem., 8:1–67, 1965.
44. Saunders, D. R., and Dawson, A. M.: The absorption of oleic acid in the bile fistula rat. Gut, 4:254–260 (Sept.) 1963.
45. Schaffner, F., Klion, F. M., and Latuff, A. J.: The long term use of cholestyramine in the treatment of primary biliary cirrhosis. Gastroenterology, 48:293–298 (March) 1965.
46. Scheinberg, I. H., and Sternlieb, I.: Wilson's disease. Ann. Rev. Med., 16:119–134 (Feb.) 1965.
47. Schoenfield, L. J., Sjövall, J., and Perman, E.: Bile acids on the skin of patients with pruritic hepatobiliary disease. Nature, 213:93–94 (Jan. 7) 1967.
48. Scott, A. J., and Khan, G. A.: Partial biliary obstruction with cholangitis producing a blind loop syndrome. Gut, 9:187–192 (April) 1968.
49. Seawright, A. A., and McLean, A. E. M.: The effect of diet on carbon tetrachloride metabolism. Biochem. J., 105:1055–1060, 1967.
50. Sharp, H. L., Carey, J. B., Jr., White, J. G., et al.: Cholestyramine therapy in patients with a paucity of intrahepatic bile ducts. J. Pediat., 71:723–736 (Nov.) 1967.
51. Sherlock, S.: Primary biliary cirrhosis (chronic intrahepatic obstructive jaundice). Gastroenterology, 37:574–586 (Nov.) 1959.
52. Smallwood, R. A., Williams, H. A., Rosenoer, V. M., and Sherlock, S.: Liver-copper levels in liver disease: studies using neutron activation analysis. Lancet, 2:1310–1313 (Dec. 21) 1968.
53. Vahouny, G. V., Kothari, H., and Treadwell, C. R.: Specificity of bile salts protection of cholesterol ester hydrolase from proteolytic inactivation. Arch. Biochem., 121:242–244 (July) 1967.
54. Walker, C. O., and Combes, B.: Biliary cirrhosis induced by chlorpromazine. Gastroenterology, 51:631–640 (Nov.) 1966.
55. Walshe, J. M.: Current therapeutics. 192. Penicillamine. Practitioner, 191:789–795 (Dec.) 1963.
56. Webling, D. D., and Holdsworth, E. S.: Bile salts and calcium absorption. Biochem. J., 100:652–660 (Sept.) 1966.
57. Williams, R. T.: Patterns of excretion of drugs in man and other species. In Wolstenholme, G. E., and Porter, R. (eds): Drug Responses in Man. Boston, Little, Brown and Company, 1966, pp. 71–82.
58. Williams, R. T.: The fate of foreign compounds in man and animals. Pure Appl. Chem., 18:129–141, 1969.
59. Zaki, F. G., Carey, J. B., Jr., Hoffbauer, F. W., et al.: Biliary reaction and choledocholithiasis induced in the rat by lithocholic acid. J. Lab. Clin. Med., 69:737–748 (May) 1967.

605 Commonwealth Avenue
Boston, Massachusetts 02215

Obscure Chest Pain as a Symptom of Reflux Esophagitis

Robert E. Crozier, M.D., James A. Gregg, M.D., and Mamigon M. Garabedian, M.D.

Regurgitation, heartburn, dysphagia, and chest pain are classic symptoms of esophagitis. Usually the chest pain is mild and is described by the patient as a substernal or epigastric discomfort while swallowing or when bending over or lying down. In a few patients, however, the chest pain may be severe, constant, or protracted and unrelated to eating, and may suggest the presence of coronary artery disease. In such patients it becomes necessary to document or discard the possible esophageal origin of pain by the use of esophagoscopy or acid perfusion-motility or both. A group of 11 such patients, 9 of whom were known to have hiatus hernia, were studied by us in this fashion, and 8 of these patients were found to have esophagitis as the source of their severe or protracted chest pain.

PATHOPHYSIOLOGY

Prolonged reflux of gastric acid or bile into the esophagus eventually leads to esophagitis. Esophagitis is seen most commonly in association with hiatus hernia of the sliding type with or without shortening of the esophagus. More than 90 per cent of all hiatus hernias are of the sliding type. The few remaining hernias are of the paraesophageal type, which are usually without symptoms from reflux apparently because the esophagogastric junction is fixed below the diaphragm, and the lower esophageal sphincter remains competent. Associated with the inflammatory reaction, which is predominantly in the lower end of the esophagus, may be a motor disturbance secondary to the esophagitis. These effects come about because incompetency of the lower esophageal sphincter permits reflux of gastric contents into the esophagus.

Some of our older concepts thought to play a vital role in maintaining competency of the sphincter have recently been challenged. Traditionally it has been held that normal sphincter pressure was dependent on maintaining the high pressure zone in a position straddling the diaphragm by the action of the diaphragmatic hiatus, phrenoesophageal ligaments, right crus of the diaphragm, the omental attachments of the stomach, and the attachments of the esophagogastric junction to the preaortic fascia. It has been reasoned that in the presence of a sliding hiatus hernia these anchoring mechanisms are defective and with upward displacement of the vestibule the lower esophageal sphincter pressure is lowered and reflux occurs. In separate articles, Cohen and Harris[4] and Lind et al.[10] reported that competence of the sphincter is not related to the presence or absence of a hiatus hernia. While we agree that hiatus hernias do not *always* lead to incompetence of the sphincter and reflux, it still is evident clinically that most cases of reflux esophagitis are associated with sliding hernias. Secretin, whose effect on the lower esophageal sphincter is opposite to that of gastrin, lowers the lower esophageal sphincter pressure, and there is good evidence that this action results because of its inhibitory effect on gastrin.[8]

Two other factors, which have not received widespread support, have been suggested as barriers to reflux. One is the "pinchcock" effect of the diaphragmatic hiatus, and the other is the acute angle (angle of His) formed by the joining of the infradiaphragmatic portion of the esophagus with the stomach, thereby producing a flap valve effect.

Cigarette smoking[7] has recently been demonstrated to have an inhibitory effect on lower esophageal sphincter pressure. This possibly explains why a patient with an incompetent sphincter may have a flare-up of symptoms with smoking.

Hormonal control of lower esophageal sphincter pressure has recently been shown to be affected by the release of gastrin, the action of which is to increase sphincter pressure,[3] an action apparently not dependent on the vagus nerve.[2] Alkalinization of the gastric contents of a patient with heartburn as a result of acid reflux has the added feature of increasing the lower esophageal sphincter pressure through the gastrin mechanism and thereby has a preventive as well as a therapeutic effect on heartburn.

SYMPTOMS

Regurgitation, heartburn, dysphagia, and chest pain are the symptoms most commonly encountered with esophagitis. Of these, heartburn or pyrosis is perhaps the most persistent and bothersome to the patient, who will describe it as a sensation of burning along the course of the esophagus or in the epigastrium during the act of swallowing or immediately after eating. Many mechanisms for the cause of pyrosis have been described. However, it is presently believed that heartburn results either from the inflammatory reaction of esophagitis or esophageal motor disturbance, or both.

While dysphagia usually results from esophageal stricture or a lower esophageal ring, it may be a result of esophagitis without these anatomic obstructions.

The mild degree of chest discomfort or pain seen with hiatus hernia presumably results from the inflammatory reaction of esophagitis. However, the more severe and protracted chest pains experienced by our patients probably result from disordered motility in addition to the inflammatory reaction. In some patients the possible role of mechanical factors as a result of postprandial distention of the intrathoracic stomach must be considered.

METHODS OF EXAMINATION

There are several tests or procedures which can be employed successfully to help in determining what part, if any, esophagitis plays in those situations in which the source of chest pain is unclear.

Acid Perfusion

Acid perfusion is perhaps the single most helpful technique now available to diagnose chest pain secondary to esophagitis. When the esophagus is perfused with 0.1 normal hydrochloric acid, there is little or no distress to the patient. In the patient with esophagitis, however, such perfusion will reproduce the chest symptoms for which the patient sought attention. Such a positive result will be seen in 95 per cent of patients with esophagitis. If results are negative, one should look other than at the esophagus as a source of pain. When the symptoms are produced by this test, they can be abolished promptly by solutions of 0.1 normal sodium bicarbonate, 0.9 normal sodium chloride, or a few ml. of 2 per cent pontocaine solution.

Esophageal Motility

Esophageal motility studies (manometry) tell us the resting pressure in the lower esophageal sphincter and the adaptive competence of the lower esophageal sphincter to externally applied abdominal pressure. Normal pressures in the lower esophageal sphincter and normal adaptive responses generally prevent gastroesophageal reflux.[1, 4, 10] In general, the lower the pressure in the lower esophageal sphincter, the more likely reflux will be present. Finally, it also tells us the position of the lower esophageal sphincter in relation to the diaphragm and the nature of the deglutition waves and the presence of esophagitis. Motility disturbances in the distal portion of the esophagus corresponding to the area of inflammation are often present.[11] The most common motility disturbance is that of nonperistaltic contractions of normal amplitude. In a few cases, the amplitude of these contractions may be abnormally high or low.

Endoscopy

Endoscopy can now be performed easily with a multitude of fiberoptic instruments, which make the procedure a much safer one than with the rigid and semirigid instruments which were used before the last few years. This test supplies us with information which is supplemental to the tests mentioned previously. Endoscopy reveals the extent and severity of the inflammatory process in the esophagus as well as the presence of any inflammatory disease or ulceration in the stomach or duodenum.

It is desirable to have biopsy confirmation of endoscopic observations, particularly in those instances where the inflammatory reaction is described as slight, since some observer error may be present in this situation. When esophagitis is moderate to marked, the correlation is excellent. Visual observations at the time of endoscopy do not correlate well with the histology of the esophageal biopsy specimen where the esophagitis appears minimal or where there is no visible inflammatory reaction in patients with severe heartburn. Biopsy specimens in these situations frequently show significant inflammatory reaction.[13-16]

Similarly one may have, as occurred in 2 of our patients, visual evidence of mild esophagitis with no histologic evidence of esophagitis. Lack of correlation is probably the result of several factors. Sampling errors probably play a large role in the lack of correlation, particularly when biopsy specimens are taken through a fiberscope in which the sample size is very small, and there may be considerable difficulty in directing the biopsy forceps at the desired inflammatory area. In addition, taking biopsies on a tangential plane poses considerable difficulties at times.

Recently, the presence of inflammatory cells alone as a criterion for esophagitis has been questioned in view of what appeared a more promising criterion to the authors, this being the ratio of the depth of the stratified zone of the esophageal epithelium to the basal zone.[9] Using the Rubin biopsy capsule which takes a much larger piece of tissue than the fiberscope biopsy, the authors were still only able to obtain 85 per cent correlation between the visual and histologic evidence of esophagitis in patients with severe heartburn. Where esophagitis was present, in only 75 per cent of cases in which two biopsies were taken were both abnormal, again verifying the problem with sampling error when mild esophagitis is present which frequently assumes a patchy nature. Thus, lack of biopsy confirmation should not necessarily change the reliability of the endoscopist's direct observations.

Six patients, who were included in this study, were examined endoscopically. Initially this was done with the Olympus EF-1 fiberesophagoscope. Later when the end-viewing panendoscopes became available, patients who were examined also underwent concurrent endoscopic examinations of the stomach and duodenum (American Cystoscope Makers, Inc. 7089A or 7986). This is a practice we do routinely in all patients with esophageal disease since we have found a rather high incidence of associated inflammatory disease in these three organs.

SELECTION OF PATIENTS

Eleven patients, 9 of whom were known to have sliding hiatus hernias, were studied because clinically it was impossible to diagnose the origin of their chest pain. Of the 2 patients without a hernia, one (Case 10) was studied by perfusion-motility because repeated resting and electrocardiographic tracings produced negative results, and the possibility of esophageal pain was entertained. The other patient (Case 11) was examined by esophagoscopy because he had had a 4 year history of almost constant, at times severe, chest pain, and all tests in the past had been negative. Table 1 briefly describes the clinical features and findings in the 11 patients studied.

FINDINGS

Endoscopic Findings

Endoscopy in the form of esophagoscopy with or without gastroscopy and duodenoscopy was performed on 6 patients. Esophagitis was diagnosed, either macroscopically or microscopically, in 5 of the 6 patients so studied. Two of these patients, who on endoscopic examination were thought to have mild esophagitis, had negative results on microscopic examinations, probably for reasons discussed earlier.

Superficial gastritis was diagnosed either macroscopically or microscopically in all 3 patients on whom gastroscopy was performed. However, biopsy revealed negative findings for one of the patients who was thought to have gastritis at endoscopy.

Duodenitis was discovered in the 3 patients on whom duodenoscopy was performed.

Acid Perfusion-Motility

Acid-perfusion studies were performed on 9 patients, and 6 were found to have an abnormal response, indicating esophagitis. Ten patients had esophageal motility examinations; of these, 7 had an abnormal result consistent with the diagnosis of esophagitis.

Composite Results

Eight of the 9 patients with known hiatus hernia had evidence of esophagitis by endoscopy or acid perfusion-motility or both. Of these 8 patients, 1 patient had coexistent esophagitis and duodenitis and 2 patients had esophagitis, gastritis, and duodenitis.

The 1 patient (Case 3) who clinically was thought to have an asymptomatic hiatus hernia was described at endoscopy as having mild esophagitis, but the biopsy results were negative, as were the results of acid perfusion-motility.

The 2 patients without hernias (Cases 10 and 11) revealed normal findings by either endoscopy or by acid perfusion-motility.

DISCUSSION

The incidence of severe or protracted chest pain resulting from esophagitis of hiatus hernia is not uncommon and may be difficult to distinguish from the pain of coronary insufficiency or infarction. In a series of 105 symptomatic hiatus hernias reported by one of us[5] (R.E.C.), the incidence of coronary-like or angina-like symptoms was slightly less than 9 per cent. Palmer,[12] in a series of 1011 patients with hiatus hernia, subacute esophagitis, and esophageal stricture, found 13 per cent who

Table 1. *Observations in 11 Patients with Obscure Chest Pain*

CASE, AGE, AND SEX	CLINICAL OBSERVATIONS*	ENDOSCOPY	PERFUSION-MOTILITY	FINAL CLINICAL DIAGNOSES**
1 41 M	Constant substernal pains; upper GI tract, slight esophageal reflux; no hernia seen by x-ray by us but reported elsewhere	Esophagitis	+,–***	Functional GI disorder with reflux esophagitis; psychoneurosis
2 64 F	Rather constant substernal pain for 2 months which patient said differed from angina	Esophagitis; duodenitis	+	Hiatus hernia with esophagitis; angina pectoris
3 39 F	One episode of severe epigastric pain extending into right chest; cardiac work-up, negative	Esophagitis	Not done	Chest wall syndrome; asymptomatic hiatus hernia
4 37 M	Chest and epigastric pain; recurrent hiatus hernia	Esophagitis; gastritis; duodenitis	+	Functional GI disorder; recurrent hiatus hernia with mild esophagitis, gastritis, and duodenitis
5 43 M	"Tearing" chest pain when under tension; cardiac work-up, negative	Not done	+	Hiatus hernia with esophagitis

6 74 F	Severe chest pain when bending over; known angina of exertion	Not done	+	Angina pectoris; hiatus hernia with mild esophagitis
7 58 F	Substernal pain for 2 months	Not done	+	Hiatus hernia with esophagitis
8 56 M	One episode of severe chest pain; epigastric pain for several months	Not done	+	Hiatus hernia with esophagitis
9 43 M	Constant upper abdominal and chest pain not responding to antacid therapy	Esophagitis; gastritis; duodenitis	Not done	Hiatus hernia with esophagitis, gastritis, duodenitis and duodenal ulcer
10 70 M	Recurrent bouts of substernal pain; cardiac work-up, negative; no hernia seen on x-ray	Not done	–	Coronary heart disease
11 40 M	Constant chest pain, 4 years; cardiac work-up, negative; temporary relief of pain by bowel movement	Gastritis	–	Functional GI disorder

*Hiatus hernia demonstrable by x-ray unless specified otherwise.

**Listed in order of importance.

***Test negative first time; positive when repeated.

sought medical attention because of acute chest pain that simulated angina pectoris or myocardial infarction. Of 301 patients who were initially thought to have angina pectoris, Delmonico et al.[6] found 40 with esophagitis. Twelve of the latter group were found to have the shortened esophagus type of hiatus hernia and on surgical correction obtained relief of symptoms.

The patient having classic symptoms of angina pectoris and having no symptoms from the associated hiatus hernia should present no problem in diagnosis. When the patient has both typical angina and also chest pain which is atypical, there may be difficulty in knowing if all the chest pain is coronary in origin or if the esophagus can also be incriminated. This, in some patients, may be very hard to differentiate especially if the atypical type of chest pain is similar to the anginal pain in its distribution.

In a few instances the pain of esophageal origin may radiate to the neck, jaws, and arms in a manner identical to that of anginal pain, although it does not occur secondary to physical activity. Fortunately two such pain patterns do not usually begin concurrently, and the intelligent patient is usually able to distinguish between them. The principal problem occurs in differentiating nonexercise-induced pain of coronary origin from that resulting from the esophagus. In this situation a vigorous diagnostic approach consisting of barium swallow, acid perfusion-motility, resting and exercise electrocardiography, and possibly coronary angiography may be necessary.

For example, one of our patients (Case 2) had had classical symptoms of angina for years that could be recognized readily and controlled with nitroglycerine. Another type of chest pain developed subsequently which the patient was able to distinguish from angina, and our studies indicated this was the result of esophagitis. The esophageal pain responded well to an antacid program.

The second patient (Case 6) had severe angina of exertion and excitement and also had similar, but less severe chest pain when bending over and lying down. It was uncertain what influence if any the hernia was having in her case. The tests were limited to esophageal motility which showed a pattern of disordered motility consistent with esophagitis. However, the response to antacid therapy was poor, suggesting that the major problem may have been coronary artery disease.

The third patient (Case 10) had a long history of chest pain suggesting the possibility of angina, but our cardiologist could not make a definite diagnosis. Repeated resting and exercise cardiograms gave negative results, so the possibility of esophageal pain was considered even though no hernia was seen. Roentgenology, endoscopy, and acid perfusion-motility studies proved to be within normal limits, virtually eliminating the esophagus as the source of chest pain. With this knowledge available, our cardiologist finally concluded that the patient probably had angina.

Another patient (Case 8) had had several months of mild to moderate epigastric and low middle anterior chest pain which followed no pattern, and one attack of severe chest pain which initially was thought to be the result of myocardial infarction. Serial electrocardiograms and enzyme studies did not confirm this diagnosis. The acid perfusion-motility studies were positive, indicating esophagitis. It was also concluded that the episodes of milder, daily chest distress were the result of the esophagitis. The single acute episode of severe chest pain was thought to represent acute esophageal spasm secondary to the esophagitis.

It is noteworthy that 6 of the 8 patients with esophagitis had almost constant daily chest pain for weeks or months without relief. One often associates nonmalignant organic gastrointestinal disease with periodicity rather than chronicity such as one encounters with "attacks" of peptic ulceration, pancreatitis, cholecystitis, and so forth. One should remember though that esophageal pain, like that of peptic ulceration and intra-abdominal inflammatory disease, may assume a chronic nature, lasting months or longer with little remission, and should not mislead the physician into diagnosing a functional disorder as the cause of symptoms. This is not to say that esophagitis may be intermittent with periods of relative calm, but often the distress tends to "hang on" for weeks with daily flare-ups.

Three of the 6 patients who had endoscopy were found to have superficial gastritis or duodenitis or both in association with esophagitis. The significance and pathogenesis of this associated inflammatory disease is not clear. However, in 1 of our patients (Case 9) it carried a bad prognosis, as his response to the antacid program was not good, and surgical correction of the hernia and ulcer was required. We have also found a number of other patients, not included in this report, who had associated inflammatory disease of the esophagus, stomach, and duodenum with or without ulceration and believe this association is not uncommon.

CONCLUSIONS

Chest pains associated with esophagitis may be chronic and at times severe and often are difficult to distinguish from coronary artery disease. Whenever possible, endoscopy should be performed when esophagitis is suspected, to determine its extent and severity and also to discover if associated inflammatory disease is present in the stomach and duodenum. Acid perfusion tests have been the single most helpful technique in diagnosing chest pain arising from esophagitis.

Esophageal motility is a method of documenting the competency of the lower esophageal sphincter and also gives information regarding motor activity in the esophagus. The motility pattern has little influence on the medical management of the patient with known esophagitis, but it is helpful to the surgeon in deciding what type of surgical repair of the hernia will be most beneficial to the patient.

Inflammatory disease of the stomach and duodenum in association with esophagitis is probably more common than appreciated. Our patients with obscure chest pain resulting from esophagitis responded as readily to antacid therapy as did patients with usual symptoms of esophagitis. Whenever one encounters a patient whose symptoms do not respond favorably to the medical regimen, coronary angiography should be considered.

REFERENCES

1. Atkinson, M.: Hiatus hernia. Brit. Med. J., 4:218–221 (Oct. 28) 1967.
2. Castell, D. O.: Changes in lower esophageal sphincter pressure during insulin-induced hypoglycemia. Gastroenterology, 61:10–15 (July) 1971.
3. Castell, D. O., and Harris, L. D.: Hormonal control of gastroesophageal-sphincter strength. New Eng. J. Med., 282:886–889 (April 16) 1970.
4. Cohen, S., and Harris, L. D.: Does hiatus hernia affect competence of the gastroesophageal sphincter? New Eng. J. Med., 284:1053–1056 (May 13) 1971.
5. Crozier, R. E., and Jonasson, H.: Symptomatic esophageal hiatus hernias. Study of 105 patients. Arch. Intern. Med., 113:737–743 (May) 1964.
6. Delmonico, J. E., Jr., Black, A., and Gensini, G. G.: Diaphragmatic hiatal hernia and angina pectoris. Dis. Chest, 53:309–315 (March) 1968.
7. Dennish, G. W., and Castell, D. O.: Inhibitory effect of smoking on the lower esophageal sphincter. New Eng. J. Med., 284:1136–1137 (May 20) 1971.
8. Hansky, J., Soveny, C., and Korman, M. G.: Effects of secretin on serum gastrin as measured by immunoassay. Gastroenterology, 61:62–68 (July) 1971.
9. Ismail-Beigi, F., Horton, P. F., and Pope, C. E.: Histological consequences of gastroesophageal reflux in man. Gastroenterology, 58:163–174 (Feb.) 1970.
10. Lind, J. F., Cotton, D. J., Blanchard, R., et al.: Effect of thoracic displacement and vagotomy on the canine gastroesophageal junctional zone. Gastroenterology, 56:1078–1085 (June) 1969.
11. Olsen, A. M., and Schlegel, J. F.: Motility disturbances caused by esophagitis. J. Thorac. Cardiovasc. Surg., 50:607–612 (Nov.) 1965.
12. Palmer, E. D.: The hiatus hernia-esophagitis-esophageal stricture complex. Twenty-year prospective study. Amer. J. Med., 44:566–579 (April) 1968.
13. Schuman, B. M., and Rinaldo, J. A.: Relative frequency of esophagitis and gastritis in patients with symptomatic hiatus hernia. Gastrointest. Endosc., 12:14–16 (Feb.) 1966.
14. Siegel, C. I., and Hendrix, T. R.: Esophageal motor abnormalities induced by acid perfusion in patients with heartburn. J. Clin. Invest., 42:686–695 (May) 1963.
15. Skinner, D. B., and Booth, D. J.: Assessment of distal esophageal function in patients with hiatus hernia and/or gastroesophageal reflux. Ann. Surg., 172:627–637 (Oct.) 1970.
16. Winans, C. S., and Harris, L. D.: Quantitation of lower esophageal sphincter competence. Gastroenterology, 52:773–778 (May) 1967.

605 Commonwealth Avenue
Boston, Massachusetts 02215

Retrograde Cannulation of the Ampulla of Vater

A Preliminary Report

James A. Gregg, M.D.

Examination of the duodenal bulb and the duodenum beyond this with a variety of end-on viewing panendoscopes is now possible, and many reports have testified to the usefulness of direct duodenal visualization in diagnosis, particularly of disease of the duodenal bulb and the periampullary area. Most good endoscopists now perform an examination of the duodenal bulb as part of the routine endoscopic examination, even when the examination is done primarily for esophageal or gastric disease. The side-viewing duodenoscopes, the Olympus JF-B and Machida FDS, however, are not used as frequently. They are still, however, the only instruments with which endoscopic examination of the third and fourth parts of the duodenum, and occasionally beyond, can be performed, and with which cannulation of the ampulla of Vater can be carried out for retrograde dye studies of the pancreatic and biliary ducts. Cannulation was first introduced by McCune et al.[12] in 1968; since that time considerable experience has been obtained by a number of investigators,[4, 10, 11, 13, 15, 17, 19] primarily in Japan, and more recently in Germany by Classen and Demling[2, 4, 5] and in this country by Shinya[17] and Vennes.[20] I have recently succeeded in cannulating the ampulla of Vater and obtaining satisfactory pancreatograms and cholangiograms. Our preliminary experience with this procedure is reported here.

PREPARATION OF THE PATIENT

The patients are prepared for upper gastrointestinal endoscopy as previously described.[6] In addition, atropine sulphate, 0.6 mg., is administered intramuscularly 20 minutes before the procedure.

The Olympus JF-B duodenoscope is easily introduced into the esophagus with the patient lying on his left side. The instrument is introduced as far as the pylorus, which is initially viewed in the head-on position. Subsequently, the procedure is essentially that described previously by

Oi.[14] The tip of the instrument is then straightened to view the lesser curvature aspect of the pylorus, and the instrument is easily advanced into the duodenal bulb. After the bulb is visualized, the instrument is introduced as far as the angulus between the second and third parts of the duodenum and then rotated 180° to bring the angulus into full view. This may present a confusing picture to the neophyte, who may suddenly find two lumens with which to cope, but the correct way to advance the instrument is easily determined after a few tries.

The instrument should then be advanced only 1 to 2 cm. further beyond the angulus, at which point the papilla of Vater should be visible on the posterior medial wall. Occasionally, a secondary papilla may also be seen within 1 to 2 cm. of the main papilla. A considerable number of endoscopies must be performed with this instrument before the papilla can be recognized in all patients. Generally, the papilla assumes three forms, as previously described,[1, 10] of which the papillary and hemispherical are the most common (Table 1). Least commonly encountered is a situation in which virtually no papilla is visible, and the ampulla is seen as a small orifice surrounded by a crinkled-appearing red area, projecting 1 to 2 mm. from around the orifice of the ampulla. The finding of a bile stain in a small area on the posterior medial wall of the duodenum frequently aids in identifying the ampullary orifice, as does finding folds in this area that run other than in the usual circular orientation. With the Olympus JF-B, I have not found it necessary to inject cholecystokinin intravenously to visualize the ampullary orifice, and, indeed, the presence of a large amount of bile in the duodenum near the papilla is not desirable since it will impair visibility.

When the papilla is located, ganglionic blockade with propantheline bromide (Pro-Banthine) or more anticholinergics may need to be administered intravenously if any duodenal contractility is present. It is extremely important at this stage that there be no duodenal motility. Next, the controls on the instrument are rotated so that the papilla is approached head on. In almost all instances this is accomplished with the patient still lying on the left side.

The plastic cannula is then inserted through the biopsy channel and the cannula deflector moved upward to see the cannula tip. If the orientation of the tip of the cannula to the ampullary orifice is not optimal after further manipulation of the controls, it is best to pull the cannula back into the duodenoscope and withdraw the duodenoscope into the first part of the duodenum, rotate it slightly, and reinsert it to the level of the papilla. Frequently, this will change the angle of entry sufficiently so that the cannula can be introduced easily into the papilla. If the cannula does

Table 1. *Shape of the Papilla of Vater*

TYPE	NUMBER	PER CENT
Papillary	38	52.1
Hemispheric	27	37.0
Flat	8	10.9
Total	73	

enter the ampulla at the wrong angle, the tip of the cannula will abut against one of the walls of the ampulla and satisfactory studies of the ductal system will not occur after dye injection. Next, the cannula is filled with 60 per cent urografin by syringe to remove any air bubbles from the cannula so that air will not be injected into the ductal system. The syringe is left attached with 4 to 5 ml. of urografin remaining. The cannula is then inserted as close as possible to the papilla and, if respiration is causing too much movement of the duodenal wall, the patient is asked to hold his breath momentarily. The cannula is then inserted into the ampulla as far as it will go easily. In many instances, this is only a few millimeters.

Next, 3 to 4 ml. of 60 per cent renografin is injected through the cannula over a period of 5 to 10 seconds. Spot films of the periampullary area are taken after the injection of renografin, 2 ml., and again immediately after the injection of the entire amount with the patient still in the left lateral decubitus position or slightly in the oblique position. The patient is immediately placed in the supine position, and additional films of the area are taken. It is important to obtain films in both positions since the information gained from one film frequently complements the other. Occasionally, the catheter may become dislodged as the patient is turned but this generally makes no difference if the dye has already been injected. Films taken minutes later frequently show prompt emptying of the dye from the ductal system. If good dye studies are obtained, the instrument is removed; if not, the procedure may be repeated. Although fluoroscopic observation of the injection of dye is desirable, it is not necessary, and fluoroscopy rarely is needed (after some experience) to insert the duodenoscope to the level of the ampulla.

RESULTS

Initially problems were encountered in locating the papilla of Vater but the papilla was seen in the last 25 patients examined. These results are similar to the 86 to 98 per cent visualization of the papilla reported by others.[2, 4, 9, 19] Of the 73 patients in whom I have seen the papilla with the Olympus JF-B, it was principally hemispherical or papillary in shape although changes from hemispherical to papillary shape were occasionally encountered. This observation is similar to that of others.[3, 7, 8, 12, 16, 18] I have not, however, encountered a situation in which a hemispherical or papillary configuration changes to a planar configuration or vice versa. In my experience and that of others the planar configuration has been encountered least frequently. An accessory papilla with an orifice too small to cannulate was seen within 1.5 cm. of the main papilla in three instances. In addition, duodenal diverticula in close proximity to the papilla were noted just inferior to the ampulla in several other patients. The orifice varied from 1 mm. to almost as large as the diameter of that of the duodenum. Of the last 25 patients endoscoped with this instrument, cannulation was attempted in 16 and successfully accomplished in 12 patients. In one instance, it was not possible to insert the cannula into the papilla for technical reasons; in another patient, it was impossible to decrease duodenal motility adequately to maintain the catheter in the ampulla despite premedication with atropine and propantheline bromide, 55 mg., injected intravenously just before the attempted cannulation. In a third patient, too much anticholinergic agent and propantheline bromide were given; tachycardia and wretching developed, and the procedure had to be discontinued.

In the fourth failure, cannulation was attempted in a woman with chronic relapsing pancreatitis of several years' duration, 10 days after she experienced an acute episode of pancreatitis. The papilla was noted to be red and indurated (papillitis) and the cannula would not enter a narrowed ampullary orifice.[10] It would have been desirable to biopsy the papilla but, unfortunately, this was not done and the patient will return for a repeat attempt at cannulation.

In the remaining 12 patients, the position of the cannula within the papilla was judged to be poor in 2; dye injection in these patients confirmed this since the dye immediately returned to the duodenum around the cannula. In 4 patients in whom the position of the cannula was judged to be good, dye was injected and satisfactory studies of the pancreatic duct were obtained. The common bile duct was satisfactorily visualized in 2 patients and the main pancreatic duct in all. In three patients, smaller pancreatic ducts including the duct of Santorini, were also seen. In the remaining 6 patients having no known pancreatic or biliary disease, catheter placement was judged excellent, but no dye was injected because of the possible risk of inducing pancreatitis. It was felt that in this group of 6 patients excellent pancreatocholangiograms would have been possible had dye been injected. The time required for the procedure varied from 10 to 50 minutes but generally 20 to 30 minutes was sufficient after successfully completing cannulation in several patients.

COMPLICATIONS

No complications were encountered from duodenoscopy with the Olympus JF-B in more than 100 examinations. In the small group of patients in whom cannulation was performed, none complained of any abdominal pain after the procedure. Serum amylase determinations were obtained prior to and at varying times up to 24 hours after the cannulation. The serum amylase level rose slightly but remained normal in all patients who underwent pancreatography, but no rise occurred in the patients in whom the papilla was cannulated but no dye was injected. Since most serum amylases were drawn 20 to 24 hours after the procedure, the principal rise that usually occurs earlier, may have been missed. Transient, usually asymptomatic, increases in serum amylase values have been reported in other studies[10, 11, 20] and, on occasion, this has been associated with transient abdominal pain that apparently has been of no consequence.[4] The only untoward result of our procedure was 1 patient (a failure) who was over-medicated with anticholinergics which required discontinuation of the procedure before attempted cannulation.

REPORTS OF CASES

Case 1

A 56 year old man was admitted to the hospital because of constant lower dorsal pain extending into the upper abdomen and associated with weight loss of two months' duration. Physical examination showed the weight was 135 lbs. and blood pressure 120/80 mm. Hg. Except for evidence of recent weight loss, the examination was otherwise unremarkable.

Pertinent laboratory studies showed hemoglobin, 14.3 gm. per 100 ml.; alkaline phosphatase, 60 I.U.; serum glutamic oxaloacetic transaminase, 20; and serum bilirubin, 0.3 mg. per 100 ml. Preoperative serum amylase levels were within normal limits. Roentgenogram of the gallbladder and barium study of the upper gastrointestinal tract were within normal limits. Selective celiac angiography showed tumor encasement of the main hepatic artery and the gastro-duodenal artery. The splenic vein was occluded and collateral venous return was marked.

The patient was gastroscoped with the American Cystoscope Makers, Inc. (A.C.M.I.) 7089A endoscope. Apart from superficial gastritis in the body of the stomach, the examination to and including the duodenal bulb was negative. The Olympus JF-B was inserted and retrograde pancreatocholangiography was carried out. The common bile duct was totally normal, but the main pancreatic duct showed marked irregularity of its inferior margin extending several centimeters into the body of the pancreas. The findings were interpreted as being the result of tumor involvement (Fig. 1).

Several days later laparotomy confirmed the finding of carcinoma of the body and tail of the pancreas with patency of the common bile duct.

Case 2

A 60 year old man was admitted to the hospital because of recurrent cholangitis that had begun after a cholecystectomy for cholelithiasis 2 years previously.

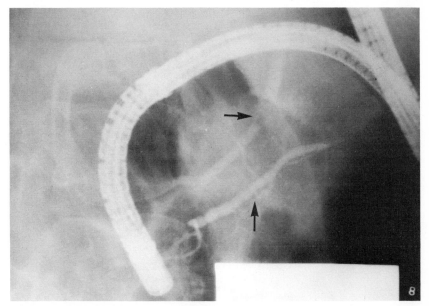

Figure 1. Retrograde pancreatocholangiogram showing irregularity of the main pancreatic duct owing to tumor invasion. The filling defects in the common duct are due to air bubbles inadvertently injected during the procedure.

On physical examination, the vital signs were normal, but the patient was noted to be slightly jaundiced. Physical examination was within normal limits except for abdominal surgical scars.

Pertinent laboratory studies showed hemoglobin, 11.2 gm. per 100 ml.; sedimentation rate, 100 mm. per hour (Westergren); alkaline phosphatase, 1,310 I.U.; serum glutamic oxaloacetic transaminase, 42 units; serum bilirubin, 2.2 mg. per 100 ml. total; serum amylase was normal. Barium study of the upper gastro-intestinal tract showed questionable extrinsic pressure on the antrum from the enlarged pancreas, and an intravenous cholangiogram did not visualize the biliary tract.

The patient was examined with the Olympus JF-B gastroscope and findings were normal. The patient then underwent cannulation of the ampulla of Vater. Excellent films of the pancreatic duct showed stenosis of the mid portion of the main duct to 50 per cent of its usual caliber. No filling of the bile ducts was observed (Fig. 2).

At laparotomy, the patient was found to have had cholecystectomy and hepaticoduodenostomy which had stenosed; the stenotic area was reconstructed. The pancreas appeared normal. The pancreatic duct was not probed.

DISCUSSION

Indications for cannulation of the ampulla of Vater are many and as a result of this procedure great diagnostic inroads should be made into diseases of the pancreas and biliary system without the use of surgery. Of particular importance will be evaluation of the pancreatic ductal system for stones, strictures, and, hopefully, for much earlier detection of periampullary and pancreatic carcinomas. In 2 of our patients, the use of this procedure was helpful in diagnosing both a partial stenosis of the main pancreatic duct in 1 patient, and malignant involvement of the main pancreatic duct in the other patient. Retrograde visualization of the

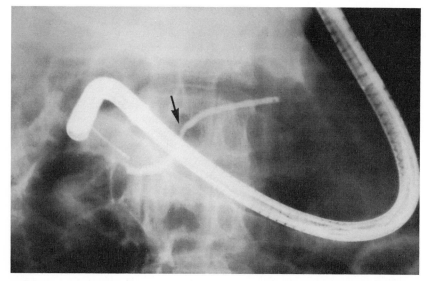

Figure 2. Retrograde pancreatogram showing partial stenosis of the main pancreatic duct in the head of the pancreas.

bile ducts has also been found helpful in the differential diagnosis of jaundice.[3, 5, 9, 19] Generally, the biliary tract has been visualized less well than the pancreatic ducts. Frequently only the common duct and not the hepatic or intrahepatic ducts is seen. Good cholangiograms that show visualization of the hepatic ducts and gallbladder have occasionally been obtained. At the present time this procedure appears to be safer although more difficult to perform than intravenous cholangiography for visualization of the common duct.

With this procedure, the pancreatic duct appears to fill in preference to the common bile duct.[4, 10] This is probably in part because the common channel is not present in a large number of cases or because the cannula selectively enters the pancreatic duct. A similar finding occurs in surgery—a probe introduced into the ampulla through the opened duodenum enters the pancreatic rather than the common duct in 80 per cent of cases. Improved methods of deflecting the tip of the cannula will hopefully be available in the near future to allow selective cannulations of either the pancreatic or biliary ductal systems. A Seldinger catheter introduced through the biopsy port of the instrument may prove helpful for this purpose.

SUMMARY

Preliminary experience with catheterization of the ampulla of Vater using the Olympus JF-B duodenoscope has been presented. After some experience, it is possible to recognize the ampulla of Vater in all cases. Cannulation was satisfactorily performed in 12 of the last 16 patients examined, and the percentage of successful cannulations should increase with more experience. When satisfactory dye studies were obtained, visualization was accomplished primarily of the pancreatic duct and to a lesser extent the common bile duct with the injection of 3 to 4 mm. of renografin. Several examples of retrograde dye studies of the pancreatic and biliary ducts are presented. No complications were encountered in this group of patients other than transient elevation of the serum amylase values in several instances.

REFERENCES

1. Ashizawa, S., and Shindo, S.: Endoscopic examination of the duodenum. Second World Congress of Gastrointestinal Endoscopy, Rome and Copenhagen, 1970.
2. Classen, M.: Progress report. Fibroendoscopy of the intestines. Gut *12*:330–338 (April) 1971.
3. Classen, M., Koch, H., and Demling, L.: Duodenitis. Frequency and significance. Bibl. Gastroent. 9:48–69, 1970.
4. Classen, M., et al.: Duodenoscopy. Abstracts of the American Society of Gastrointestinal Endoscopy, Miami, Florida, May 11, 1971. (Unpublished data.)
5. Demling, L., and Classen, M.: Duodenojejunoscopy. Endoscopy 2:115–117, 1970.
6. Garabedian, M., and Gregg, J. A.: Esophageal endoscopy. Surg. Clin. N. Amer. *51*:641–647 (June) 1971.
7. Hara, Y., and Ogoshi, K.: Clinical use of duodenal fiberscope (Olympus), duodenum and pancreatocholedochography through it. Second World Congress of Gastrointestinal Endoscopy, Rome and Copenhagen, 1970.

8. Kasugai, T.: Pancreato-cholangiography under fiber-duodenoscopy. Abstracts of the American Society of Gastrointestinal Endoscopy, Miami, Florida, May 11, 1971. (Unpublished data.)
 9. Kasugai, T., Ito, K., Kuno, N., and Aoki, J.: Studies on endoscopic examination of the duodenum. Second World Congress of Gastrointestinal Endoscopy, Rome and Copenhagen, 1970.
10. Kasugai, T., Kuno, N., Aoki, A., et al.: Fiberduodenoscopy: analysis of 353 examinations. Gastroint. Endosc. *18*:9–16 (Aug.) 1971.
11. Kozu, T., Oi, I., Suzuki, S., and Takemoto, T.: Fiberduodenoscopic observation on the dynamics of the duodenal papilla. Endoscopy 2:99–102, 1970.
12. McCune, W. S., Shorb, P. E., and Moscovitz, H.: Endoscopic cannulation of the ampulla of Vater: a preliminary report. Ann. Surg. *167*:752–756 (May) 1968.
13. Oi, I: The valvular protrusion of the papilla of Vater. EECO Congress, Munich, Germany, 1970.
14. Oi, I.: Endoscopy of the small intestine – with emphasis on the current condition of duodenal endoscopy. Stomach and Intestine 4:469, 1968. Cited by Shindo, et al., 1970.
15. Oi, I., Kobayashi, S., and Kondo, T.: Endoscopic pancreatocholangiography. Endoscopy 2:103–106, 1970.
16. Oi, I., et al.: Endoscopy of the duodenum overall. Clin. Med. *19*:307, 1970. Cited by Shindo, et al., 1970.
17. Shinya, H., et al.: Duodenal fiberoscopy. Abstracts of the American Society of Gastrointestinal Endoscopy, Miami, Florida, May 11, 1971. (Unpublished data.)
18. Sohma, S., Kidokoro, T., and Takezoe, T.: Clinical application of a duodenofiberscope. Second World Congress of Gastrointestinal Endoscopy, Rome and Copenhagen, 1970.
19. Takagi, K., Ikeda, S., Nakagawa, Y., et al.: Retrograde pancreatography and cholangiography by fiber duodenoscope. Gastroenterology *59*:445–452 (Sept.) 1970.
20. Vennes, J.: Personal communication.

605 Commonwealth Avenue
Boston, Massachusetts 02215

Management of the Climacteric and Postmenopausal Woman

Robert W. Cali, M.D.

At the turn of this century, life expectancy was still under 50 years of age. It has only been during the last half century that women have lived long enough to make the medical profession aware of the multiple problems presented by the climacteric period in a woman's life. Menopausal and postmenopausal women are, and will continue to be, encountered in large numbers. Today, such women are the subject of a controversy, the center of which is the alleged need for, safety, and value of prolonged hormone therapy.

The current gynecologic literature, both professional[15] and popular,[31] has led to a dichotomy of opinion in the proper management of these patients. It has been said that a girl becomes a woman when estrogen and progesterone arrive; when they depart, she is a woman by courtesy only, in reality, a castrate.[34] This philosophy has generated the notion that the menopause is a quasi pathologic entity, a deficiency disease which requires treatment with hormones until the end of life. This stands in sharp contrast to a consideration of the climacteric as a normal physiologic point in the life of a woman, which in the majority of patients requires no endocrine therapy. The impact of this opposing philosophy on the public and a large segment of the medical profession has resulted in muddled thinking and subsequently muddled therapy.

It is the purpose of this paper to outline an intelligent approach to the management of the climacteric and the postmenopausal patient. The entity under discussion should be guided by a rational and purposeful plan, which of necessity requires a basic knowledge of the physiology, endocrine changes, and symptomatology of the climacteric.

Etymologically, the term climacteric means rung of a ladder or climax—a step which every woman must take as she passes from the cradle to the grave. It is a phase of adjustment to the waning potential of the ovary, which takes place over a period of years and is the counterpart of puberty. The menopause, the counterpart of the menarche, is only one of a train of symptoms that marks the climacteric and refers only to the cessation of menstruation. This occurs when two, three, or more decades of life remain. The age at which the menopause usually appears is approximately 50. Some women may stop menstruating at age 35, and others may continue to 55, both limits being unusual. Climacteric, the period of transition, covers approximately 15 years between 45 and 60 years of age. It is a regressive process, resulting in an imbalance in the endocrine system, which causes symptoms requiring treatment in 25 per cent of patients. A premature menopause, one that takes place before the age of 40, occurs in about 8 per cent of women. This may create a problem in differential diagnosis, and an organic cause must be assiduously sought to account for the cessation of ovarian function and the amenorrhea which results.

PHYSIOLOGIC AND ENDOCRINE CHANGES

The key physical change is permanent and irreversible atrophy of the ovaries. The ovaries are gradually depleted of primordial follicles, a process which begins at puberty. Senescence of the ovaries, the basic fault, is accompanied by a corresponding decline in the vital hormones, estrogen and progesterone. Once the ovarian hormones decrease, the feedback mechanism which they previously had with the anterior pituitary gonadotropic hormone, follicle-stimulating hormone (FSH), is disrupted, and large amounts of gonadotropins appear in the blood and urine. Thus, the functional life of the ovary terminates when its stock of primary oocytes is exhausted.

In the normal menstruating woman, estrogen is produced by the stromal and theca cells. Progesterone is produced by the luteinized granulosa cells following ovulation and the formation of a corpus luteum. With the cessation of ovulation, it has been established that estrogenic production in the human female does not disappear. Some estrogenic function is maintained in the majority of women for at least a 10 year period. According to the studies of Masukawa,[16] severe atrophy of the menopausal smear is found in only 25 per cent of patients within a 10 year post-menopausal period and in only 37 per cent of patients after 10 years. Twenty per cent of menopausal women continue to show estrogenic smears for approximately 10 years postmenopausally, and urinary estrogen excretion is maintained at levels compatible with those found in the early follicular phase of the cycle, 5 to 15 mcg. per 24 hours.

Studies[16, 17] of vaginal smears have shown an estrogenic effect to persist for a decade or more beyond the menopause in nearly 80 per cent of all postmenopausal women. McLennan and McLennan recently reported that about 40 per cent of menopausal women maintain moderate levels of estrogenic activity during the remaining years of life.[17] This residual estrogen is produced by the adrenal gland, the ovarian stromal cells which have the capacity for steroidogenesis, and perhaps from an unknown source yet to be determined.

Randall et al.[24] observed that the ovary was a source of a significant proportion of the estrogens affecting the tissues of a majority of women for years after the menopause. This does not necessarily imply that all estrogen is of ovarian origin. Good evidence exists that some of the estrogens are of adrenocortical origin. It has been demonstrated that urinary estrogen levels in oophorectomized women did not differ significantly from those found in women after a normal physiologic menopause.[3]

Most of the hormone synthesis in the postmenopausal ovary takes place in the ovarian stroma.[21] The normal major pathway for biosynthesis of estrogens in the ovary is the formation of cholesterol from acetate and its conversion into estrogen by way of: $\triangle^5$Pregnenolone$\rightarrow$Progesterone$\rightarrow$17α-Hydroxyprogesterone$\rightarrow\triangle^4$-Androstenedione$\rightleftarrows$Testosterone$\rightarrow$ Estradiol. A minor pathway is the conversion of cholesterol via $\triangle^5$Pregnenolone$\rightarrow$17α-Hydroxy-$\triangle^5$Pregnenolone$\rightarrow$Dehydroepiandrosterone$\rightarrow\triangle^4$ Androstenedione. These same biosynthetic pathways occur in the adrenal gland.[14]

As estrogen decreases, the pituitary hormone (FSH) increases. Urinary levels of FSH may be increased 20 to 50 times. The decrease in progesterone is certainly not as significant as its primary effects seem to be on the breast and uterus. Isreal[12] believes that the declining levels of estrogen induce a pituitary hyperactivity which results in a pluriglandular hyperfunction. The course features include a propensity for latent diabetes to become overt, and the appearance of hirsutism, both suggestive of a hyperfunction of the anterior hypophysis.[12]

SYMPTOMATOLOGY

It is perhaps pertinent to point out that only 25 per cent of all women have significant symptoms which bring them to a physician. The majority cease to menstruate, and life continues as before. There are two classic symptoms of the menopause, namely, vasomotor instability, characterized by the hot flush, and menstrual irregularities. Two other important symptoms which occur are the psychological changes and senescent vaginitis. The claim has been made that osteoporosis and the increased incidence of coronary atherosclerosis in the postmenopausal woman is the result of estrogen deficiency.

Vasomotor Instability

The hot flush or flash is pathognomonic of the menopausal syndrome, as it occurs only in this instance. They may occur from 1 to 10 years, and in some patients appear before the menopause is definitely established, during the time when estrogen levels are known to fluctuate. They gradually begin as a sensation of warmth over the upper part of the chest and characteristically spread over the neck, face, and upper extremities. They appear with such suddenness that they are referred to as hot flashes, and are often followed by profuse perspiration and chilliness. The frequency and severity are subject to wide variations.

Other vasomotor symptoms include numbness and tingling, cold hands and feet, palpitations, headache, and vertigo. The precise mechanism for the vasomotor symptoms is uncertain. It may be speculated that high levels of FSH may be responsible. However, the high levels found in the urine of young amenorrheal patients with primary ovarian failure is not productive of the hot flush. It may be that the vasomotor instability is related to a disturbance of the autonomic nervous system. It has been postulated that estrogen exerts a protective action on the subcutaneous blood vessels. But again we note that ovarian dysgenesis is not associated with the hot flush. The inciting factor is as yet unknown.

Menstrual Irregularities

The menstrual disturbances that herald the menopause may be of all the recognized varieties—menorrhagia, hypomenorrhea, polymenorrhea, oligomenorrhea, and metrorrhagia. These are the endometrial manifestations of the changing endocrine status. As ovulation and luteinization disappear, the growth of follicles may proceed, allowing continued estrogen production and causing irregular episodes of bleeding as a result of irregular shedding. The continuing estrogen stimulation causes endometrial proliferation and various stages of hyperplasia. This results in break-through bleeding that is usually unpredictable in duration, frequency, and amount.

Psychological Changes

The emotional instability experienced by women during the climacteric is well documented. The specter of advancing years is dramatically and suddenly revealed to every woman. The symptom complex of nervousness, emotional instability, insomnia, fatigability, and depression is part of the menopausal syndrome. Whether a woman reacts with equanimity or anxiety will depend in part on what has occurred before. The symptoms of anxiety and depression are not the result of estrogen withdrawal but rather are functional in origin.

Senescent Vaginitis

Finally, with the withdrawal of estrogen, the glycogen-containing superficial cells of the vaginal epithelium disappear. Mucosal atrophy is reflected by alterations in the cytologic smear with an increase in the parabasal cells. The predominating symptoms of senile vaginitis are discharge, itching, burning, and dyspareunia. Not infrequently one sees a blood-tinged discharge which arouses a suspicion of malignancy. Patients with an atrophic type of vaginitis have a predominantly spotting type of bleeding. Usually a blood-tinged vaginal discharge is present and the vagina shows small foci of superficial hemorrhages. Occasionally, the T. vaginalis is found and should be treated accordingly. The symptoms of senile urethritis are frequency and nocturia unassociated with infection, which are related to a shrinking of the urethral meatus.

Osteoporosis

Currently, much is being written about osteoporosis.[4, 5, 13, 18] It has been estimated that four million persons in the United States have this disease, and four fifths of them are postmenopausal women.[8] However, there is considerable controversy about the diagnosis and treatment of this disease.

In 1941 Albright et al.[1] reported that estrogens can produce a positive calcium and phosphorus balance in elderly women with osteoporosis. The view has been held that the decrease in bone mass as seen in postmenopausal osteoporosis is the net effect of diminished secretion of gonadal hormones which favors bone formation and a normal secretion of adrenocortical hormones which favors bone resorption. On the other hand, other investigators have stated that the disorder is the result of a long-continued negative calcium balance, related to either a low calcium intake or greater calcium needs, which, in effect, results in increased bone resorption rather than decreased bone formation.[20] In addition to mineral or sex hormone deficiencies, other pathogenetic factors must be entertained, for example, lack of vitamin D, decreased physical activity, and atrophy of old age. Both points are theoretical, and prospective studies are needed to evaluate the effect of estrogen in the prophylaxis of postmenopausal osteoporosis.

Coronary Atherosclerosis

A major achievement of the recent prospective epidemiologic studies on coronary heart disease has been the quantitative delineation of the association between several abnormalities and risk of middle-age coronary disease. It has been unequivocally demonstrated that abnormalities such as hypercholesterolemia and hypertension, diabetes, and heavy cigarette smoking are associated with a severalfold increase in risk of coronary disease of middle age. Obesity has similarly been indicted, also positive family history of premature (before age 60) vascular disease, hypothyroidism, renal damage, sedentary living, and certain personality-behavior problems. The overwhelming evidence indicates the disease is multifactorial in causation, with diet as a key essential etiologic factor.

It has been observed that the onset of the climacteric and the diminution of estrogen production coincide with the rapid and progressive increase of atherosclerosis and coronary heart disease.[29] It has been stated that estrogens are of value in the prevention of atherosclerosis in postmenopausal women.[11, 23, 26, 28, 35] On the other hand, Novak and Williams,[22] in a study of autopsy specimens, reported no difference in the incidence of atherosclerosis in castrated women and in control subjects.

It is generally accepted that elevated cholesterol levels and cholesterol to phospholipid (C/P) ratios are indicators of coronary disease. In the Framingham study,[29] men or women in whom coronary heart disease developed had C/P ratios at the time of entry into the study which were not different from those of individuals who remained free of the disease for 12 years. Thus, even if estrogens can lower the C/P ratio, this does not mean that such treatment reduces the risk of subsequent development of the disease. Further, data concerning the incidence of coronary atherosclerosis in bilaterally oophorectomized women and postmenopausal subjects remain controversial.[25]

As one reviews the evidence for and against the possible role of endogenous estrogen in the pathogenesis of coronary heart disease it becomes apparent that there are some factors apart from estrogen which are responsible for the relative freedom of women from coronary heart disease as compared with men. While it is beyond the scope of this paper to present all the arguments for and against, suffice it to say that proof of the efficacy of long-term estrogen replacement as a means of preventing heart diseases is lacking.

CANCER AND ESTROGEN

The question which has caused some concern is whether or not prolonged estrogen therapy can predispose or incite the development of cancer. Again, on the basis of present data the only correct and honest answer is that we do not know. Despite the clinical and experimental work which has been done in this area, dogmatic conclusions cannot be made.

Breast cancer in the human female can be altered by changing the hormonal environment in which the tumor is growing. In premenopausal women, ovarian ablation will often cause remission of metastatic breast cancer. However, the administration of estrogens to postmenopausal women causes remission of breast cancer in a certain number of patients. On the basis of this we may conclude that breast cancer is dependent on certain hormonal factors during its late stages, but it gives us no information that these factors necessarily operate during the preclinical stages.

The statistical evidence which has been advanced in support of the arguments that estrogen has not increased the incidence of breast cancer must be examined carefully.[6, 33]

Some evidence exists that a pathogenetic relationship exists between the hormone status of the patient and the development of endometrial cancer.[7, 30] It has been possible to produce experimentally carcinoma of the endometrium by means of prolonged estrogen therapy.[19] We cannot ignore the association between prolonged and uninterrupted estrogen stimulation, endometrial hyperplasia, and carcinoma.[2] Further, it has recently been reported that there is a statistically significant relationship between the maternal ingestion of diethylstilbestrol during pregnancy and the development of vaginal adenocarcinoma in the offspring exposed.[10]

The relationship between long-term estrogen administration and its association with cancer requires further clarification. Our knowledge is limited. The entire question of carcinogenesis remains to be clarified. Until such time as that occurs, it would seem wise to use estrogen with caution.

THERAPY

General Measures

It must be remembered that we are dealing with a patient whose complaints may not be of menopausal origin. The physician should be cognizant that the climacteric symptoms can shield organic disease. It is important to distinguish between the physical, psychosomatic, and degenerative processes which may occur. The patient's headache, nervousness, low backache, and left-sided abdominal pain deserve proper evaluation.

Psychological Problems

The only treatment necessary for a large proportion of menopausal patients is reassurance and physician education. Our society has led us to believe that a woman's role is a biological one, whose primary function is sexual, reproductive, and childbearing. As the woman observes the cessation of menses, she becomes acutely aware of factors which threaten her ego and which subsequently precipitate anxiety and depression: decrease in sexual capacity, loss of reproductive function, a shrinking social circle of friends, and departure of her children. Her husband is usually occupied with his career, and more often than not his libido and potency are reduced. In addition, she is exposed to a society which has placed emphasis on the desirability of youthfulness, femininity, and sensuality through all channels of communication. Such a patient is not in need of psychiatric care; nor are estrogens the answer.

The feeling of well being which is lacking is not related to estrogen deficiency. To encourage her in her pursuit of eternal youth, to delude her into thinking that she has found it in the form of estrogen, and to allow her to believe that she will assume her previous role in life by the consumption of these estrogens is akin to medical chicanery. The physician must bring the problem into perspective for the patient, reestablish her self-esteem as a social and sexual partner, and inform her that the end of menstruation and appearance of hot flashes do not spell the end of her femininity. Interest, reassurance, and interpretation of the clinical features of the climacteric will go far in controlling the psychogenic factors precipitated by the menopause. The use of a mild tranquilizer will be of some help.

I have found that it is at this time in life that women most often raise the questions of decreased libido, lack of orgasm, and frigidity. The function of the ovary in the human has little to do with libido and orgasm. The sexual relationship between the climacteric woman and her husband is decided in the earlier years of marriage. Any of the problems which appear at this time no doubt existed before, but the patient is now more cognizant of them than ever before. The climacteric should not be held culpable, and estrogen will not be the solution. The idea that a postmenopausal woman loses her ability to respond sexually is nothing more than a cultural fallacy. Finally it must be mentioned that a certain number of patients arrive at the menopause with prepsychotic personalities, those who have had a lifetime of maladjustment. In these patients the menopause may trigger full-blown psychoses, but it is not the cause.

Estrogen Therapy

The only symptoms which improve with estrogen therapy are vasomotor symptoms, insomnia, senescent vaginitis, and dysfunctional bleeding. In treating the hot flush, the aim of good therapy is to control symptoms as rapidly as possible with as little medication as possible and to discontinue treatment as soon as possible. There is no need for the parenteral administration of estrogen. It is painful, expensive, and unpredictable.

In the patient with an intact uterus the smallest oral dose should be administered in cyclic fashion, 21 to 25 days a month. Whether one employs a daily dose of 0.625 mg. of conjugated equinine estrogen, 0.25 mg. of stilbestrol, or 0.02 mg. of ethinyl estradiol is unimportant. Stilbestrol, 0.1 mg., will usually control vasomotor symptoms and rarely causes endometrial bleeding. Larger doses may result in breakthrough bleeding. The aim is to achieve sub-bleeding doses and at the same time control the vasomotor symptoms. If a patient has no uterus, estrogen is initiated on a constant daily basis. The dosage should be titrated, starting with a small dose. If one begins with large doses and then decreases the amount, the incidence of troublesome bleeding is increased. The endpoint of successful therapy is the absence of hot flashes and night sweats.

A number of authors use the vaginal cytogram as a means of determining adequate estrogen replacement.[32] The vaginal smear, not the patient, is treated. This method evaluates the karyopyknotic index (KI) or percentage of superficial cells in the total population of squamous cells exfoliated from the vaginal wall, and the maturation index (MI), or percentage of cells from each of the three squamous cell layers (parabasal, intermediate, and superficial). Thus, an MI of 100/0/0 would indicate a complete absence of estrogen. However the maturation count is too limited and too arbitrary. It is the result of an interplay between estrogen and other hormones and subject to extraneous factors. The clinical response to therapy is a much better guide to treatment.

If we are dealing with a premenopausal patient who is still menstruating and who is experiencing hot flashes, hormonal therapy may be instituted. This is the patient in whom premenstrual tension, edema, and dysmenorrhea are exaggerated. The proper treatment consists of the administration of cyclic estrogen or cyclic estrogen-progesterone therapy. The use of anovulatory doses of estrogen, for example, stilbestrol, 1 mg. daily for 21 days beginning on the first day of the menstrual flow, will result in regular cycles, control hot flashes, and have the added bonus of contraception as the pituitary gonadotropins are suppressed. Alternative therapy can be accomplished through the cyclic use of estrogen and progesterone, for example, 16 days of ethinyl estradiol, 0.1 mg., and 5 days of megestrol acetate, 5.0 mg., and ethinyl estradiol, 0.1 mg. The commercially available oral contraceptives will achieve the same purpose; however, in view of the present controversy surrounding the pill and the long train of associated symptoms, it is best to avoid their use in the patient approaching the climacteric.

There is no need for other steroids in the treatment of the postmenopausal woman. Androgens are poor substitutes, and the amount required to alleviate symptoms approximates virilizing doses. Furthermore, androgen does not decrease the incidence of bleeding, nor will it retard osteoporosis. It may have a place in patients having severe mastodynia while taking estrogen therapy. In these patients the customary dose of estrogen may be halved and 5.0 mg. tablet of methyltestosterone may be administered for several months. Progesterone plays no significant role in the physiology of the menopause. Estrogens should be administered to the young surgical castrate and to patients with a premature menopause.

Menopausal and Postmenopausal Bleeding

Irregular bleeding (dysfunctional bleeding) is related to anovulation, continuing estrogen stimulation of the endometrium, proliferation, and hyperplasia with subsequent breakthrough bleeding that is unpredictable in duration, frequency, and amount. The patient must have a thorough evaluation, and one must be reasonably certain that the bleeding is not the result of carcinoma and is functional in origin. The most rational approach to the problem of anovulation and irregular bleeding is through the cyclic administration of a progestational agent. Medroxyprogesterone acetate, 10 mg. daily for 4 days every 4 weeks, will generally insure regular endometrial sloughing. Again, if the patient is having severe vasomotor symptoms, one may use an estrogen in the form of stilbestrol, 1.0 mg. daily for 21 days. This will prevent ovarian function through the suppression of pituitary gonadotropins, and the patient will bleed cyclically.

Exogenous Estrogen and Bleeding

Uterine bleeding during the menopausal phase and postmenopausal period in a patient receiving estrogen therapy must be viewed with suspicion. It should not give the physician a false sense of security. Provided that the pelvic examination and Papanicolaou smear are normal and the patient ceases to bleed within 10 days after the withdrawal of estrogen therapy, she may be observed carefully. We have found it worthwhile to treat patients who give a history of estrogen-related bleeding with a course of medroxyprogesterone acetate, 10 to 20 mg. daily for 3 days, the so-called chemical curettage. Such patients are allowed 2 weeks of withdrawal bleeding after which persistence is considered an indication for dilatation and curettage.

Postmenopausal bleeding is particularly troublesome and must be presumed to be of uterine origin until proved otherwise. Bleeding as a result of estrogen administration and a blood-tinged vaginal discharge secondary to severe atrophic vaginitis are common causes of genital bleeding in the postmenopausal period. By definition, postmenopause means the absence of any bleeding for 1 year. In years past, postmenopausal bleeding was of malignant origin in the majority of patients.

Today a reversal of incidence has taken place, and the majority of postmenopausal bleeding investigated by curettage is of benign origin. In a study from our clinic involving 335 patients, pelvic malignancy accounted for 20 per cent and benign causes for 80 per cent of postmenopausal bleeding[9] (Table 1). This study showed that the commonest cause of bleeding was exogenous estrogen (26.6 per cent), followed by no identifiable cause (23.3 per cent). The other important categories showed corpus carcinoma, 13.4 per cent, and atrophic vaginitis, 9.8 per cent.

The low incidence of malignancy in postmenopausal bleeding is the

Table 1. *Analysis of Cause Among 335 Cases of Initial Postmenopausal Bleeding**

LESION	PROBABLE CAUSE		POSSIBLE CAUSE, NUMBER	INCIDENTAL FINDING, NUMBER
	Number	Per cent		
No cause found (includes atrophic endometrium, and so forth)	78	23.3	0	0
Recent estrogen therapy	89	26.6	16	5
Urethral caruncle	4	1.2	5	4
Atrophic vaginitis	33	9.8	28	4
Cervical polyps	14	4.2	9	6
Cervicitis and cervical erosion	8	2.4	2	13
Endometrial polyps	23	6.8	22	6
Endometritis and pelvic inflammatory disease	0	0.0	1	1
Endometrial hyperplasia	11	3.3	12	12
Leiomyoma of uterus	1	0.3	1	42
Trauma	7	2.1	6	0
Carcinoma of vagina	3	0.9	0	0
Carcinoma of bladder to vagina	1	0.3	0	0
Epidermoid carcinoma of cervix	13	3.9	0	0
Adenocarcinoma of cervix	1	0.3	0	0
Adenocarcinoma of endometrium	38	11.3	0	0
Adenoacanthoma of endometrium	4	1.2	0	0
Carcinosarcoma of uterus	3	0.9	0	0
Carcinoma of ovary	3	0.9	0	1**
Carcinoma of tube	1	0.3	0	0
Leukemia	0	0.0	1	0
Totals	335	100.0	103	94

*From Hawwa, Z. M., et al.: Postmenopausal bleeding. Lahey Clin. Found. Bull., *19*:63 (April–June) 1970.

**Incidental to endometrial carcinoma.

result of increasing use of estrogens, decrease in the number of patients with carcinoma of the cervix, and cancer prevention crusades. Thus, it is our policy to treat apparent estrogen-related bleeding with a brief course of a progestin, and if no bleeding occurs beyond the 2 weeks allowed for withdrawal bleeding, such patients are cautiously observed. In the event of further bleeding, curettage is performed. Patients who are obese, diabetic, or hypertensive are more likely to have a malignancy.

Senescent Vaginitis

The absence of estrogen is the basic cause of the atrophy, and the administration of estrogen will restore the vaginal epithelium to its former thickness. There is an increase in the glycogen content of the epithelial cells, and the normal flora returns. The best method is to administer an estrogen-containing cream, nightly for 2 weeks, after which a maintenance dose is employed twice weekly. An alternative approach is the use of stilbestrol suppositories, 0.5 mg. nightly, for several months. It is generally not necessary to employ oral estrogen in the control of senile vaginitis.

Osteoporosis and Atherosclerosis

So long as we are relatively ignorant of the aging process, we are not in a position to forestall the inevitable changes—osteoporosis and atherosclerosis. The efficacy of long-term estrogen replacement in the prevention of these degenerative processes has not been fully substantiated.

CONCLUSION

The proper aim of therapy is to facilitate the transition during the climacteric and not to eliminate it. Therapy must be directed at the patient—not the menopause, the vaginal cytogram, or chronologic age. Hormones should be used only when indicated to control distressing vasomotor symptoms, dysfunctional uterine bleeding, and senile vaginitis. It must be remembered that the climacteric and menopause are normal physiologic events in the life of a woman and are not pathologic states. Our limited knowledge of potential side effects of long-term hormone therapy and lack of accurate statistical information as to its need in the prevention of degenerative processes should discipline us in our enthusiasm for flooding all of our senior female population with hormones. It is naive to assume that in estrogen we have found the elixir of youth. Probably the most important aspects of management comprise reassurance, sympathy, understanding, and explanation.

REFERENCES

1. Albright, F., Smith, P. H., and Richardson, A. M.: Postmenopausal osteoporosis. Its clinical features. J.A.M.A., 116:2465–2474 (May 31) 1941.
2. Bromberg, Y. M., Liban, E., and Laufer, A.: Early endometrial carcinoma following prolonged estrogen administration in an ovariectomized woman. Obstet. Gynec., 14:221–226 (Aug.) 1959.
3. Bulbrook, R. D., and Greenwood, F. C.: Persistence of urinary oestrogen excretion after oophorectomy and adrenalectomy. Brit. Med. J., 1:662–666 (March 23) 1957.
4. Davis, M. E., Lanzl, L. H., and Cox, A. B.: Detection, prevention and retardation of menopausal osteoporosis. Obstet. Gynec., 36:187–198 (Aug.) 1970.
5. Dunn, A. W.: Senile osteoporosis. Geriatrics, 22:175–180 (Nov.) 1967.
6. Greenblatt, R. B., Barfield, W. E., and Jungck, E. C.: The treatment of the menopause. Canad. Med. Assoc. J., 86:113–114 (Jan. 20) 1962.
7. Gusberg, S. B.: Precursors of corpus carcinoma estrogens and adenomatous hyperplasia. Amer. J. Obstet. Gynec., 54:905–927 (Dec.) 1947.
8. Henneman, P. H.: Postmenopausal osteoporosis. Clin. Obstet. Gynec., 7:531–544 (June) 1964.
9. Hawwa, Z. M., Nahhas, W. A., and Copenhaver, E. H.: Postmenopausal bleeding. Lahey Clin. Found. Bull., 19:61–70 (April-June) 1970.
10. Herbst, A. L., Ulfelder, H., and Poskanzer, D. C.: Adenocarcinoma of the vagina. Association of maternal stilbestrol therapy with tumor appearance in young women. New Eng. J. Med., 284:878–881 (April 22) 1971.
11. Higano, N., Robinson, R. W., and Cohen, W. D.: Increased incidence of cardiovascular disease in castrated women. Two-year follow-up studies. New Eng. J. Med., 268:1123–1125 (May 16) 1963.
12. Israel, S. L.: Diagnosis and Treatment of Menstrual Disorders and Sterility. New York, Hoeber Medical Division, Harper and Row Publishers, 1967, 638 pp.
13. Jowsey, J.: Microradiography of bone resorption. In Sognnaes, R. F. (ed.): Mechanism of Hard Tissue Destruction. Washington, American Association for the Advancement of Science, Publication No. 75, 1963, p. 447.

14. Kistner, R. W.: Gynecology: Principles and Practice. Chicago, Year Book Medical Publishers, Inc., 1965, 654 pp.
15. Kupperman, H. S., Wetchler, B. B., and Blatt, M. H.: Contemporary therapy of the menopausal syndrome. J.A.M.A., 171:1627–1637 (Nov. 21) 1959.
16. Masukawa, T.: Vaginal smears in women past 40 years of age with emphasis on their remaining hormonal activity. Obstet. Gynec., 16:407–413 (Oct.) 1960.
17. McLennan, M. T., and McLennan, C. E.: Estrogenic status of menstruating and menopausal women assessed by cervicovaginal smears. Obstet. Gynec., 37:325–331 (March) 1971.
18. Meema, H. E., Bunker, M. L., and Memma, S.: Loss of compact bone due to menopause. Obstet. Gynec., 26:333–343 (Sept.) 1965.
19. Meissner, W. A., Sommers, S. C., and Sherman, G.: Endometrial hyperplasia, endometrial carcinoma, and endometriosis produced experimentally by estrogen. Cancer, 10:500–509 (May-June) 1957.
20. Nordin, B. E.: The pathogenesis of osteoporosis. Lancet, 1:1011–1015 (May 13) 1961.
21. Novak, E. R., Goldberg, B., Jones, G. S., et al.: Enzyme histochemistry of the menopausal ovary associated with normal and abnormal endometrium. Amer. J. Obstet. Gynec., 93:669–682 (Nov. 1) 1965.
22. Novak, E. R., and Williams, T. J.: Autopsy comparison of cardiovascular changes in castrated and normal women. Amer. J. Obstet. Gynec., 80:863–872 (Nov.) 1960.
23. Oliver, M. F., and Boyd, G. S.: Effect of bilateral ovariectomy on coronary-artery disease and serum-lipid levels. Lancet, 2:690–694 (Oct. 31) 1959.
24. Randall, C. L., Birtch, P. K., and Harkins, J. L.: Ovarian function after the menopause. Amer. J. Obstet. Gynec., 74:719–729 (Oct.) 1957.
25. Randall, C. L., Paloucek, F. P., Graham, J. B., et al.: Causes of death in cases of preclimacteric menorrhagia. Amer. J. Obstet. Gynec., 88:880–897 (April 1) 1964.
26. Stamler, J., Pick, R., Katz, L. N., et al.: Effectiveness of estrogens for therapy of myocardial infarction in middle-age men. J.A.M.A., 183:632–638 (Feb. 23) 1963.
27. Struthers, R. A.: Post-menopausal oestrogen production. Brit. Med. J., 1:1331–1335 (June 9) 1956.
28. Sznajderman, M., and Oliver, M. F.: Spontaneous premature menopause, ischemic heart-disease, and serum-lipids. Lancet, 1:962–965 (May 4) 1963.
29. Thomas, H. E., Kannel, W. B., Dawber, T. R., et al.: Cholesterol-phospholipid ratio in the prediction of coronary heart disease. The Framingham Study. New Eng. J. Med., 274:701–705 (March 31) 1966.
30. Wallach, S., and Henneman, P. H.: Prolonged estrogen therapy in postmenopausal women. J.A.M.A., 171:1637–1642 (Nov. 21) 1959.
31. Wilson, R. A.: Feminine Forever. Philadelphia, J. B. Lippincott Co., 1965, 224 pp.
32. Wilson, R. A., Brevetti, R. E., and Wilson, T. A.: Specific procedures for the elimination of the menopause. Western J. Surg., 71:110–121 (May-June) 1963.
33. Wilson, R. A.: The roles of estrogen and progesterone in breast and genital cancer. J.A.M.A., 182:327–331 (Oct. 27) 1962.
34. Wilson, R. A., and Wilson, T. A.: The fate of the nontreated post-menopausal woman: A plea for maintenance of adequate estrogen from puberty to the grave. J. Amer. Geriat. Soc., 11:347–362 (April) 1963.
35. Wuest, J. H., Dry, T. J., and Edwards, J. E.: Degree of coronary atherosclerosis in bilaterally oophorectomized women. Circulation, 7:801–809 (June) 1953.

605 Commonwealth Avenue
Boston, Massachusetts 02215

The Future of Tumor Immunology

B. Cinader, Ph.D., D.Sc., F.R.I.C., F.R.S.C.

In the next decade, progress in cancer-control will depend to a considerable extent on a multidisciplinary approach and on an intimate combination of available diagnostic and therapeutic methods at every stage of patient care. Immunology should have a role to play in various aspects of detection, treatment, and control: early diagnosis, identification and assessment of the patient's disease, evaluation and selection of chemotherapeutic agents, evaluation of short and long term consequences of excision therapy, appropriate regulation of body defense mechanisms, and preventive treatment. The use of immunologic methods of treatment depends on several assumptions, and we shall examine, in the course of this review, the available evidence for an evaluation of our prospects in terms of meeting the requirements for each of these objectives.

TUMOR ANTIGENS

The first assumption, and the most basic one, is that in and on tumor cells, there are several antigens which are characteristic of the tumor. The first indications of tumor-specific antigens were obtained from transplantation of tumors into pre-immunized syngeneic animals. The technique was limited to animal experiments, but subsequently introduced methods of analysis were applicable to patients. Such methods have greatly extended our knowledge of human and animal tumors, and there is now good evidence for the existence of multiple macromolecular differences between tumor cells and normal cells. There appear to be embryonic antigens which are released by tumors into the circulation and others which can only be detected in tumor tissue. Embryonic tumor antigens have been demonstrated in several types of human tumors (Table 1), in virally transformed cells, and in carcinogen-induced tumors of mice and rats (SV-40 transformed cells,[11, 41, 55] Mc-induced sarcomas,[10, 21] and DAB-induced hepatomas[2, 10]). Antigens have also been

---

*Professor in the Department of Medical Cell Biology, Medical Biophysics and Pathological Chemistry, and Director of the Institute of Immunology, Medical Faculty and School of Graduate Studies, University of Toronto

Table 1. *Tumor-Dependent Embryonic Antigens of Patients with Neoplastic Disease*

TUMOR	ANTIGEN Designation	ANTIGEN Localization	SPECIFICITY	HUMORAL ANTIBODY IN PATIENT	REFERENCES
Adenocarcinomas of digestive system (esophagus, stomach, small bowel, colon, rectum, pancreas, liver)	Carcinoembryonic (CEA)	Cell membranes (glycocalix) and serum	100% depending on the antigen-preparing and the sensitivity range of the test	70% with localized cancer; 60% with metastatic dissemination	77, 78, 128, 189, 194
Hepatomas (mouse and man)	Alpha₁-fetoprotein	Tumor cells and serum	Also found in 10% of testicular tetra-blastomas and in 50% of pyridoxine-deficient baboons	—	2, 65, 67, 187
Malignant tumors of children with nephroblastoma, neuro-blastoma, tetratoma, hepatoma, lymphosarcoma, reticulum cell sarcoma, osteogenic sarcoma, cerebral tumors	Alpha₂H-ferroprotein	Serum	81% of children with malignant tumors; 8% of children with non-cancerous disease	—	25

Various malignant tumors	Regan alkaline phosphatase isozyme (Placental alkaline phosphatase)	Tumor cells	4–5% of patients with various malignant tumors	—	177
Gastric cancer	Fetal sulfoglycoprotein antigen	Gastric juice	96% of gastric cancers; 10% of normals and patients with non-cancerous gastric pathology	—	83
Many different malignant tumors	Heterophile fetal antigen	Saline extract of tumor (71%); sera (9%)	Absent from normal sera but present in 75% benign tumor tissues and 4% non-neoplastic tissue; human antibody cross-reacts with fetuses of many mammals	0.8% of patients with antigen	58

revealed by means of antibodies found in the circulation of patients after tumor excision or in the serum of pregnant women or pregnant animals, and by suitably absorbed antisera from immunized normal rabbits or from immunized rabbits which were rendered tolerant to tissue extracts.

The first tumor antigens were demonstrated by rejection of syngeneic tumors. The conclusions based on this type of test remain essentially as I summarized them in 1962 and 1963,[35, 36] and are given in Table 2.

In addition to and distinct from virus-induced transplantation antigens, there are virus coat antigens which may also be expressed on the cell membrane. Furthermore, there are other viral antigens (core antigens) which are not necessarily found in the viral coat. These antigens are less readily detected in tumor cells induced by DNA viruses, than in tumor cells induced by RNA viruses and are demonstrable on both the membrane from which virus buds and, in soluble form, in the cytoplasm. Some of the core antigens of the RNA viruses are intraspecies specific (i.e., the same for all neoplasms of the same species) and others are interspecies specific (common to mammalian though not to avian tumors).[13, 71, 72, 159] One particularly intriguing core antigen is RNA-dependent DNA polymerase (inverse transcriptase). Sera from rats bearing transplantable tumors, induced by murine C-type viruses, contain an inhibitor of this enzyme activity. Antibodies, raised by immunization of rabbits with partially purified murine leukemia virus polymerase, cross-react with polymerases of other mammalian C-type RNA-containing tumor viruses. In short, the polymerases from different mammalian

Table 2. *Tumor-Specific Antigens*

Chemical carcinogens
  3-Methyl cholanthrene
  1,2,5,6-Dibenzanthracene
  9,10-Dimethylbenzanthracene
  3,4,9,10-Dibenzpyrene
  3,4-Benzpyrene
  p-Dimethylaminoazobenzene
Physical agents
  Films: Millipore filter
          Cellophane
  Radiation: Ultraviolet
                  Strontium-90
	"Individualistic" tumor antigens — Distinct tumor antigens for each tumor

DNA viruses
  Adenovirus 12, 18
  Polyoma
  SV 40
  Shope papilloma
 	
RNA viruses
  Mammary — tumor agents
  Leukemia viruses
    Grass, Graffi
    Moloney, Rich
    Rasucher, Friend
  Rous (Schmidt Ruppin)
	Group antigens — Tumor antigens are similar for tumor induced by the same virus or by related viruses

tumor viruses are antigenically related.[1] This may be a first indication that antibodies against animal virus may be of value in the detection of human tumor viruses.

Most of the evidence on virus-induced transplantation antigens is still confined to animal systems; however, evidence for disease specific immunity and antibody are now available for Burkitt's lymphoma,[98, 117, 150] melanoma,[125, 126, 137, 139, 146] neuroblastomas of infancy,[93] osteogenic sarcoma,[63, 135, 136] bladder tumors,[23] and Hodgkin's disease.[151] Whether the common human antigens are embryonic in origin or are coded in the viral genome is known only in the case of the carcinoembryonic antigens of adenocarcinomas of the digestive system. Even in the case of Burkitt's lymphoma, the viral origin of the disease remains uncertain, the identity of the virus controversial, and the control of the common antigen unknown.[98, 150]

Diagnostic and Screening Tests

Two groups of techniques, based on (1) the humoral and (2) the cell-mediated immune responses, are available for the detection of "new" antigens. Circulating antigens can be detected by standard immunochemical methods such as double diffusion in agar but most readily by an extremely sensitive radioimmunoassay as is illustrated by the radioimmunoassay for carcinoembryonic antigen.[189] The presence of antigens which are not released in appreciable quantities can be shown in tumor tissue by means of fluorescent staining with appropriate antisera,[80] or by cytotoxic tests.[182] Furthermore, colony inhibition tests can help to reveal additional antigenic relationships[95] and blocking, and cytotoxicity tests can extend this analysis. With patient sera, one can, in this way, demonstrate, as has been done in the case of human melanomas, antigenic similarities between tumors[95, 139] as well as the existence of "individual" antigens characteristic of each individual tumor.[84] Only the first group of techniques (Table 3) offers hope for early diagnosis, but it is limited to antigens which appear in the circulation.

Some of the antigens, which do not circulate, may be revealed by demonstrating the presence of circulating antibody against already discovered tumor-specific antigens. In this context, antibodies against "individualistic" tumor antigens are irrelevant since they are obviously not suitable for diagnostic purposes. Antibodies against embryonic antigens can be detected most readily by circulating antibody but this will have to be studied extensively before its diagnostic use in females can be relied upon. Antibodies could also be used to explore the association of putative human tumor viruses with a given disease and to detect unknown human tumor viruses by the reactivity of patient sera with known animal tumor viruses. The already mentioned cross-reactivity of DNA-dependent RNA polymerase illustrates this point.

The puzzling presence of SV40 neutralizing antibodies in United States and North Indian residents without history of polio immunization[160-162] and the presence in some human milks of particles physically identical with mouse mammary tumor viruses[156] are tantalizing indications of possibilities that may exist in this area for determining virus/tu-

Table 3.   *Techniques for the Detection of Human Tumor Antigens*

| | | IMMUNE REAGENTS | |
TECHNIQUE	SOURCE OF TUMOR ANTIGENS	Type	Source
Precipitin (e.g., Ouchterlony, radio-immunoassay, etc.) Fluorescent staining	Fluids (serum, gastric juice, tissue extracts, etc.) Tissues	Antibody	Sera from: (1) Tumor-bearers after excision or spontaneous recovery (2) Multiparous females (3) Immunized normal animals and animals tolerant to normal tissue
Colony inhibition Cytolytic	Tissues	Lymphoid cells	Tumor-bearers

mor association and, ultimately, to base diagnostic tests on these associations. It is perhaps worthwhile to mention an obvious and foreseeable limitation to this approach. This limitation is best illustrated by the experience with the herpes-like Epstein-Barr virus (EBV) which has been suggested as the causative agent of Burkitt's lymphomas, infectious mononucleosis, carcinoma of the posterior nasal space, and sarcoidosis.[97, 98, 102, 143, 150]

It turns out that 70 to 85 per cent of normal adults have antibodies against EBV[75, 123] and if a proven tumor virus should be so widely distributed and so nonspecific in its action, detection of a virus-antibody will clearly have little or no diagnostic value except, possibly, in terms of fluctuation in titers of the virus antibody. If a tumor virus really turned out to be universally distributed, early diagnosis of disease would have to depend on transplantation antigens or embryonic antigens.

A simple method for the detection of transplantation antigens and of an active state of cellular immunity would greatly add to the range of diagnostic possibilities. Current methods are not suitable for routine hospital use and the development of a quick and simple assay is an important objective in the search for a wide-range of diagnostic tests.

We have so far discussed diagnostic tests which, when used in combination, may have discriminatory power and hence great diagnostic potential. For screening we need a technique which does not necessarily discriminate between different types of cancer but by which tumor-bearers can be distinguished from tumor-free individuals. There are some intriguing developments in this direction, based on a lipid, ceramiside-lactoside (cytolipin H), which is found in high concentration only in the membrane of tumor cells and in trophoblastic tissue. These lipids combine with a serum globulin (T-globulin) in the serum of cancer patients and pregnant women at delivery. This globulin is not detected in the serum of patients with other diseases or in the serum of normal individuals.[184, 185] The detection of T-globulin could serve as a diagnostic test. Coded serum samples from 520 patients were tested for the presence of T-globulin and good correlation between the presence of cancer and the presence of T-globulin was established.[186] The predictive value of the test remains to be examined.

In summary, embryonic antigens, virus coat and core antigens, tumor transplantation, general membrane and cytoplasmic antigens, and antibodies directed against them, have been detected in a sufficient variety of animal and human cancers to justify the hope for a battery of tests which will allow the early detection of tumors and possibly even their identification. The large number of tumor tests which in the past have appeared like brilliant stars and have disappeared into oblivion like spent fireworks have justly hardened us against excessive optimism. However, our present knowledge of tumor antigens provides a very different background for research and implementation from that available a decade ago, and the resulting tools are immediately applicable to enumeration and detection of embryonic antigens. One can now foresee a development in these areas which is analogous to the development of our knowledge of blood group substances in the decade between 1929 and 1940. An immediate transition from fundamental to screening work, i.e., to applied research, is conceivable and indeed desirable. This is not a task for investigators motivated by an interest in fundamental problems. Rapid progress will depend on the establishment and support of appropriate diagnostically oriented groups of serologists, clinical immunologists, and pathologists.

Application of Diagnostic Tests

Once it has become possible, detection of disease before it becomes clinically observable will reveal tumors which progress to clinical disease as well as tumors which may regress. The relative frequency of these two types of tumors is unknown. The advantages of early treatment must, therefore, be subjected to clinical trials so that a distinction can be made between spontaneous regression and cure caused by early treatment.

One can foresee a much more rapid implementation of tumor-antigen detection in the realm of surgical practice. Here additional sensitive techniques for determining the extent of tumor growth and the involvement of draining lymph nodes by locally injected, radioactively labelled, specifically purified antibodies could provide extremely rapid objective assessment of the extent of local tumor spread. The last tumor cell or the distant metastasis will obviously not be detected by this approach, but the extent of local surgical intervention might become a little less intuitive. Furthermore, tumor antigens in the circulation and the corresponding antibodies could become a guide to determining the consequences of surgical treatment, of chemotherapy and of the resurgence of disease.

Finally, it seems quite likely that the types of tumors will ultimately be characterized by a sufficiently large number of antigens to permit a classification of disease which takes into account distinctive macromolecular diversity and which would thus create a much more refined classification of tumors. The refined molecularly based disease classification will clearly provide a much improved method for patient-selection and thus a narrowing of the statistical range of the consequences of therapeutic intervention.

In stressing the roads which are open to applied research, I may have given the impression that there is no need in this area for fundamental investigations. Nothing is further from the truth or from my view of it. Many examples could be given and the need to understand the nature of "individualistic" tumor cell antigens may serve as one. This is an extremely puzzling phenomenon and though there is little to be hoped for with regard to diagnostic purposes, an insight into the control of these antigens may have much to teach us about tumerogenesis.

IMMUNOTHERAPY

I would like to turn next to immunotherapy and thus to the consequences of a second assumption, that some tumor antigens evoke an immune response which has the potential of destroying the tumor. In this context, we must distinguish between tumor antigens which are in the cytoplasm, and hence inaccessible to the immune apparatus, and antigens which are on the cell surface.

The Membrane of Tumor Cells

So far I have dealt with tumor antigens in general but it has no doubt become apparent to the reader that many antigens which are common to a particular type of tumor are found in or on membranes. These include embryonic host antigens as well as virus-directed transplantation antigens. The difference between the tumor cell membrane and the normal membrane is quite extensive and is not confined to the acquisition of antigens. There is a loss of antigens in chemically induced tumors, a reduction in the concentration of normal transplantation antigens, and also a general rearrangement of normal macromolecules. Changes in distribution and density of normal membrane macromolecules may be exemplified by differences in the interaction of normal and transformed cells with carbohydrate-binding proteins such as concavalin A,[106, 164] soybean agglutinin,[127, 158] and glycoprotein from wheat germ.[26] In short, these substances combine with membrane sites which are more accessible in transformed cells than they are in normal cells, and we may conclude that the position and/or density of these binding sites must be altered in the course of malignant transformation. Furthermore, it appears that malignant transformation is associated with a change in the position of amino acid and carbohydrate transport sites in relation to the binding sites for concavalin A.[107] Whether or not these binding sites are antigenically altered remains to be seen. It is known that lipids are extensively changed in tumor cells. These changes may affect the distribution of other antigens and in themselves are known to result in lipid-determined antigenic changes.[32, 155, 163]

We have already seen that transplantation experiments, colony inhibition assays, and immunofluorescent staining have provided ample evidence that in addition to deletion, rearrangement, and density changes of normal membrane components, tumor membranes contain antigens which are distinct from normal membrane-components. We will now evaluate the validity of our assumption that these tumor antigens on membranes evoke an immune response which affects the progress of tumor-growth.

Immunologic Surveillance

There is some indirect evidence that the incidence of clinical cancers would be much greater were it not for the surveillance by the immune system. It is perhaps easiest to support this statement by a list of arguments. There is: (1) a high incidence of tumors in cases of inborn errors of the cell-mediated immune apparatus,[7] (2) an increased incidence of tumors in thymectomized animals which are infected by tumor viruses or tumor cells, (3) an increase in the minimal number of tumor cells required for tumor take after immunization, (4) a high incidence of cancer in immunosuppressed patients, and (5) a difference in immunologic parameters between animals infected with the same virus, but having a regressing or progressing tumor.

Spontaneous regression, which has been repeatedly observed in human tumors can be observed in experimental systems and clearly appears to be an immune phenomenon. The tumor-controlling effects of immunity are most strikingly illustrated by infection with rapid tumor-inducing viruses such as Yaba virus in monkeys, Shope fibroma and papilloma virus in rabbits, and Rous sarcoma virus in fowl. A few days after virus inocculation, tumor masses appear, grow rapidly at first, and later disappear. Animals which recover from the primary tumor do not develop tumors after a second injection.[8]

On the basis of this type of experiment, it appears most likely that many tumors may regress before they cause irreparable damage and that clinical cancer is due to the minority of tumors which escape control by the immune system. In fact, children with inborn errors of the immune system, especially with defects of cell-mediated immunity, show an increased tendency to develop malignancy, often of the lymphoreticular system.[7] Furthermore, a very high incidence of reticulum-cell sarcomas and other tumors is observed in patients who receive immunosuppressive treatment after renal transplantation.[152]

If immunity plays a role in cancer-control, one would assume that immunization with membrane components of the cancer cell would reduce the incidence of cancer in the immunized population. I suggest that there is already a population available, consisting of individuals who have been left unimmunized or have been immunized to varying extents with embryonic antigens which are found on tumors. This population consists of women who are childless or who have borne children and appear to have acquired immunity to many embryonic antigens. Thus, women represent such a population with "built-in" controls. Indeed, if one compares cancer incidence in sites other than secondary and primary sex organs, one finds that the incidence of disease in males is usually higher than in females.[206] Thyroid tumors are a striking exception to this general rule.

Cancer of the intestine is among the few cancers with a similar incidence among men and women. This is not attributable to a general failure in cellular immunity, since cytocidal properties of peripheral lymphocytes from patients with digestive system cancer could be demonstrated by the colony inhibition test.[91] However, carcinoembryonic antigen (CEA) does not stimulate lymphocyte transformation of blood lymphocytes from patients with CEA,[103] so that it is possible that cancers of the colon have more than one antigen in common and that the embryonic antigen, CEA, does not provoke cellular immunity. At any rate, cancer of the intestine and of the thyroid are exceptions to the correlation between cancer incidence and sex.

It does not necessarily follow that all antigenic differences result in a strong immunological response. Indeed, we know that in tissue transplantation some groups of antigens induce much more potent responses than others and we shall return to this question in our discussion of preventive immunization. Here, the question is posed whether embryonic antigens are targets of tumor destruction.

To answer this question, we need to examine cancer incidence in terms of parity. It should be possible to make such figures available in the not too distant future. Until then, we must remain in doubt whether *any* difference between men and women can ever be attributed to a single factor. It is clearly desirable that cancer registries should create the conditions for the collection of data which may help us to decide on the value of actively induced immunity to embryonic antigens and on the prospects of making the world a little safer, at least for men.

The sex-dependent cancer incidence must remain a weak link in our otherwise fairly compelling chain of evidence for an important role of the immune apparatus in limiting the development of tumors.

In short, tumors are immunogenic, and both humoral and cellular responses occur. These responses exercise an effective control of potential or nascent tumors, though they are not the only mechanism involved in control.[171]

It seems justified to conclude that immunologic surveillance is an important limiting factor in tumor incidence. Does immunologic surveillance retard tumors when they have progressed to become clinically recognizable neoplasms? Are the components of the immune response still responsive when a tumor has escaped this surveillance? If they are, there would be a continuous high level of tumor antigens and antibody as well as tumor-directed cellular immunity.

Tumor Growth in the Face of Surveillance

It may be assumed that of all tumors which develop, only some go on to progressive development and cannot be controlled by the immune system. The possible reasons for this progressive development of the tumor may be found in a variety of causes. I shall list them in the temporal order of their impact but confine my discussion to those items which are most relevant to a consideration of therapy. Such problems as the relative immunogenicity of various tumor antigens and the genetic control of immunological responsiveness will be omitted here to be discussed in the section on preventive measures:

(1) genetic predisposition of the tumor patient;

(2) selection of tumors for weakly immunogenic transplantation antigens;

(3) inhibition of effective cellular immunity by humoral immunity;

(4) induction of tolerance by an overwhelming antigenic load, released at the final stages of disease.

I want to deal with the inhibition of effective immunity and then consider two approaches to immunological potentiation: (1) induced change in the balance between humoral and cellular immunity by a regulatory interference with the production of enhancing (or blocking) humoral antibody and (2) nonspecific stimulation of the immune apparatus by such agents as BCG.

Tumors which break through control mechanisms seem to coexist with tumor-directed humoral and cellular immunity. We have already considered the evidence for humoral immunity. The evidence for cellular immunity is based on colony-inhibition assays by which it can be shown that most tumor patients have lymphoid cells which can inhibit growth of the patient's tumor cells. Thus, a tumor patient has, at the same time, tumor tissue which is localized, tumor cell components and tumor antigens which are disseminated throughout the blood space and the lymphatics, host cells which are immune to some of the tumor antigens and antibody which is directed against them. The question arises why the immunological instrumentarium does not dispose of the tumor. This type of failure is probably not unique to the immunological relation between tumor and tumor host and may be analogous to the relation between fetus and mother.[195] If so, it will find an explanation for its evolutionary and survival value in a need for the coexistence between mother and this particular natural graft. The phenomenon of enhancement (i.e. antibody-mediated promotion of tumor growth) provided the first clue that humoral antibody may somehow abrogate effective tumor immunity.[112, 113]

At this stage, it must be stated unequivocally that the best available *in vivo* evidence on enhancing and on cytotoxic antibody in organ transplantation leads to the conclusion that IgM fractions of antibody provoke rejection and that IgG fractions are enhancing.[68, 138] The same conclusion can be drawn from work on tumor enhancement in mice.[17, 109, 181]

The Hellströms provided an experimental system[117] which may be relevant to an understanding of the permissiveness for tumor growth in the presence of tumor-directed humoral and cellular immunity. They showed that the serum of tumor-bearing animals can block the in vitro activity of immune lymphocytes which are capable of inhibiting growth of tumor cells (colony inhibition) in the absence of added serum. Sera from animals in which a tumor has regressed do not block.[89] The blocking factor may constitute a powerful mechanism for escape from efficient lymphocyte-mediated cellular immunity if the blocking sera has the same effect in vivo as in vitro. There is some evidence that this may be so.

In vivo tumor growth is increased in animals which have been injected with blocking serum after tumor isografting and is inhibited after injection with a serum which has been selected for its in vitro capacity to counteract serum blocking activity.[91, 167] I have already indicated that an active but ineffective immune state may not be confined to the tumor host relationship. It may in fact underlie several aspects of the phenomenon which we designate as immunologic tolerance and may involve active interaction between host and graft. The chimeric state in tissue-tolerant animals[192, 193] and the mutual tolerance of parabiotic animals[81] may owe their existence to antibody-mediated protection of the chimeric state against cell-mediated immunity. Low dose tolerance to defined antigens may also involve an active immune state and the participation of antibody.[51] It is tempting to speculate that in all these cases, T cells may be kept inactive by antigen-antibody complexes, attached to T cell-receptors. If such inhibition occurs it may be, at least partly, reversible. Strong cytotoxic effects of lymphocytes can be demonstrated during the latency period and long before a tumor can be detected,[168] and yet immunization with tumor cells during the latency period has a significant prophylactic effect.[49, 79]

Some therapeutic implications of these speculations are obvious. The transition from speculation to a framework of established facts is therefore important. We need to know the extent to which antibody affects the immune apparatus directly and the extent to which it prevents the immune response by blocking access of killer cells to antibody-coated tumor cells. The nature of blocking antibody remains to be explored. Does *any* tumor-specific antibody block, depending only on its absolute quantity? Is a particular immunoglobulin sub-class blocking (possibly one that is non-complement-fixing? Is blocking dependent on specificity (i.e. does the antibody have to be directed against the same antigen as the immune lymphocyte)? And finally is blocking partially or entirely dependent on quality and quantity of antibody? No doubt precise answers to these questions will be available in a year or two. There is some evidence that a serum fraction of a molecular weight below that of antibody can potentiate the blocking activity of immunoglobulin and this might turn out to be a first clue to the mechanism of blocking by antigen-antibody complexes.[92, 169]

Immunotherapy by Attempts to Remove Antibody-Interference with Cellular Immunity

It seems reasonable to assume that there is a stage, before disease has become disseminated but at which tumors are recognized clinically, in which tumor growth could be retarded or could even be arrested if host interference with cellular immunity could be eliminated. The strategy of this approach will become more subtle and less intuitively inspired when the mechanism of blocking is finally understood. Until then we can only base our proposal on a number of experimental models which arose from the analysis of blocking and which have been conceived in these research contexts. I shall mention two types of potential therapy which are not feasible at the moment, but could be implemented after some technical objectives have been met. I mention them because they need fundamental research with a well-defined goal, but in addition would involve a major investment in biological engineering in order to obtain reasonably large quantities of human tumor specific antigens.

I have already mentioned animal experiments in which administration of unblocking serum was found to delay the development of tumors.[91, 167] Indeed, there are reports of occasional regression of malignant melanomas after injection with serum from patients with spontaneous regressions.[180, 188] It is surely desirable to remove this clinical phenomenon from the realm of the anecdotal since a feasible trial can be visualized with some chance of a successful, i.e. definitive, conclusion. One would have to culture melanoma cells on a large scale, purify the common melanoma antigen, ascertain that it is free of virus and of nucleic acid, prepare antibodies in male volunteers, screen the antibodies by colony-inhibition assays or by a similar test of the future and employ the selected unblocking serum in clinical trials. There are alternative strategies, but they are less promising. I shall mention them because they illustrate general approaches which have already become technically feasible or might become practicable.

Removal of blocking antibody from the patient's serum by physical means, as might be achieved by passage of blood over immunoabsorbent columns, would be feasible[190] if appropriate isolated tumor antigens were available. However, this is unlikely to be effective since the antibody would be rapidly replaced by new synthesis.

Specific inhibition of antibody-formation by the injection of antigen-antibody complexes or antibody before or after surgery or tumor lysis may be expected to have long lasting inhibitory effects on antibody formation as we have already found for Rh antibody production in the therapy of erythroblastosis fetalis. This approach is not practicable in tumor treatment since it might lead to simultaneous inhibition of cellular immunity. This type of strategy must therefore be dismissed, unless it turns out that the thresholds for the inhibition of cellular and humoral immunity are vastly different.

Other possibilities for the differential inhibition of antibody formation might become practicable. If blocking antibodies turn out to be a special subclass of immunoglobulins, it might become possible to find a way to suppress them with antibody directed against this particular subclass. This has already been demonstrated in the newborn infant[34, 54] and it is conceivable that ways could be found to achieve it in the adult. There have been recent reports that starvation reduces the humoral immune response without reducing the cellular immune response;[174] if these reports are confirmed we may have a new approach to the potentiation of tumor resistance.

It is clearly not useful to continue an enumeration of possibilities since the exact nature of the mechanism of antibody-mediated blocking has to be known before such speculation can become cogent. The foregoing paragraph simply serves to indicate that we have some information which needs to be extended and which could lead to therapeutic applications. In short, we need more precise information on the relation between inhibition of cellular immunity, on the one hand, and the properties of blocking antibody or the blocking antigen-antibody complexes, on the other. Once this information has been obtained, a number of therapeutic options will become available. It is, however, already clear that the availability of appropriate human tumor antigens is essential for progress in further therapeutic exploration. This need became apparent when we discussed diagnosis and thus reasons for applied programs for isolation of tumor membrane components come from many different objectives.

A deviation of the immune response from humoral to cellular immunity is one of the obvious therapeutic objectives if the view is held that a tumor-bearing individual has an active immune apparatus which has lost its effectiveness by "internal" cancellation. Ultimately, this will almost certainly turn out to be an oversimplification, and a profound analysis of regulation, in the widest sense, is needed. The need for this analysis is common to the management of tumors, transplantation, autoimmune diseases, and atopic diseases, etc. Here, in terms of medical relevance, is the most important target-area for future immunologic research.

It was originally suggested that tolerance for tumor antigens may be involved in tumor growth[35, 36] and we have seen, in the foregoing discussion, that this view must now be revised. As so often in the history of science, it is becoming apparent that what was thought of as a single phenomenon is, in fact, to be subdivided according to mechanism. Enhancement and low dose tolerance may be related or even identical phenomena. If they involve antibody-mediated inhibition, it occurs in T cells and is maintained only as long as antibodies circulate. High dose tolerance, on the other hand, represents failure directly induced by antigen, may not depend on antibody, is probably induced by soluble but not by cell-bound antigens,[33, 114, 131, 132] and, if at all, might occur in the very late stages of disseminated disease, but not in the localized disease which we are considering at this point.

It is generally believed that the cellular immune response depends on thymus derived cells (T cells) and that antibody is formed by bone marrow derived cells (B cells) with the cooperation of T cells. Our strategy, therefore, involves either induction of high dose B cell tolerance under conditions which avoid or circumvent T cell tolerance. The first of these alternative courses has major technical difficulties, since the threshhold for T cell tolerance seems to be lower than the threshhold for B cell tolerance, except under special circumstances.[110] Perhaps we can find another way of potentiating the effectiveness of a blocked immune system.

Circumvention of tolerance can be induced with cross-reactive molecules.[35, 37, 39, 179, 196] In low dose tolerance, this will affect the activity of T cells much more profoundly than the activity of the uninhibited B cells. Activation of T cells may be achieved before significant inhibition by tumor-specific antibodies occurs. For this reason, immunization with chemically modified tumor cells may appear as a promising approach.[35, 36]

A particularly attractive version of this approach is available in skin cancers which can be treated locally with chemical skin-sensitizers after the patient has been sensitized. Under these circumstances, delayed hypersensitivity (and not soluble antibody) is induced, presumably by "skin" macromolecules with which the chemical skin sensitizer combines.[116] It has been reported that squamous skin cancers were rejected after the affected skin area was painted. Some of the experiments that have been undertaken along these lines have involved diazotization,[35, 36, 38, 47] acetylation,[154] enzyme alteration,[14] skin application of 2-4 dinitrochlorobenzene,[116] freezing,[140, 172] and heating.[30]

Animal experiments have shown that immunization with physically or chemically modified tumor cells heightens immune surveillance, as judged by the number of tumor cells which produce a given mortality.[154] More important, in a spontaneous mouse mammary adenocarcinoma, a significant delay in tumor onset and mortality was achieved by preinjection with heat-treated syngeneic cells.[30] Thus, animal experiments provide us with evidence that preventive treatment with modified tumor cells may be rewarding and may deserve consideration when vertical transmission of a tumor virus occurs; however, the findings have no direct bearing on the question of treatment of an established, i.e. clinically detectable, tumor.

Whether the immune response to such neoplasms could be potentiated by immunization with modified tumor antigens is much less securely established. Our own results with cervical tumors have so far yielded cause for moderate optimism but not a significant difference between treated and untreated patients.[38] Others have reported anecdotal findings which gave them cause for great optimism which we could not share. The results of skin application[116] and of in situ freezing of tumors of the prostate (cryosurgery[140, 172]) are suggestive of a pathway which may have promise in the management of certain tumors but needs confirmation and extension. It is clear that this type of intervention is most promising if it occurs when the tumor mass has been reduced by surgery, chemotherapy, or radiation therapy; but it only holds promise if the excision therapy is so arranged as to leave the immune system intact. We shall discuss this point as it applies to chemotherapy in the section on nonspecific stimulation.

Immunotherapy Based on Direct Increase of Cellular Immunity

If cellular immunity is the effective tumor-destroying process, it might be thought possible to cure tumors by transfer of cells from individuals with spontaneous regressions. Furthermore, it might seem conceivable that cellular immunity could be freed of antibody-mediated inhibition by an increase in the number of cells which are primed to make an appropriate response. For these reasons, adaptive transfer of allogeneic leukocytes from individuals immunized with or recovered from an analogous tumor has been, to many investigators, an attractive approach.[46, 105, 120, 141, 180] So far, the results of these trials hold out little hope for success.

There are two reasons for doubting the potential of this approach. Allogeneic leukocytes would be rapidly rejected and hence would have little chance to survive and destroy the tumor. If this were overcome, and the life span of the leukocytes could be prolonged, say by a process of enhancement (i.e. with specific antibodies directed against HL-A),[24] graft-versus-host reactions might affect normal tissue as much as tumor tissue. This danger might be minimized by tissue matching or by isolation of tumor-specific cells, using suitable fractionation techniques. The long term future of this approach may depend on the isolation of mediators which are responsible for the aggressiveness of the leukocyte and on the direct employment of such substances. It might become possible to produce these substances from large scale tissue culture of established cell lines. Finally, it may be that we can potentiate the immune response by activation of *autologous* leukocytes. In fact, it has been found possible to render cells aggressive by activation with phytohemagglutinin;[31, 69, 157] we shall return to this question and to its pitfalls when we deal with transfer factor.

The above discussion might be summarized by the slogan: "In tumor immunity the T cell is good and the B cell and its products are bad!" Like many slogans, this one would elevate a partial insight to the level of unwarranted certainty and would impede our inclination to explore those observations further which are in discord with the slogan. There are indications that humoral antibody has some value in tumor control and that cells other than the T cell can contribute to tumor resistance. We shall first look into the possibility that antibodies, directed against tumor specific antigens, may cause tumor destruction and thus may be involved in tumor control.

Antibody as a Direct Tool of Immunotherapy

I have presented evidence that IgM antibody can contribute to the rejection of transplants (p. 811). The immunotherapeutic potential of antibody has been referred to in the discussion of antibody interference with cellular immunity (p. 811); however, I want to consider now some aspects of antibody-therapy which are not dependent on interference with enhancement. Can antibody bring about complement-mediated tumor destruction or is there a failure of in vivo complement-activation?

Both IgG and IgM human antibodies, directed against sarcomas, are regularly found in patients who do not have widespread disease.[59] The IgM antibodies fixed complement, and trypsinized human sarcoma cells from an established cell line can be lysed with these antibodies.[200] However, many human sera fail to lyse cells in the presence of human complement alone, but do so if rabbit complement is added to the test system.[201] Thus some human antibodies can fix complement but do so inefficiently. Nevertheless, there is good reason for the assumption that some, albeit not all antibodies, can lyse human tumor cells. There are other examples of cytotoxic tumor antibodies; for instance, antibodies directed against human melanoma.[126] Finally, in animals with Maloney virus sarcomas, cytotoxic antibodies are found in the blood of animals which have rejected tumors, whereas the blood of animals with progressing tumors contains blocking antibodies which do not fix complement. The cytotoxic antibody in experimental animal disease and clinical human disease is present only during limited periods.[64, 126, 169] In short, it appears as though some types of antibody can activate homologous complement more readily and that other antibodies may fail to do so, and that only those antibodies which can activate complement may contribute to cell death.

I shall now turn to a consideration of therapeutic application of these antibodies (1) in treatment of solid tumors and (2) in treatment of residual tumor after excision. I apologize in advance for some repetitiveness in the following paragraphs in which a temptation to explore therapeutic possibilities is balanced by the fear that harm could be done unless we can better evaluate all immunologic consequences of our intervention.

Cytotoxic antibodies may have a limited and peripheral effect on the size of a solid tumor. Their appearance may, therefore, cause a temporary improvement; but this may be counterbalanced by increased release of tumor antigen, the resulting formation of antigen-antibody complexes, and the consequent depression of the cellular immune response. Events might take a different course if ways could be found to facilitate access to and spread through a tumor mass. I have suggested in an earlier review that this might be achieved by passive administration of antibody through regional perfusion,[36] with access to tumor cells further facilitated by pharmacologic agents which increase permeability. Trials of this type must be postponed until we understand the mechanism of enhancement and, in particular, until we know whether or not antigen-antibody complexes are involved. Otherwise, this would constitute an unjustifiable procedure since antigen-antibody complexes may ultimately appear in the general circulation and so reach and possibly inhibit cellular immunity. Should it be proved that enhancement, in fact, does depend on antigen-antibody complexes, regional perfusion could be followed by removal of complexes from the general circulation with immunoabsorbent columns.[190] Such a procedure would be useless for the removal of actively synthesized antibody, and might even lead to increased synthesis, but would clearly be quite effective in removing passively administered antibody.

Whereas there appears to be little prospect that antibody treatment of solid tumors may become a method of excision, it is conceivable that antibody treatment after surgical, chemotherapeutic or x-ray excision could become an adjunct to conventional treatment.

One would assume that the above mentioned antigen-antibody triggered chain of events might not occur *after* removal of the tumor mass. Under these circumstances, the central therapeutic objective would be the prevention of the spread of cells through the lymphatic and vascular system. Thus, the total tumor mass would be very small, consisting of single cells and minute tumor nodules; antibody-mediated cell lysis would thus occur more readily and the relatively small quantity of circulating antigen-antibody complexes might not have a major depressant effect on cellular immunity. Furthermore, the formation and spread of metastases may be limited by cytotoxic antibody and, therefore, might be favorably affected by passively administered cytotoxic antibody. Passive administration of antibody, even as a step toward excision of residual tumor, can only be envisaged when we have defined the parameters of enhancement. This condition may be met in the not too distant future as the results of ongoing investigation become available.

Antibody might be employed to bring about appropriate local concentration of chemotherapeutic agents in tumor tissue, and without damage to normal cells. It could serve to deliver any toxic substance which retains toxicity when covalently linked to an antibody molecule. The validity of this approach has been demonstrated with antibodies directed against mumps antigens and with monkey kidney cells which had acquired the antigen after infection with mumps virus. The antibody was conjugated with diphtheria toxin and the infected kidney cells were lysed by the toxin carried to their surface by the antibody.[133] Similarly, chlorambucil and radioactive iodine could be carried to Ehrlich ascites cells.[76] If heterologous specifically purified antibody were used, it might not only deliver and concentrate toxic substances, but, in addition, might direct delayed hypersensitivity to the cells coated with the foreign immunoglobulin.

There is a long way between the demonstration of therapeutic possibility and a practicable method of treatment. In the example under discussion, the main hurdle is the provision of large quantities of specific and purified antibody. Some problems of antibody therapy have been discussed in the preceding pages, as has the need for production of large quantities of purified tumor (embryonic) antigens. If this were undertaken, it would allow the preparation of heterologous antibodies, purification by immunoabsorbents, and thus the production of considerable quantities of specifically purified antibodies for conjugation with appropriate chemotherapeutic substances.

The therapeutic use of antibodies against human tumor viruses is currently not worth detailed consideration, since it would depend on unequivocal identification of such viruses. Once this is achieved, some viruses might be found to cause tumors after short incubation periods. Were this found to be the case, antibody, administered passively to individuals at risk, might be a desirable measure of public health.

In short, it is premature to conclude that antibody cannot increase the effectiveness of tumor surveillance. On the other hand, it is established beyond doubt that antibody depresses the impact of the cellular immune apparatus in many situations. It seems possible that passive antibody-administration may have a therapeutic role to play, but it is clear that this type of experimental intervention is not warranted until the border line between conditions favoring complement mediated cell-destruction and conditions favoring enhancement can be clearly delineated.

Immunotherapy by Nonspecific Stimulation of the Immune Apparatus

I shall now turn to the second process, dependent on macrophages, which I have mentioned in expressing some caution against premature adoption of a rigid view that the effect of the T cell is "good" and that the products of the B cell are harmful. There is evidence that the macrophages and possibly the accessory cells (A cells) may be involved in tumor destruction. This view is based on tumor inhibition with peritoneal exudates[149] and the inhibition of pulmonary metastases (methylcholanthrene tumors) with thoracic duct lymph but *not* with thoracic duct lymphocytes.[183] Furthermore, Takeda has shown that a soluble product, which passes a millipore filter, is capable of instructing macrophages alone and of stimulating them to destroy methylcholanthrene tumors.[170, 183] While the potential of specific activation of macrophages has yet to be explored, the involvement of nonspecific activation of macrophages has been a long-standing theme of immunotherapy.

An example of this nonspecific activation is the augmentation by BCG of the macrophages' bacteriolytic power and the effect of lysosomal labilizers in enabling macrophages to convert antigens to greater immunogenicity.[53, 173, 191] In vivo, such substances may affect several components of the immune apparatus. In vitro experiments with cell fractions are needed to disentangle the complexity of the in vivo situation. At any rate, stimulation by nonspecific factors, i.e., substances which enhance immunity to structurally unrelated antigens, has been demonstrated with a large number of microorganisms, subcellular fractions obtained from microorganisms, and macromolecules such as nucleic acid and synthetic polynucleotides, and DNA digests.[204] In fact, it is quite likely that all antigens exercise an effect which augments the responsiveness of the immune apparatus[203] only the magnitude of the effect being different for different substances.

It is clearly tempting to consider treatment with the most potent stimulating substances for nonspecific augmentation of tumor resistance. Indeed, the incidence of spontaneous tumors can be reduced by pretreatment with BCG[148] or with a methanol-extracted residue of BCG.[197] Tumor induction by carcinogens has been delayed by pretreatment with BCG[148] and polyinosine polycytidylic acid (poly I:C).[73] In general, it seems that the effectiveness of the nonspecific stimulators is greatest before tumor growth and before tumor implantation, though synthetic nucleotides, such as polyinosinic polycytidylic acid, reduced tumor incidence *after* tumor grafting.[19, 20, 124] It has recently been reported that direct injection of BCG into established intradermal tumor nodules of guinea pigs resulted in tumor regression and prevented the formation of metastases.[205] It remains to be seen whether this effect is general or is confined to skin tumors or to certain anatomic sites. The latter may be the case if inhibition of tumor growth is dependent on the site of the delayed hypersensitivity reaction.

Under clinical conditions, it would seem unlikely that nonspecific stimulation of the immune response could achieve more than a reduction of tumor growth and as a consequence, such treatment would have to be combined with some form of chemotherapy. Since chemotherapy is often immunosuppressive, one is faced with the problem of a possible antagonism of treatments.

It is already apparent that various chemotherapeutic agents differ in their effect on the outcome of nonspecific stimulation. Combined pretreatment with BCG and methyl-hydrazine was less effective than chemotherapy alone[9] whereas cyclophosphamide (6 days after tumor implantation) potentiated the effect of the nonspecific stimulator *C. parvum,* given 12 days after implantation.[202] Systematic exploration of these different interactions with the same tumor systems might have a great deal to teach us, not only about the interactions which I have mentioned, but also about the choice of chemotherapeutic reagents.

There is good evidence that the stimulating agents, which I have mentioned, potentiate the immune apparatus and inhibit tumor growth. The following arguments support the view that they inhibit tumor growth through potentiation of the immune apparatus:

1. Some agents can induce immunosuppression *and* induce tumors. In some cases, nonspecific stimulators can overcome both effects.[144, 176]

2. Poor immunologic responses in old or young animals are accompanied by greater tumor incidence, and this can be compensated for by nonspecific stimulation.[175, 199, 204]

3. Nonspecific stimulators such as *B. pertussis, C. parvum,* and lactic dehydrogenase virus (L.D.V.) prevent induction of immunological tolerance.[22, 130, 153]

In general, nonspecific stimulation affects cellular immunity as well as humoral immunity, and systematic exploration of the relative extent of the augmentation is clearly necessary to assure optimization of these factors and for the design of rational immunotherapy.

We have, so far, dealt with animal experiments in which pretreatment with nonspecific stimulants has been tested, the interaction with immunosuppressant has been examined, and evidence for the immunological nature of the nonspecific stimulation has been obtained. We shall now examine clinical trials of nonspecific stimulation.

The possibility of nonspecific stimulation as an avenue of tumor treatment arose from clinical and epidemiologic observations on the relatively low incidence of cancer in tuberculin-positive patients.[86, 104, 142]

There are many clinical observations which may be taken to support the view of an association between tuberculin sensitivity and neoplastic disease. For instance, in one group of leukemic patients, the number of individuals giving positive skin tests to a battery of antigens was only slightly higher in patients than it was in a control group. But the incidence of responders to PPD showed a marked difference: it was 33 per cent in patients and 79 per cent in the normal group.[56]

Though tuberculin is the best known, there are many types of bacterial antigens which can induce potentiation of the immune apparatus. "Colytoxins," mixtures of beta-hemolytic streptococci and Candida albicans, have been used to provide this type of stimulation. More recently, and against a background of animal experimentation, nonspecific stimulation with BCG, combined with chemotherapy, has been used in the treatment of human leukemia.

So far, the results of these studies have been contradictory. A very optimistic evaluation of a trial in France[129] has not been confirmed by those who repeated the treatment in England.[74] A further trial has to be completed before the value of this particular version of nonspecific stimulation can be decided. Whatever the outcome of this study, systematic examination of the effects of nonspecific stimulation on the production of various classes of immunoglobulins on the production of blocking and unblocking antibody, on cellular immune response, and on macrophage activity may be rewarding. A study of the interaction between chemotherapeutic reagents and nonspecific stimulation may not only help in devising a strategy for combined therapy but may increase our understanding of the clinical effects of chemotherapy.

Nonspecific stimulation may have some role to play in immunotherapy and the precise nature of this role will emerge from an analysis of the relevant parameters of the immune response and of the cellular mechanism of nonspecific potentiation. Brave short cuts into immunotherapy may not hasten our progress toward this goal unless they are so designed as to permit evaluation of several parameters of the humoral and cellular response.

Many of the immunotherapeutic pathways which I have so far discussed have been considered for several decades and have been redesigned as more fundamental information became available. Next, I shall briefly consider pathways for which the conceptual basis is fairly new or where feasibility has only recently become apparent. I have already mentioned mediators of cellular immunity and I shall not elaborate on them, since the identity and in vivo effects of these reagents are still so controversial that a detailed discussion of their therapeutic potential would be too speculative to have predictive value. I shall confine myself to a list of putative factors (Table 4)[108] and to a brief discussion of two of them.

Table 4. *Putative Mediators of Cellular Immunity*[108]

Factors released upon interaction with antigen	Migration inhibitory factor (MIF)
	Macrophage spread inhibitory factor
	Macrophage aggregating factor
	Skin-reactive factor
	Products of antigen recognition (PAR)
	Lymphotoxin
	Cloning inhibitory factor
	Proliferation inhibitory factor
	Inhibitor of DNA synthesis
	Chemotactic factors
	Blastogenic factors
	Interferon
Factors pre-existent in cells	Transfer factors
	Lymph node permeability factor
	Cytophilic antibody
Direct lymphocyte-target cell cytotoxicity	Killer cell

Transfer Factor and Interferon

The prospects for the utilization of transfer factor, of interferon, and of interferon-inducers are summarized in Table 5. Any prediction as to the potential of transfer factor must await the outcome of current clinical trials. The employment of interferon-inducers involves little risk to the patient. Some interferon-inducers are nonantigenic and nontoxic; others, such as the toxic poly I:C, seem to be nonspecific stimulators of the immune system as well as being interferon inducers.[20] A broad range of tumor-controlling mechanisms may be stimulated by such compounds and they deserve clinical attention.

The short duration of interferon action and the ineffectiveness of interferon vis á vis some herpes-like viruses limits its potential usefulness. Its effectiveness in the control of vertically transmitted virus deserves further investigation in view of recent indications that interferon may be transmitted through the placenta.[119] In the preceding pages we have considered various strategies for immunologic tumor destruction; we must now turn to tumor-dependent inhibitions of immunity.

We have, so far, assumed normal responsiveness of each component of the immune system. This assumption may not always be valid and there are indications of some depression of the antibody response of animals infected with leukemia viruses and of patients in the late stages of their disease.

Debilitation of the Immune Apparatus by Tumor Virus and Tumor Growth

Infection of susceptible mice with RNA murine leukemia viruses, resulting in malignant proliferative disease, is accompanied by nonspecific inhibition of the immune response to many antigens. In the case of infection with Freund leukemia virus, it was suggested that the viruses compete with antigen for stem cells which would normally differentiate into AFC.[27, 165] From recent work, it seems that cells producing virus can-

Table 5. *The Therapeutic Potential of Transfer Factor and Interferon*

FACTOR	SITE OF ACTION	SOURCES Allogeneic	Exogeneic	DURATION OF EFFECT	POSSIBLE APPLICATION	DIFFICULTIES IN APPLICATION
Transfer factor[122,147]	Cell-mediated	Can cross species barriers[3,5,6,48]		Prolonged	Following tumor removal	Population of susceptible cells may be decreased in tumor patients[60,96] though it may increase after tumor excision[4]
Interferon	Wide range of cells	Species-specific	Antigenic and species-limited range of action	Few days (longest duration in nonliving cells)	To limit spread of certain viruses and to protect the newborn[119]	Poor effect against herpes virus group Only effective when given prior to or within a few hours of virus infection Effect is of short duration Repeated application required (procurement-problems)
Interferon-inducers[101]	Wide range of cells	Synthetic nonantigenic sources (e.g., I:C)		Short (as for interferon)	To limit spread of certain viruses and to protect the newborn[119]	As for interferon, but repeated application does present procurement problems

not be induced to make antibody,[45] and that the susceptibility to suppression is greatest in the response against antigens to which the animals have been exposed prior to infection.[145] This may be a fairly general phenomenon, since Rauscher leukemia virus has been found to replicate more vigorously in the spleen of germ-free mice previously immunized with sheep erythrocytes than it does in un-immunized germ-free controls.[29] In this situation, sensitization with virus antigen might pave the way for intensified virus infection. If such a situation existed in any human disease, interferon treatment might deserve much more attention than I have given it in the preceding discussion.

Generalized immune suppression is not confined to tumors induced by recognized viruses. It appears to occur also in mice bearing methylcholanthrene tumors and results in a decrease of T cell functions as manifested in graft-versus-host reaction and responsiveness to PHA stimulation. It is difficult to distinguish between a direct depressive effect of the carcinogen, of a cell product, and of immunologic "exhaustion" by a continuous flood of tumor antigens.[85, 170] However, irrespective of the mechanism by which this process works, it imposes limitations on the design for immunotherapy. This is a further reason for the previously advanced argument for cooperative treatment, since removal of the tumor mass is required before effective immunologic potentiation can be undertaken. The extent of immunodepression in cancer patients varies with the disease and its progress and it is clearly one variable that needs further exploration within narrowly defined patient groups.

PREVENTIVE IMMUNIZATION AND VACCINATION

I have left preventive aspects of tumor control to the end of my considerations since this is one area in which major obstacles can be anticipated and even limited progress will be slow. There are several types of immunization, aimed at limiting: growth of tumor cells, virus multiplication, or both. Types of antigens which might be used include embryonic and virally induced antigens, and mutant tumor virus (infective), inactivated virus (noninfective), subviral component, and passenger virus.

As you will see from this list, the formidable practical difficulties of immunization with viruses will deflect me at various points of the argument, from vaccination, in the classical sense, to immunization with tumor tissue antigens, with viral-coat fragments, and with virally controlled membrane antigens. Immunization with such substances has already been considered in this review, when post excision treatment was discussed. Nevertheless, it may be useful to re-examine the general problem in a new context since the immune status of the patient, after extensive exposure to tumor antigens, is presumably quite different from that of the individual who is free of clinical cancer.

All membrane antigens may be regarded as potential transplantation antigens, though their capacity to induce a rejection varies over an enormous range and some antigens are so weakly immunogenic that their contribution to rejection escapes detection if other more potent transplantation-antigens are on the same membrane. This is already illus-

trated in that carcinogen-induced antigens are considered as "individualistic" antigens in some cases and common, or group, antigens in others.
Two examples are MC[10, 21] and DAB.[2, 10] Both findings are well documented and reflect differences in the techniques by which "individualistic" and common antigens are detected. In some instances, the "individualistic" antigens were found by transplantation experiments, and the
common antigens by fluorescent staining with recovery antibodies. In
other words, the "individualistic" antigens invoked a much more potent
rejection reaction than did the group antigens. This is fortunately not
always the case since many common group-antigens of tumors have been
found by staining with fluorescent antibody as well as by transplantation
techniques.

The question which we must raise in this connection concerns (1)
the molecular attributes which distinguish weak from strong transplantation antigens, and, ultimately, (2) the processes by which a weak
transplantation antigen can be converted to a rejection-inducing antigen
(Table 6). Even in tissue transplantation-oriented research the first of
these questions has not been answered definitively and the second is obviously not being asked. The strong tissue-transplantation antigens may
well be outside the "scale of strength" of tumor antigens, but it may be
worthwhile to scan a list of the factors which have been considered in attempts to relate antigenic strength to molecular and genetic parameters
(Table 6).

Among the experimental factors cited in Table 6, the most important
is the cumulative effect of weak transplantation antigens. Thus pre-im-

Table 6. *Processes Which May Determine "Strength"*
of Transplantation Antigens

PROCESS	ARGUMENTS FOR INVOLVEMENT OF PROCESS
Antigen density on membrane[12, 15, 40, 50, 99, 198]	Substantial differences in (a) distribution of transplantation antigens in different tissues (HL-A2 more abundant in spleen than in kidney or heart), and (b) intensity of rejection of different tissues with the same histocompatibility. Weak tissue antigens can become important to rejection through their cumulative differences.
Genetic control of host responsiveness in terms of:	
Structure of antigens of host and recipient (individual variation)[82, 100]	Interallelic combination rather than donor or recipient phenotype determines intensity of rejection. Humoral response is controlled by genes in or near main transplantation-antigen locus.
Number of antigen-sensitive cells (interspecies variation)[166]	In immunized animals, the number of cells reactive with strong transplantation antigens is greater than that reactive with other cellular antigens (particularly xenogenic grafts).

munization with antigen cocktails (or intact killed cells), rather than immunization with single isolated antigens, optimizes the prospects of vigorous rejection. The outcome of immunization is clearly complicated by the intervention of already mentioned additional factors such as (1) cytotoxic antibodies (IgM), (2) enhancing antibodies (IgG and/or AgAb complexes) and tolerance, and (3) nonspecific immunosuppression. If active immunization is intended, we need to learn the process by which cellular immunity and the formation of nonenhancing cytotoxic antibodies is preferentially induced. In what follows, I shall not stress these problems further.

In the foreseeable future, preventive immunization with embryonic tumor antigens may become possible, particularly if it should turn out that natural immunization during pregnancy provides some protection. It may not be advisable to immunize premenopausal women with the embryonic antigens. There is no sex barrier to immunization with virus-dependent transplantation antigens. We, therefore, need to know whether or not a common human tumor antigen is embryonic. There is some evidence that tumor free relatives of cancer patients have a much higher incidence of antibodies against the tumor of the patient than does the general population.[61, 62] This could be taken as a first criterion for a human tumor antigen being *not* embryonic and hence – probably – virally controlled. Antigens of this type could be used for immunization of members of sibships with a high incidence of breast cancer. Trials for the effectiveness of such immunization would require a long period for evaluation even in high incidence families and would be beset by doubts of the planners, probably unjustified, that enhancement may be induced.

There is one further point in the transplantation results of Table 6 which deserves consideration. The immune responsiveness to some individual determinants is controlled at a locus which is linked to the locus for the strong transplantation antigens. If this is widely applicable to antigens and if it can be extended to the cellular immune response, it may be an important factor in the effectiveness of immune surveillance. Exploration of connections between transplantation antigens and resistance to tumor might ultimately have predictive value. It might allow us to anticipate whether an individual patient will benefit from immunization with a particular tumor antigen. In the case of Hodgkin's disease, there appears to be an association between the disease and HL-A8, 4c and possibly also A1.[44, 111, 115] By comparision with the normal population, an increase of the incidence of transplantation specificity A8 is found in patients having Hodgkin's disease for more than 5 years.[63] Thus it is conceivable that resistance or even immune responsiveness to some tumors is closely linked to the HLA transplantation locus. However, it will require much further work to determine the nature of the mechanisms by which the inception or progress of the disease is dependent on the HL-A genetic region. Several different factors may be involved and the observed association could be further complicated by heterogeneity of the disease-entity.[134] This may result in a decrease or increase of more than one HL-A-specificity by comparison with the healthy population.

Several different factors of disease induction and progression may be linked to the HLA genetic region:

(1) susceptibility to disease-induction (for instance susceptibility to virus infection), and immunological resistance to the tumor cell which either (2) prevents the development of clinical disease or (3) retards the appearance and progress of clinical disease. Observations linking HL-A specificities to inception, duration, and progression should be of great value in the development of a therapy which allows for the genetic differences between patients. To unravel the cause and effect of HL-A involvement may take much longer than the empirical use of data.

To many of us, protection with isolated membrane antigens appears inferior to vaccination. Is it possible to provide long lasting protection by immunization with tumor viruses? In principle this can be achieved and in Marek's disease, a common lymphoproliferative disease of domestic chickens, an attenuated, cell-associated vaccine has been developed and applied in field trials. In 3 out of 4 trials, the incidence of disease was significantly lower in vaccinated than in unvaccinated animals.[16] Why, then, the pessimism that was expressed in the opening sentences of this section? Let us assume that the identification, isolation, and cultivation of human tumor viruses were achieved. We are now faced with several formidable hurdles. Can we assume that cytopathogenic effects provide a sufficiently reliable test for safety or a vaccine? If not, how do we prove that an attenuated virus or even a heat-killed virus is being tested adequately in an experimental animal? For this purpose, a species would have to be found which is more susceptible to human virus than is man. With animals of this type, we would have to demonstrate that the vaccine could be attenuated, or so treated as to give essentially zero tumor incidence. Thus, it might be necessary to think in terms of 50,000 animals. This would be completely unrealistic if the sensitive species turned out to be primates. Human tissue culture might replace the experimental animal but it is difficult to conceive that a Public Health Service would be prepared to guarantee complete safety of an attenuated virus tested in tissue culture alone. Clearly, the safest vaccine, and the one most readily acceptable for testing, would not be an inactive virus, but subviral components or virus-induced antigens, free of nucleic acid. Let us add to our house of cards by assuming that this problem were solved. How are we to demonstrate the usefulness of this vaccine?

Human tumors caused by viruses with short latent periods are the only ones for which a vaccine could be developed and could be tested for safety and effectiveness without following up unrealistically large control and experimental groups. These conditions exist in Burkitt's lymphoma and acute childhood leukemia since the majority of tumors occur in children under the age of 10. It might perhaps be best to quote here Higginson and his colleagues on a vaccine against Burkitt's lymphoma:[99] "Even in this case, it would be necessary to follow a population of 50,000 for at least 5 to 7 years in order to determine whether the disease is related to the Epstein-Barr virus (EBV), even assuming a short latent period between virus infection and disease. The period [of follow-up] will have to be lengthened or the size of the population will have to be increased if the latent period is found to be longer or irregular. Such a study would also indicate whether or not the titers against EBV are meaningful in terms of immunity, since if cancer only occurs in children with high titers it would be assumed that a successful vaccine cannot be developed whose potential effectiveness is based on titer." Thus, there is, at this moment, only one disease which offers us a reasonable possibility for examining a tumor vaccine. However, the problem of undertaking such a study in underdeveloped countries with limited cancer registration and follow-up systems are certainly quite formidable. Superficially it may appear that the testing of an EBV vaccine is no more difficult than it was to test BCG vaccine or poliomyelitis vaccine. Nevertheless, there are many important differences in the incidence of the diseases, the country in which they could be tested, and the ease with which the safety of the two vaccines could be established.

There is little doubt that other virus-induced diseases will not have the same relatively favorable conditions for testing as just discussed in the case of Burkitt's lymphoma. In any situation in which viruses are relatively nonspecific cancer-inducing agents and in which only a small proportion of the infected population develops cancer after a long and variable latent period, it would require a very large number of individuals who would have to be followed for several decades.[99]

I have already cited presumptive evidence for the existence of vertical transmission of virus or virus genomes from parents to offspring. It has now been reported that mammalian ova can be infected with the small DNA tumor viruses and that even sperm can take up tumor virus (Simian virus 40) and can, at fertilization, transfer it to ova.[18, 28] It is thus clear that vertical transmission can occur through ova and sperm. Vertically transmitted viruses would be present but would not cause disease until changes in host susceptibility or the host's infection with a passenger virus would result in oncogenic expression. It is clear that such circumstances, i.e., a large number of infected individuals, a relatively low proportion of diseased individuals, and a varying period before onset of disease, would magnify the already formidable problems of establishing the value of a vaccine. I can see only one promising set of circumstances: If a helper virus were involved in the oncogenic expression of the tumor virus, it *might* be possible to vaccinate with killed helper virus particles.

It is clear that we need to consider possibilities of eradication of vertically transmitted viruses which do not depend on vaccination and it is for this reason that I have introduced a consideration of interferon into an earlier part of this paper.

If the outlook for vaccination is rather bleak, effective immunization after infection has occurred may afford better prospects for success. We know from animal experiments that this can be done with massive doses of virus or of virus-induced antigens.[57, 70, 118, 121] Trials of vaccine given late during the latent period and capable of increasing the individual's immunity against natural infection would not be subject to the same formidable hurdles as those discussed before. This would be an acceptable substitute for classical vaccination, if serologic tests of adequate sensitivity could be developed to identify infected individuals. I have indicated in the first section of this paper that conditions are favorable for the development of such tests.

At the present time, an anticancer virus vaccine can be visualized only for a very limited range of disease entities and under circumstances which depart from classical vaccination in terms of the nature of antigen and in the time of administration. It would be most injudicious to assume or to create the impression that a tested cancer virus vaccine, corresponding to those vaccines used in communicable diseases, could be available within the next decade. Indeed, it seems improbable that classical vaccination will become a practical method for the majority of virally caused tumors.

SUMMARY

Neoplastic cells differ from normal adult cells in antigenic composition. Some tumor antigens are specific for the disease entity, others for the embryonic origin of the tissue in which the tumor arises; yet others are specific for oncogenic virus regardless of the species or tissue involved. Some tumor antigens have a universal distribution, others are restricted to a tumor type and a third group are characteristic of individual tumors. The occurrence of tumor antigens and of tumor-directed antibody in the serum have now been described for a considerable number of neoplasms. Antibodies to embryonic antigens are found not only in the serum of tumor patients but also in the serum of pregnant women. Sera from multiparous syngeneic females have been used to detect embryonic antigens in animal tumors. With appropriate controls for the detection of normal transplantation and tissue antigens, this approach is applicable to the human situation and, in conjunction with fluorescent staining, would extend our knowledge of the range and distribution of embryonic antigens in human neoplasms. Indications of tumor-specific immunity are found in disease-free members of patients' families. Tumor antigens, antibodies and cellular immunity may provide a means for both the early detection and molecular classification of disease. Radioactivity labelled tumor antibodies could be employed for the assessment of tumor spread in surgery. Circulating tumor antigens and antibodies may allow a precise assessment of the consequences of tumor excision. It is now important to establish laboratories in which all existing tests for tumor antigens can be utilized on patient material and in which distribution of embryonic antigens in a wide variety of different tumors can be determined with batteries of sera from multiparous women.

Pregnancy induces immunity to embryonic antigens, which are found on tumor cells. Consequently, the assessment of the conditions for effective implementation of immunotherapy would be greatly aided by statistical information on the relation between parity and tumor incidence; it is hoped that tumor registries will be adapted to provide this information. Basically, immunotherapy could be developed (1) by interference with enhancement, for instance by using unblocking antisera; (2) by potentiation of immune responsiveness with chemically or physically altered tumor antigens; (3) by nonspecific stimulation of the immune response; (4) by employment of mediator of cellular immunity such as transfer factor; (5) by means of factors which interfere with virus replication such as interferon. There are no immediate prospects for effective tumor vaccination and the formidable obstacles in the way of such a preventive approach are discussed in detail.

ACKNOWLEDGMENTS

The author's thanks are due the Medical Research Council and the National Cancer Institute of Canada for long-standing grant support and to the Ontario Cancer Treatment and Research Foundation for the financing of clinical trials of immunotherapy. Dr. R. A. MacBeth (Department of Surgery, University of Alberta, Edmonton), Dr. D. L. Morton, (NIH, Bethesda, Maryland), Dr. Leo Sachs (Department of Genetics, The Weizmann Institute of Science, Rehovot, Israel), Dr. H. O. Sjögren (Fred Hutchinson Cancer Center, Seattle, Washington), Dr. R. T. Smith (University of Florida, Gainesville, Florida), and Dr. D. J. Yashphe (Department of Immunology, Hebrew University, Hadassah Medical School, Jerusalem, Israel) have provided reprints of reviews and of original articles and their help is gratefully acknowledged.

REFERENCES

1. Aaronson, S. A., Parks, W. P., Scolnick, E. M., and Todaro, G. J.: Antibody to the RNA-dependent DNA polymerase of mammalian C-type RNA tumor viruses. Proc. Nat. Acad. Sci., 68:920–924, 1971.
2. Abelev, G. I.: Study of antigenic structure of tumors. Acta U.I.C.C., 19:80–82, 1963.
3. Adler, W. H., Takiguchi, T., Marsh, B., and Smith, R. T.: Cellular recognition by mouse lymphocytes in vitro. I. Definition of a new technique and results of stimulation by phytohemagglutinin and specific antigens. J. Exper. Med., 131:1049–1078, 1970.
4. Adler, W. H., Takiguchi, T., and Smith, R. T.: Phytohemagglutinin unresponsiveness in mouse spleen cells induced by methylcolanthrene sarcomes. Cancer Res., 31:864–867, 1971.
5. Alexander, P., Bensted, J., Delorme, E. J., Hall, J. G., and Hodgett, J.: The cellular immune response to primary sarcomata in rats II. Abnormal responses of nodes draining the tumour. Proc. Roy. Soc. Lond. B., 174:237–251, 1967.
6. Alexander, P., Delorme, E. J., Hamilton, L. D. G., and Hall, J. G.: The role of immunoblasts in host resistance and immunotherapy of primary sarcomata. Advances Cancer Res., 13:1–37, 1970.
7. Alexander, J. W., and Good, R. A.: Immunobiology for Surgeons. Philadelphia, W. B. Saunders, 1970.
8. Alison, A. C.: Immune responses to virus-induced tumors. Proc. Roy. Soc. Med., 62:956–958, 1969.
9. Amiel, J. L., and Béradet, M.: Essais de traitements de la leucémie E$_a$G2 associant chimiothérapie et immunothérapies actives non spécifiques et spécifiques. Rev. franç. clin. biol., 14:685–688, 1969.
10. Baldwin, R. W., Glaves, D., and Pimm, M. V.: Tumor-associated antigens as expressions of chemically-induced neoplasia and their involvement in tumor-host interaction. Progress in Immunology. New York, Academic Press, 1:907–920, 1971.
11. Baranska, W., Koldovsky, P., and Koprowski, H.: Antigenic study of unfertilized mouse eggs: cross reactivity with SV40-induced antigens. Proc. Nat. Acad. Sci., 67:193–199, 1970.
12. Barker, C. F., and Billingham, R. E.: Comparison of the fates of A$_g$-B locus compatible homografts of skin and hearts in inbred rats. Nature (London), 225:851–852, 1970.
13. Bauer, H., and Janda, H. G.: Group-specific antigen of avian leukosis viruses. Virus specificity and relation to an antigen contained in Rous mammalian tumor cells. Virology, 33:483–490, 1967.
14. Bekesi, G., St.-Arneault, G., and Holland, J. F.: Increased immunogenicity of leukemia L-120 cells after vibrio cholerae neuraminidase treatment. Proc. Amer. Assoc. Cancer Res., 12:47, 1971.
15. Berah, M., Hors, J., and Dausset, J.: A study of HL-A antigens in human organs. Transplantation, 9:185–192, 1970.
16. Biggs, P. M., Payne, L. N., Milne, B. S., Churchill, A. E., Chubb, R. C., and Powell, D. G.: Field trials with an attenuated cell associated vaccine for Marek's disease. Vet. Rec., 87:704–709, 1970.
17. Bloom, E. T., and Hildemann, W. H.: Mechanisms of tumor-specific enhancement versus resistance toward a methyl-cholanthrene-induced murine sarcoma. Transplantation, 10:321–333, 1970.

18. Brackett, B. G., Baranska, W., Sawicki, W., and Kiprowski, H.: Uptake of heterologous genome by mammalian spermatozoa and its transfer to ova through fertilization. Proc. Nat. Acad. Sci., 68:353–357, 1971.

19. Braun, W., Lampen, J. O., Plescia, O. J., and Pugh, L.: Effects of nucleic acid digests on spontaneous and implanted tumors of C3H mice. In Conceptual Advances in Immunology and Oncology, Symposium on Fundamental Cancer Research, Anderson Hospital and Tumor Institute, 1962. New York, Hoeber Med. Div. Harper and Row, Inc., 1963, p. 450.

20. Braun, W.: New approaches to immunology as potential adjuncts to chemotherapy. In Proceedings of the Sixth International Congress of Chemotherapy, Tokyo. Vol. 1, 1961, pp. 17–26.

21. Brawn, R. J.: Possible association of embryonal antigen(s) with severe primary 3-methylcholanthrene-induced murine sarcomas. Int. J. Cancer, 6:245–249, 1970.

22. Brooke, M. S.: Conversion of immunological paralysis to immunity by endotoxin. Nature (Lond.), 206:635–636, 1965.

23. Bubenik, J., Pearlmann, P., Helmstein, K., and Moberger, G.: Immune response to urinary bladder tumours in man. Int. J. Cancer, 5:39–46, 1970.

24. Buckely, R., Rowlands, D. T., Jr., quoted by R. T. Smith, in Potential for immunologic intervention in cancer. In Amos, B., ed.: Progress in Immunology. New York, Academic Press, 1971, pp. 1115–1129.

25. Buffe, D., Rimbaut, C., Lemerle, J., Schweisguth, O., and Burtin, P.: Presence d'une ferroproteine d'origine tissulaire, 1' α_2H, dans le serum des enfants porteurs de tumeurs. Int. J. Cancer, 5:85–87, 1970.

26. Burger, M. M.: A difference in the architecture of the surface membrane of normal and virally transformed cells. Proc. Nat. Acad. Sci., 62:994–1001, 1969.

27. Ceglowski, W., and Friedman, H.: Suppression of the primary antibody plaque-response of mice following infection with Friend disease virus. Proc. Soc. Exper. Biol. Med., 126:662–666, 1967.

28. Cell Biology Correspondent. Vertical transmission, Nature:230:83, 1971.

29. Cerny, J., McAlack, R. F., Ceglowski, W. S., and Friedman, H.: Divergence between immunosuppression and immunocompetence during virus-induced leukemogenesis. Proc. Nat. Acad. Sci., 68:1862–1865, 1971.

30. Check, J. H., Childs, T. C., Brady, L. W., Derasse, A. R., and Fuscaldo, K. E.: Protection against spontaneous mouse mammary adenocarcinoma by inoculation of heat-treated syngeneic mammary tumor cells. Int. J. Cancer, 7:403–408, 1971.

31. Cheema, A. R.: Local tumor immunotherapy with in vitro activated autochtonous lymphocytes. Proc. Amer. Assoc. Canc. Res., 12:46, 1971.

32. Cheema, P., Yogeeswaran, G., Morris, H. P., and Murray, R. K.: Ganglioside patterns of three morris minimal deviation hepatomas. FEBS Letters, 2:181–184, 1970.

33. Chiller, J. M., Habicht, G. S., and Weigle, W. O.: Cellular sites of immunological unresponsiveness. Proc. Nat. Acad. Sci., 65:551–556, 1970.

34. Chou, C.-T., Cinader, B., and Dubiski, S.: Allotypic specificity and hemolytic capacity of antibodies produced by single cells. Int. Arch. Allergy, 32:583–616, 1967.

35. Cinader, B.: Acquired tolerance, autoantibodies and cancer. Canada. Med. Assoc. J., 86:1161–1165, 1962.

36. Cinader, B.: Perspectives and prospects of immunotherapy. Autoantibodies and acquired immunological tolerance. In Canadian Cancer Conference. New York, Academic Press, 1963, vol. 5, pp. 279–318.

37. Cinader, B., and Dubert, J. M.: Acquired immune tolerance to human albumin and the response to subsequent injections of diazo human albumin. Brit. J. Exper. Path., 36:515–529, 1955.

38. Cinader, B., and Meakin, J. W.: Immunisation of patients with a diazotised extract of their own tumor. In Annual Report of the Ontario Cancer and Treatment Research Foundation, 1965–1967, and 1971 (in press).

39. Cinader, B., St. Rose, J. E. M., and Yoshimura, M.: The effect of cross-reacting antigens on the tolerant state. J. Exper. Med., 125:1057–1073, 1967.

40. Cochrum, K. C., and Kountz, S. L.: Histocompatibility antigens of human lymphocytes and kidney cells. Fed. Proc. 29:No. 2, Abstract No. 1465, 1970.

41. Coggin, J. H., Ambrose, K. R., and Anderson, N. G.: Fetal antigen capable of inducing transplantation immunity against SV40 hamster tumour cells. J. Immunol., 105:524–526, 1970.

42. Collins, F. M., and Mackaners, G. B.: The relationship of delayed hypersensitivity to acquired antituberculous immunity. I. Tuberculin sensitivity and resistance to reinfection in BCG-vaccinated mice. Cell Immunol., 1:253–265, 1970.

43. Collins, F. M., and Mackaners, G. B.: The relation of delayed hypersensitivity to acquired antituberculous immunity. II. Effect of adjuvant on allergenicity and immunogeneity of heat killed Tubercle Bacilli. Cell Immunol., 1:266–275, 1970.

44. Coukell, A., Bodmer, J. G., and Bodmer, W. F.: HL-A types of forty four Hodgkin's patients. Transplant. Proc., 3:1291, 1971.

45. Cremer, N. E., Taylor, D. O. N., and Lenette, E. H.: Quantitation of immunoglobulin – and virus – producing cells in rats infected with Moloney leukemia virus. J. Immunol., *107*:689–697, 1971.
46. Curtis, J. E.: Adoptive immunotherapy in the treatment of advance malignant melanoma. Proc. Amer. Assoc. Canc. Res., *12*:52, 1971.
47. Czajkowski, N. P., Rosenblatt, M., Cushing, E. R., Vazquez, J., and Wolf, P. L.: Production of active immunity to malignant neoplastic tissue. Cancer, *19*:739–749, 1966.
48. Deckers, P. J., and Pilch, Y. H.: Transfer of tumor immunity with RNA (Abstract). Proc. Amer. Assoc. Canc. Res., *12*:24, 1971.
49. Deichmann, G. I., and Kluchareva, T. E.: Prevention of tumour induction in SV_{40}-infected hamsters. Nature, *202*:1126–1128, 1964.
50. De Planque, B., Williams, G. M., Siegel, A., and Alvarez, C.: Comparative typing of human kidney cells and lymphocytes by immune adherence. Transplantation, 8:852–860, 1969.
51. Diener, E., and Feldman, M.: Antibody mediated suppression of the immune response *in vitro*. II. A new approach to the phenomenon of immunological tolerance. J. Exper. Med., *132*:31–43, 1970.
52. Dore, J. F., Marholev, L., Colas de la Noue, H., DeVassal, F., Motta, R., Hrsak, I., Seman, G., and Mathe, G.: New antigens in human leukemia cells and antibody in the serum of leukemic patients. Lancet, 2:1396–1398, 1967.
53. Dresser, D. W.: Effectiveness of lipid and lipidophilic substances as adjuvants. Nature (Lond.), *191*:1169–1171, 1961.
54. Dubiski, S., Chou, C.-T., and Cinader, B.: Allotypic specificity as a marker of cells and cell receptors; antigen recognition and antibody production. *In* Cohen, S., Cudkowicz, G., and McCluskay, R. T.: Cellular Interactions in the Immune Response. Second International Convocation Immunol., Buffalo, New York, S. Karger, 1971, pp. 140–152.
55. Duff, R., and Rapp, F.: Reaction of serum from pregnant hamsters with surface of cells transformed by SV40. J. Immunol., *105*:521–523, 1970.
56. Dupuy, J. M., Kourilsky, F. M., Fradelizzi, D., Feingold, N., Jacquillat, A., Bernard, J., and Dausset, J.: Depression of immunologic reactivity of patients with acute leukemia. Cancer, 27:323–331, 1971.
57. Eddy, B. E., Grubbs, G. E., and Young, R. D.: Tumor immunity in hamsters infected with adenovirus type 12 or simian virus 40. Proc. Soc. Exper. Biol. (N.Y.)*117*:575–579, 1964.
58. Edynak, E. M., Old, L. J., Vrana, M., and Lardis, M.: A fetal antigen in human tumours detected by an antibody in the serum of cancer patients (Abstract). Proc. Amer. Assoc. Cancer Res., *11*:22, 1970.
59. Eilber, F. R.: Immunologic and immunotherapeutic studies: human sarcomas. Ann. Intern. Med., *74*:595–599, 1971.
60. Eilber, F. R., and Morton, D. L.: Impaired immunologic reactivity and recurrence following cancer surgery. Cancer, 25:362–367, 1970.
61. Eilber, F. R., and Morton, D. L.: Immunological studies of human sarcomas: additional evidence suggesting an associated sarcoma virus. Cancer, 26:588–596, 1970.
62. Eilber, F. R., and Morton, D. L.: Sarcoma-specific antigens: detection by complement fixation with serum from sarcoma patients. J. Nat. Cancer Inst., *44*:651–656, 1970.
63. Falk, J., and Osoba, D.: HL-A antigens and survival in Hodgkin's disease. Lancet, 2:1118–1120, 1971.
64. Fefer, A.: Immunotherapy and chemotherapy of Moloney sarcoma virus-induced tumours. Canc. Res., 29:2177–2183, 1969.
65. Fetoproteins. (Editorial.) Lancet, *1*:397–398, 1970.
66. Fink, M. A., Karon, M., Rauscher, F. J., Malmgren, R. A., and Orr, H. C.: Further observations on the immunofluorescence of cells in human leukemia. Cancer, *18*:1317–1321, 1965.
67. Foy, H., Kondi, A., Linsell, C. A., Parker, A. M., and Sizaret, P.: The α_1-fetoprotein test in hepatocellular carcinoma. Lancet, *1*:411, 1970.
68. French, M. E., and Batchelor, J. R.: Immunological enhancement of rat kidney grafts. Lancet, *1*:1103–1106, 1969.
69. Frenster, J. H., and Rogoway, W. M.: Immunotherapy of human neoplasms with autologous lymphocytes activated *in vitro*. *In* Harris, J. H.: Proceedings of the Fifth Leukocyte Culture Conference, 1970, pp. 359–373.
70. Friend, C., and Rossi, G. B.: Transplantation immunity and the suppression of spleen colony formation by immunization with murine leukemia virus preparations (Friend). Int. J. Cancer, *3*:523–529, 1968.
71. Geering, G., Aoki, T., and Old, L. J.: Shared viral antigen of mammalian leukaemia viruses. Nature, 226:265–266, 1970.
72. Geering, G., Hardy, W. D., Old, L. J., de Harven, E., and Brodey, R. S.: Shared group specific antigen of murine and feline leukemia viruses. Virology, 36:678–680, 1968.
73. Gelboin, H. V., and Levy, H. B.: Polyinosinic-polycytidylic acid inhibits chemically induced tumorigenisis in mouse skin. Science, *167*:205–207, 1970.

74. General Discussion of the Fifth Annual Brook Lodge Conference on Immunologic Intervention, Kalamazoo, Michigan. New York, Academic Press, 1972.
75. Gerber, P., and Birch, S. M.: Complement-fixing antibodies in sera of human and non-human primates to viral antigens derived from Burkitt's lymphoma cells. Proc. Nat. Acad. Sci., 58:478–484, 1967.
76. Ghose, T., and Nigam, S.: Effect of radioisoline and chlorambucil conjugated antibodies on the growth of Ehrlich ascites carcinoma. Proc. Can. Fed. Biol. Soc., 14:127, 1971.
77. Gold, P.: Circulating antibodies against carcinoembryonic antigens of the human digestive system. Cancer, 20:1663–1667, 1967.
78. Gold, P., and Freedman, S. O.: Specific carcinoembryonic antigens of the human digestive system. J. Exper. Med., 122:467–481, 1965.
79. Goldner, H., Girardi, A. J., Larson, V. M., and Hilleman, M. R.: Interruption of SV_{40} virus tumorigenesis using irradiated homologous tumor antigen. Proc. Soc. Exper. Biol. Med., 117:851–857, 1964.
80. Goldstein, G.: Immunofluorescent detection of human antibodies reactive with tumor. Ann. N.Y. Acad. Sci., 177:279–285, 1971.
81. Good, R. A.: Presentation at the Fifth Annual Brook Lodge Conference on Immunologic Intervention, Kalamazoo, Michigan. New York, Academic Press, 1972.
82. Graff, R. J., Silvers, W. K., Billingham, R. E., Hildemann, W. H., and Snell, G. D.: The cumulative effect of histocompatibility antigens. Transplantation, 4:605–617, 1966.
83. Häkkinen, I., and Viikari, S.: Occurrence of fetal sulphoglycoprotein antigen in the gastric juice of patients with gastric diseases. Ann. Surg., 169:277–281, 1969.
84. Hamilton Fairley, G., Lewis, M. G., Ikonopisov, R. L., Nairn, R. C., and Alexander, P.: Detection of tumor specific immune reactions in human melanoma. Ann. N.Y. Acad. Sci., 177:286–289, 1971.
85. Hanna, M. G., Jr., Walburg, H. E., Tyndall, R. L., and Snodgrass, M. J.: Histoproliferative effect of Rauscher leukemia virus on lymphatic tissue. II. Antigen-stimulated germfree and conventional BALB/c mice. Proc. Soc. Exper. Biol. Med., 134:1132–1141, 1970.
86. Haybittle, J. L.: Mortality rates from cancer and tuberculosis. Brit. J. Prev. Soc. Med., 17:23–28, 1963.
87. Hellström, I., Evans, C. A., and Hellström, K. E.: Cellular immunity and its serum-mediated inhibition in Shope virus-induced rabbit papillomas. Int. J. Cancer, 4:601–607, 1969.
88. Hellström, K. E., and Hellström, I.: Cellular immunity against tumor antigens. Advances Cancer Res., 18:167–223, 1969.
89. Hellström, K. E., and Hellström, I.: Immunologic defenses against cancer. Hosp. Prac., 5:45–61, 1970.
90. Hellström, K. E., and Hellström, I.: Immunological enhancement as studied by cell culture techniques. Ann. Rev. Microbiol., 24:373–398, 1970.
91. Hellström, I., and Hellström, K. E.: Colony inhibition studies on blocking and non-blocking serum effects on cellular immunity to Moloney sarcomas. Int. J. Cancer, 5:195–201, 1970.
92. Hellström, I., Hellström, K. E., Evans, C. A., Heppner, G. H., Pierce, G. E., and Yang, J. P. S.: Serum-mediated protection of neoplastic cells from inhibition by lymphocytes immune to their tumor-specific antigens. Proc. Nat. Acad. Sci., 62:362–368, 1969.
93. Hellström, I., Hellström, K. E., Pierce, G. E., and Bill, A. H.: Demonstration of cell bound and humoral immunity against neuroblastoma cells. Proc. Nat. Acad. Sci., 60:1231–1238, 1968.
94. Hellström, I., Hellström, K. E., Pierce, G. E., and Yang, J. P. S.: Cellular and humoral immunity to different types of human neoplasms. Nature, 220:1352–1354, 1968.
95. Hellström, I., Sjögren, H. O., Warner, G., and Hellström, K. E.: Blocking of cell-mediated tumor immunity by sera from patients with growing neoplasms. Int. J. Cancer, 7:226–237, 1971.
96. Helson, L., Ramos, C., Oettgen, H., and Murphy, M.: DNCB reactivity in children with neuroblastoma. (Abstract.) Proc. Amer. Assoc. Cancer Res., 12:86, 1971.
97. Henle, G., Henle, W., and Diehl, V.: Relation of Burkitt's tumor-associated Herpes-Y type virus to infectious mononucleosis. Proc. Nat. Acad. Sci., 59:94–101, 1968.
98. Henle, G., and Henle, W.: Immunofluorescence in cells derived from Burkitts lymphoma. J. Bact., 91:1248–1256, 1966.
99. Higginson, J., De-The, G., Geser, A., and Day, N.: An epidemiological analysis of cancer vaccines. Int. J. Cancer, 7:565–574, 1971.
100. Hildemann, W. H.: Weak transplantation barriers. Transplant. Proc., 3:76–80, 1971.
101. Hilleman, M. R.: Interferon induction and utilization. J. Cell Physiol., 71:43–57, 1968.
102. Hirshaut, Y., Glade, P., Vieira, L. O. B. D., Ainbender, E., Dvorak, B., and Siltzbach, L.: Sarcoidosis, another disease associated with serologic evidence for herpes-like virus infection. New Eng. J. Med., 283:502–506, 1970.
103. Hollinshead, A., Glew, D., Bunnag, B., Gold, P., and Heberman, R.: Skin-reactive soluble antigen from intestinal cancer-cell-membranes and relationship to carcinoembryonic antigens. Lancet, 1:1191–1195, 1970.

104. Holmgren, I.: Försök och iaktta gelser över kancersjukas förhållande till tuberculin. Hygiea (Stockholm), 79:218, 1917.
105. Humphrey, L. J., Jewell, W. R., Murray, D. R., and Griffen, W. O.: Immunotherapy for the patient with cancer. Ann. Surg., 173:47–54, 1971.
106. Inbar, M., and Sachs, L.: Structural difference in sites on the surface membrane of normal and transformed cells. Nature, 223:710–712, 1969.
107. Inbar, M., Ben-Bassat, H., and Sachs, L.: Location of amino acid and carbohydrate transport sites in the surface membrane of normal and transformed mammalian cells. J. Membrane Biol., 1971 (in press).
108. In Vitro Methods in Cell-mediated Immunity. Bloom, B. R., and Glade, P. R., eds., New York, Academic Press, 1971.
109. Irvin, G. L., Eustace, J. C., and Fahey, J. L.: Enhancement activity of mouse immunoglobulin classes. J. Immunol., 99:1085–1091, 1967.
110. Jacobs, M. E., Gordon, J. K., and Talal, N.: Inability of the NZB/NZW F$_1$ thymus to transfer cyclophosphamide-induced tolerance to sheep erythrocytes. J. Immunol., 107:359–364, 1971.
111. Jeannet, M., and Magnin, C.: HL-A antigens in hematological malignant diseases. Transplant. Proc., 3:1301, 1971.
112. Kaliss, N.: Immunological enhancement of tumor homografts in mice. Cancer Res., 18:992–1003, 1958.
113. Kaliss, N., Molomut, N., Harris, J. L., and Gault, S. D.: Effect of previously injected immune serum and tissue on the survival of tumor grafts in mice. J. Nat. Cancer Inst., 13:847–850, 1953.
114. Kaplan, A. M., and Cinader, B.: Manuscript in preparation.
115. Kissmeyer-Nielsen, F., Jensen, K. B., Ferrara, G. B., Kjerbye, K. E., and Svejgaard, A.: HL-A phenotypes in Hodgkin's disease. Transplant. Proc., 3:1287, 1971.
116. Klein, E.: Hypersensitivity reactions at tumor sites. Cancer Res., 29:2351–2362, 1969.
117. Klein, G., Clifford, P., Klein, E., Smith, R. T., Minowada, J., Kourilsky, F. M., and Burchenal, J. H.: Membrane immunofluorescence reactions of Burkitt lymphoma cells from biopsy specimens and tissue cultures. J. Nat. Cancer Inst., 39:1027–1044, 1967.
118. Kobayashi, H., Sendo, F., Kaji, H., Shirai, T., Saito, H., Takeichi, N., Hosokawa, M., and Kodama, T.: Inhibition of transplanted rat tumours by immunization with identical tumour cells infected with Friend virus. J. Nat. Cancer Inst., 44:11–19, 1970.
119. Korsantiya, B. M., and Smorodinbev, Al. A.: Transplacental transmission of endogenous interferon in pregnant mice inoculated with influenza or Newcastle disease virus. Nature (Lond.), 232:560–561, 1971.
120. Krementz, E. T., and Samuels, M. S.: Tumor cross transplantation and cross transfusion in the treatment of advanced malignant disease. Bull. Tulane U. Med. Faculty, 26:263–270, 1967.
121. Larson, V. M., Raupp, W. G., and Hilleman, M. R.: Prevention of SV virus tumorigenisis in newborn hamsters by maternal immunization. Proc. Soc. Exper. Biol. (N.Y.), 126:674–677, 1967.
122. Lawrence, S.: Presentation at the Fifth Annual Brook Lodge Conference on Immunologic Intervention, Kalamazoo, Michigan. New York, Academic Press, 1972.
123. Levy, J. A., and Henle, G.: Indirect immunofluorescence tests with sera from African children and cultured Burkitt lymphoma cells. J. Bact., 92:275–276, 1966.
124. Levy, H. B., Law, L. W., and Rabson, A. S.: Inhibition of tumor growth by polyinosinic-polycytidylic acid. Proc. Nat. Acad. Sci. (Wash.), 62:357–361, 1969.
125. Lewis, M. G.: Possible immunological factors in human malignant melanoma in Uganda. Lancet, 2:921–922, 1967.
126. Lewis, M. G., Ikonopisov, R. L., Nairn, R. C., Phillips, T. M., Fairley, G. H., Bodenham, D. C., and Alexander, P.: Tumour-specific antibodies in human malignant melanoma and their relationship to the extent of the disease. Brit. Med. J., 3:547–554, 1969.
127. Lis, H., Sela, B. A., Sachs, L., and Sharon, N.: Specific inhibition by N-acetyl-D-galactosamine of the interaction between soybean agglutinin and animal cell surfaces. Biochim. Biophys. Acta, 211:582–585, 1970.
128. Lo Gerfo, P., Krupey, J., and Hansen, H. J.: Demonstration of an antigen common to several varieties of neoplasia. Assay using zirconyl phosphate gel. New Eng. J. Med., 285:138–141, 1971.
129. Mathé, G., Amiel, J. L., Schwarzenburg, L., Schneider, L., Cattan, A., Schlumberger, J. R., Hayat, M., and de Vassal, F.: Active immunotherapy for acute lymphoblastic leukaemia. Lancet, 1:697–699, 1969.
130. Mergenhagen, S. E., Notkins, A. L., and Dougherty, S. F.: Adjuvanticity of lactic dehydrogenase virus: Influence of virus infection on the establishment of immunological tolerance to a protein antigen in adult mice. J. Immunol., 99:576–581, 1967.
131. Mitchison, N. A.: Immunological paralysis as a dosage phenomenon. In Cinader, B., ed.: Regulation of the Antibody Response. Springfield, Illinois, Charles C Thomas, 1968, pp. 54–67.

132. Mitchison, N. A.: Perspectives of immunological tolerance in transplantation. Transplant. Proc., 3:953–959, 1971.
133. Moolten, F. L., and Cooperband, S. R.: Selective destruction of target cells by diphtheria toxin conjugated to antibody directed against antigens on the cells. Science, 169:68–70, 1970.
134. Morris, P. J., and Forbes, J. F.: HL-A in follicular lymphoma, reticulum cell sarcoma, lymphosarcoma and infectious mononucleosis. Transplant. Proc., 3:1315, 1971.
135. Morton, D. L., and Malgren, R. A.: Human osteosarcomas. Immunologic evidence suggesting an associated infectious agent. Science, 162:1278–1281, 1968.
136. Morton, D. L., Malgren, R. A., Hall, W. T., and Schidlovsky, G.: Immunologic and virus studies with human sarcomas. Surgery, 66:152–161, 1969.
137. Morton, D. L., Malgrom, R. A., Holmes, E. C., and Ketcham, A. S.: Demonstration of antibodies against human malignant melanoma by immunofluorescence. Surgery, 64:233–240, 1968.
138. Mullen, Y., and Hildemann, W. H.: Kidney transplantation genetics and enhancement in rats. Transplant. Proc., 3:669–672, 1971.
139. Muna, N. M., Marcus, S., and Smart, C.: Detection by immunofluorescence of antibodies specific for human malignant melanoma cells. Cancer, 23:88–93, 1969.
140. Myers, R. S., Hammond, W. G., and Ketcham, A. S.: Tumor-specific transplantation immunity after cryosurgery. J. Surg. Oncol., 1:241–246, 1969.
141. Nadler, S. H., and Moore, G. E.: Clinical immunologic study of malignant disease: response to tumor transplants and transfer of leukocytes. Ann. Surg., 164:482–490, 1966.
142. Nauts, H. C.: The apparently beneficial effects of bacterial infection on host resistance to cancer. Monograph No. 8, New York Cancer Res. Inst., 1969.
143. Niederman, J. C., McCollum, R. W., Henle, G., and Henle, W.: Infectious mononucleosis. Clinical manifestations in relation to EB virus antibodies. J.A.M.A., 203:205–212, 1968.
144. Nilsson, A., Revesz, L., and Stjernsward, J.: Suppression of strontium 90 induced development of bone tumors by injection with Bacillus Calmette Guerin (BCG). Radiation Res., 26:378–382, 1965.
145. Notkins, A. L., Mergenhagen, S. E., and Howard, R. J.: Effect of virus infections on the function of the immune system. Ann. Rev. Microbiol., 24:525–538, 1970.
146. Oettgen, H. F., Aoki, T., Old, L. J., Boyse, E. A., De Harven, E., and Mills, G. M.: Suspension culture of a pigment-producing cell line derived from a human malignant melanoma. J. Nat. Cancer Inst., 41:827–831, 1968.
147. Oettgen, H., Old, L. J., Farrow, J., Valentine, F., Lawrence, S., and Thomas, L.: Effects of transfer factor in cancer patients. J. Clin. Invest., 50:71a, 1971.
148. Old, L. J., Benacerraf, B., Clarke, D. A., Carswell, and Stockert, E.: The role of the reticulo endothelial system in the host reaction to neoplasia. Cancer Res., 21:1281–1300, 1961.
149. Old, L. J., Boyse, E. A., Clarke, D. A., and Carswell, E. A.: Antigenic properties of chemically induced tumors. Ann. N.Y. Acad. Sci., 101:80–106, 1962.
150. Old, L. J., Boyse, E. A., Oettgen, H. F., de Harven, E., Geering, G., Williamson, B., and Clifford, P.: Precipitating antibody in human serum to an antigen present in culture of Burkitt's lymphoma cells. Proc. Nat. Acad. Sci., 56:1699–1704, 1966.
151. Order, S. E., Porter, M., and Hellman, S.: Hodgkin's disease: evidence for a tumour-associated antigen. New Eng. J. Med., 285:471–474, 1971.
152. Penn, I., Helgrinson, C. G., and Starzl, T. E.: De novo malignant-tumors in organ transplant recipients. Transplant. Proc., 3:773–778, 1971.
153. Pinkard, R. N., Weir, D. M., and McBridge, W. H.: Factors influencing the immune response. III. The blocking effect of Corynebacterium parvum upon the induction of acquired immunologic unresponsiveness to bovine serum albumin in the adult rabbit. Clin. Exper. Immunol., 3:413–421, 1968.
154. Prager, M. D., Derr, I., Swann, A., and Cotropia, J.: Immunization with chemically modified cancer cells. Proc. Amer. Assoc. Cancer Res., 12:2, 1971.
155. Rapport, M. M.: Immunological properties of lipids and their relation to the tumor cell. Ann. N.Y. Acad. Sci., 159:446, 1969.
156. Ross, J., Scolnick, E. M., Todaro, G. J., and Aaronson, S. A.: Separation of murine cellular and murine leukaemia virus DNA polymerases. Nature New Biology, 231:163–167, 1971.
157. Schlosser, J. V., and Benes, E. H.: Immunotherapy of human cancer with phytohemagglutinin stimulated lymphocytes. Proc. Amer. Assoc. Cancer Res., 12:82, 1971.
158. Sela, B. A., Lis, H., Sharon, N., and Sachs, L.: Different locations of carbohydrate-containing sites in the surface membranes of normal and transformed mammalian cells. J. Membrane Biol., 3:267–279, 1970.
159. Shäfer, W., Anderer, F. A., Bauer, H., and Pister, L.: Studies on mouse leukemia viruses. I. Isolation and characterization of a group specific antigen. Virology, 38:387–394, 1969.

160. Shah, K. V.: Neutralizing antibodies to simian virus 40 (SV40) in human sera from India. Proc. Soc. Exper. Biol. Med., *121*:303–307, 1966.
161. Shah, K. V.: Investigation of human malignant tumors in India for simian virus 40 etiology. J. Nat. Cancer Inst., *42*:139–145, 1969.
162. Shah, K. V., Ozer, H. L., Pond, H. S., Palma, L. D., and Murphy, G. P.: SV40 neutralizing antibodies in sera of US residents without history of polio immunization. Nature, *231*:448–449, 1971.
163. Sheinin, R., Onodera, K., Yogeeswaran, G., and Murray, R. K.: Studies of components of the surface of normal and virus-transformed cells. *In* The Biology of Oncogenic Viruses. New York, American Elsevier, 1971, pp. 274–285.
164. Shoham, J., Inbar, M., and Sachs, L.: Differential toxicity on normal and transformed cells *in vitro* and inhibition of tumor development *in vivo* by concanavalin A. Nature, *277*:1244–1246, 1970.
165. Siegel, B. V., and Morton, J. I.: Serum agglutinin levels to sheep red blood cells in mice defeated with Rauscher virus. Proc. Soc. Exper. Biol. Med., *123*:467–470, 1966.
166. Simonsen, M.: On the nature and measurement of antigenic strength. Transplant. Rev., *3*:22–35, 1970.
167. Sjögren, H. O., and Bansal, S. C.: Antigens in virally induced tumours. Progr. Immunol., *1*:921–938, 1971.
168. Sjögren, H. O., and Borum, K.: Tumor-specific immunity in the course of primary polyoma and Rous tumor development in intact and immunosuppressed rats. Cancer Res., *31*:890–900, 1971.
169. Sjögren, H. O., Hellström, I., Bansal, S. C., and Hellström, K. E.: Suggestive evidence that the "blocking antibodies" of tumor-bearing individuals may be antigen-antibody complexes. Proc. Nat. Acad. Sci., *68*:1372–1375, 1971.
170. Smith, R. T., Potentials for immunological intervention in cancer. *In* Amos, B., ed.: Progress in Immunology. New York, Academic Press, 1971, pp. 1115–1129.
171. Smith, R. T., and Landy, M.: Immune Surveillance. New York, Academic Press, 1970.
172. Soanes, W. A., Gonder, M. J., Albin, R. J., Maser, M. D., and Jagodzinski, R. V.: Clinical and experimental aspects of prostatic cryosurgery. J. Cryosurg., *2*:23–29, 1969.
173. Spitznagel, J. K., and Allison, A. C.: Mode of action of adjuvants: Retinol and other lysosome-labilizing agents as adjuvants. J. Immunol., *104*:119–127, 1961.
174. Starving cancer. *In* The Sciences, New York Acad. Sci., *11*:22, 1971.
175. Stjernswärd, J.: Age-dependent tumor-host barrier and effect of carcinogen-induced immunodepression on rejection of isografted methylcholanthrene-induced sarcoma cells. J. Nat. Cancer Inst., *37*:505–512, 1966.
176. Stjernswärd, J.: Effect of Bacillus Calmette Guerin and/or methylcholanthrene on the antibody-forming cells measured at the cellular level by a hemolytic plaque test. Cancer Res., *26*:1591–1594, 1966.
177. Stolbach, L. L., Krant, M. J., and Fishman, W. H.: Ectopic production of an alkaline phosphatase isoenzyme in patients with cancer. New Eng. J. Med., *281*:757–762, 1969.
178. Strong and weak histocompatibility antigens (Ed. G. Möller). Transplant. Rev., *3*:5–102, 1970.
179. St. Rose, J. E. M., and Cinader, B.: The effect of tolerance on the specificity of the antibody response and on immunogenicity. Antibody response to conformationally and chemically altered antigens. J. Exper. Med., *125*:1031–1055, 1967.
180. Summer, W. C., and Foraker, A. C.: Spontaneous regression of human melanoma. Clinical and experimental studies. Cancer, *13*:79–81, 1960.
181. Takasugi, M., and Hildemann, W. H.: Regulation of immunity toward allogeneic tumors in mice. I. Effect of antiserum fractions on tumor growth. J. Nat. Cancer Inst., *43*:843–855, 1969.
182. Takasugi, M., and Klein, E.: A microassay for cell-mediated immunity. Transplantation, *9*:219–227, 1970.
183. Takeda, K.: Immunology of Cancer. Hokkaido University School of Medicine, Sapporo, Japan, 1969.
184. Tal, C.: The nature of cell membrane receptor for the agglutination factor present in the sera of tumour patients and pregnant women. Proc. Nat. Acad. Sci. (Wash.), *54*:1318–1321, 1965.
185. Tal, C., Dishon, T., and Gross, J.: The agglutination of tumour cells in vitro by sera from tumour patients and pregnant women. Brit. J. Cancer, *18*:111–119, 1964.
186. Tal, C., and Halperin, M.: Presence of serologically distinct protein in serum of cancer patients and pregnant women. An attempt to develop a diagnostic cancer test. Israel J. Med. Sci., *6*:708–716, 1970.
187. Tatarinov, Yu. S.: Content of embryospecific alpha-globulin in the blood serum of human foetus, new-born and adult man in primary cancer of the liver. Vop. Med. Khim., *11*:20–24, 1965.
188. Teimourian, B., and McCune, W. C.: Surgical management of malignant melanoma. Amer. Surg., *29*:515–519, 1963.

189. Thomson, D. M. P., Krupey, J., Freedman, S. O., and Gold, P.: The radio immunoassay of circulating carcinoembryonic antigen of the human digestive system. Proc. Nat. Acad. Sci., 64:161–167, 1969.

190. Uhr, J.: Presentation at the Fifth Annual Brook Lodge Conference on Immunological Intervention, Kalamazoo, Michigan. New York. Academic Press, 1972.

191. Unanue, E. R., Askonas, B. A., and Allison, A. C.: A role of macrophages in the stimulation of immune responses by adjuvants. J. Immunol., 103:71–78, 1969.

192. Voisin, G. A.: Discussion, In Wolstenholme, G. E. W., and Cameron, M. P., eds.: Transplantation, A Ciba Foundation Symposium on Transplantation, 1961. London, J. and A. Churchill, 1962, pp. 343–348.

193. Voisin, G. A., Kinsky, R. B., and Maillard, J.: Reactivité immunitaire et anticorps facilitants chez des animaux tolérants aux homogreffes. Ann. Inst. Pasteur, 115:855–879, 1968.

194. von Kleist, S., and Burtin, P.: Isolation of a fetal antigen from human colonic tumours. Cancer Res., 29:1961–1964, 1969.

195. Wegmann, T. G., Hellström, I., and Hellström, K. E.: Immunological Tolerance: "Forbidden clones" allowed in tetraparental mice. Proc. Nat. Acad. Sci., 68:1644–1647, 1971.

196. Weigle, W. O.: The immune response of rabbits tolerant to bovine serum albumin to the injection of other heterologous serum albumins. J. Exper. Med., 114:111–125, 1961.

197. Weiss, D. W.: Immunology of spontaneous tumors. In Lecam, L., and Neyman, J., eds.: Proceedings of the Fifth Berkeley Symposium on Mathematical Statistics and Probability. Berkeley, University of California Press, 1967, pp. 657–706.

198. White, E., Hildemann, W. H., and Mullen, Y.: Chronic kidney allograft reactions in rats. Transplantation, 8:602–617, 1969.

199. Wigzell, H., and Stjernswärd, J.: Age-dependent rise and fall of immunological reactivity in the CBA mouse. J. Nat. Cancer Inst., 37:513–517, 1966.

200. Wood, W. C.: Antibody in sarcoma patients cytotoxic to human sarcoma cells. In Morton, D. L., moderator: Immunological aspects of neoplasia: a national basis for immunotherapy. Ann. Intern. Med., 74:587–604, 1971.

201. Wood, W. C., and Morton, D. L.: Microcytotoxicity test: detection in sarcoma patients of antibody cytotoxic to human sarcoma cells. Science, 170:1318–1320, 1970.

202. Woodruff, M. F. A., and Boak, J. L.: Inhibitory effect of injection of Corynebacterium parvum on the growth of tumor transplants in isogenic hosts. Brit. J. Cancer, 20:345–355, 1966.

203. Wu, C.-Y., and Cinader, B.: Antigen promotion. Increase in hapten-specific plaque-forming cells after preinjection with structurally unrelated macromolecules. J. Exper. Med., 134:693–712, 1971.

204. Yashphe, D. J.: Immunological factors in non-specific stimulation of host resistance to syngeneic tumours. Israel J. Med. Sci., 7:90–110, 1971.

205. Zbar, B., and Tanaka, T.: Immunotherapy of cancer: Regression of tumours after intralesional injection of living mycobacterium bovis. Science, 172:271–273, 1971.

Segi, M., Kurihar, A. M., and Matsuyama, T.: Cancer mortality for selected sites in 24 countries. No. 5. Sendai, Japan, Tohoku University School of Medicine, 1969.

206. Segi, M., Kurihara, M., and Matsuyama, T.: Cancer mortality for selected sites in 24 countries. No. 5. Sendai, Japan, Tohoku University School of Medicine, 1969.

Institute of Immunology
University of Toronto
Toronto, Ontario
Canada

Index

Note: Page numbers of article and symposium titles are in **boldface** type.

ADRENALECTOMY, for metastatic breast cancer, 659
Adrenergic receptors, blockers of, for angina pectoris, 602–603
Alkylating agents, in dermatologic disorders, 733
Ampulla of Vater, retrograde cannulation of, **781–788**
Androgens, for metastatic breast cancer, 658
Angina pectoris, severe, treatment of, **599–609**
Antibiotics, in dermatologic disorders, 734
Antigens, tumor, 801
Antihypertensive drugs, **633–644**
Arrhythmia, atrial, paroxysmal, **611–614**
  ventricular, in ambulatory patients, **615–624**
Atrial fibrillation, paroxysmal, **611–614**
Azaribine (Triazure), in dermatologic disorders, 733
Azathioprine (Imuran), in dermatologic disorders, 732

BLEOMYCIN, 734
Blood, pressure, high. See *Hypertension*.
Bone, metastases, from breast cancer, 655
Breast cancer, metastatic, **651–664**

CARCINOMA, colorectal, investigation and treatment, **665–675**
  immunologic aspects, future of, **801–836**
  of breast, metastatic, **651–664**
Cardiac death, sudden, prevention and treatment, **625–631**
Cardioversion, for atrial fibrillation, 614
Carotid sinus stimulation, for angina pectoris, 604

Catecholamines, in Parkinson's syndrome, 696–698
Chest pain, reflux esophagitis and, **771–780**
Cholestasis, chronic, pruritus of, 762–765
Climacteric, management of, **789–800**
Clinical medicine, drug interactions in, **585–597**
  hypnotherapy in, **687–692**
Colorectal cancer, investigation and treatment, **665–675**
Coronary atherosclerosis, angina of, treatment, **599–609**
  menopause and, 793
Coronary surgery, for angina pectoris, 605
Corticosteroids, for metastatic breast cancer, 658
  for multiple sclerosis, 712

DERMATOLOGY, chemotherapy in, present status of, **725–737**
Diet, drugs and, 585–587
Digitalis, in paroxysmal atrial fibrillation, 612
Drugs, interactions in clinical medicine, **585–597**
  metabolism, 591–594
Dying patient, physician's responsibility to, **677–680**
Dysgammaglobulinemias, 752–753

EPITHELIOMAS, recurrent, chemosurgery in, **739–745**
Esophagitis, reflux, **771–780**
Estrogen, for metastatic breast cancer, 658
  in postmenopausal women, 795–797

FIBRILLATION, atrial, paroxysmal, **611–614**

837

GOITER, toxic nodular, 720–721
Graves' disease, 717–720

HYDROXYUREA (Hydrea), in dermatologic disorders, 732
Hypertension, arterial, complicated, **633–644**
Hypertensive crisis, 640–642
Hyperthyroidism, 717–724
Hypnotherapy in clinical medicine, **687–692**
Hypogammaglobulinemia, 753–754
Hyponatremia, **645–649**
Hypophysectomy, for metastatic breast cancer, 659

IMMUNOLOGIC deficiency states, **747–757**
Immunology, tumors and, **801–836**
Imuran. See *Azathioprine.*
Inderal. See *Propranolol hydrochloride.*

JAUNDICE, chronic obstructive, **759–770**

LEVODOPA, in Parkinson's syndrome, 696–698
Lithium carbonate, in manic and depressive episodes, **681–686**
Liver, metastases, from colorectal cancer, 670–673

MANIC-depressive reactions, lithium carbonate in, **681–686**
Matulane. See *Procarbazine hydrochloride.*
Menopause, management, **789–800**
Methotrexate, in dermatologic disorders, 731–732
Mohs' technique, for recurrent epitheliomas, **738–745**
Multiple sclerosis, **711–716**
Myocardial infarction, early treatment, 627–630
Myocardium, oxygen consumption, 599–600

NITRITES, for angina pectoris, 601–602
Nutrition, chronic obstructive jaundice and, 760–762

Nutrition (*Continued*)
drugs and, 585–587

ONCOVIN. See *Vincristine.*
Oophorectomy, in metastatic breast cancer, 657
Osteoporosis, in postmenopausal women, 792

PARKINSON's syndrome, **693–709**
Procainamide, for paroxysmal ventricular tachycardia, 622
Procarbazine hydrochloride (Matulane), in dermatologic disorders, 735
Propranolol hydrochloride (Inderal), in paroxysmal atrial fibrillation, 612
Pruritus, in chronic cholestasis, 762–765
Psychologic aspects of dying, **677–680**

QUINIDINE, for paroxysmal ventricular tachycardia, 622

REFLUX esophagitis, **771–780**

SKIN, disorders, chemotherapy in, **725–737**
Sodium deficiency, **645–649**
Streptonigrin, 734
Sudden cardiac death, prevention and treatment, **625–631**

THYROID gland, function, lithium carbonate and, **681–686**
Thyrotoxicosis, T-3, 721–722
Triazure. See *Azaribine.*
Tumor immunology, future of, **801–836**

VAGINITIS, senescent, 792, 798
Vater, ampulla of, retrograde cannulation of, **781–788**
Ventricular arrhythmias, in ambulatory patients, 615–624
Vincristine (Oncovin), in dermatologic disorders, 735

Time for a periodical checkup!

☐ HUMAN PATHOLOGY
Quarterly, $18.50 per year

☐ MEDICAL CLINICS
Bimonthly, $21 per year

☐ SURGICAL CLINICS
Bimonthly, $21 per year

☐ PEDIATRIC CLINICS
Quarterly, $18 per year

☐ RADIOLOGIC CLINICS
3 issues, $20 per year

☐ OTOLARYNGOLOGIC CLINICS
3 issues, $22 per year

☐ ORTHOPEDIC CLINICS
3 issues, $22.50 per year

☐ DENTAL CLINICS
Quarterly, $20 per year

☐ NURSING CLINICS
Quarterly, $12 per year

☐ VETERINARY CLINICS
3 issues, $22 per year

3 new Clinics
with an international outlook

☐ GASTROENTEROLOGY CLINICS
3 issues, $30 per year

☐ HEMATOLOGY CLINICS
3 issues, $30 per year

☐ ENDOCRINOLOGY & METABOLISM
CLINICS, 3 issues, $30 per year

Check over this list of Saunders periodicals. Thousands of your colleagues rely on the widely acclaimed *Clinics of North America* to keep them abreast of new developments. Each hardbound, illustrated issue focuses on a specific topic of current interest and concern. Use this convenient card to order the periodicals of interest to you.

Name_____

Address_____

City_____State_____ZIP_____

On the move?

Make sure that your subscription to Saunders periodicals goes with you. Fill in and mail the attached card today. Please be sure to include your new zip code. Allow one month for your change of address to be processed.

As of___/_/___send my "Clinics" issues to my new address given below.

Name_____
NEW ADDRESS_____
City_____State_____ZIP_____
OLD ADDRESS_____
City_____State_____ZIP_____

☐ MEDICAL CLINICS

☐ SURGICAL CLINICS

☐ PEDIATRIC CLINICS

☐ OTOLARYNGOLOGIC CLINICS

☐ RADIOLOGIC CLINICS

☐ ORTHOPEDIC CLINICS

☐ DENTAL CLINICS

☐ NURSING CLINICS

☐ VETERINARY CLINICS